Respiratory Control

RESPIRATORY CONTROL

Central and Peripheral Mechanisms

DEXTER F. SPECK
MICHAEL S. DEKIN
W. ROBERT REVELETTE
DONALD T. FRAZIER
Editors

THE UNIVERSITY PRESS OF KENTUCKY

This book and the meeting which initiated it were made possible
by the support of many organizations. The National Institutes of Health
provided funds through a meeting grant (NS28638). Support from
the University of Kentucky was extensive, with contributions
from Research and Graduate Studies, the Chancellor of the Medical Center,
the Dean of the Medical Center, the University Hospital administration,
and the Department of Physiology and Biophysics. We would also like to
recognize the generous contribution from Schering-Plough Corporation.
We are grateful for each of these sponsors.

Library of Congress Cataloging-in-Publication Data

Respiratory control : central and peripheral mechanisms / Dexter F.
Speck . . . [et al.], editors.
    p. cm.
Includes bibliographical references and index.
ISBN 0-8131-1788-7 (alk. paper) :
1. Respiration—Regulation.
[DNLM: 1. Respiratory System—innervation. 2. Respiratory System
—physiology. WF 102 R4349]
QP123.R44 1992
612.2—dc20
DNLM/DLC
for Library of Congress   92-13720

Contents

Part VIII Behavioral Control of Breathing

Part IX Ventilatory Control in Humans

Preface

This book is the result of an international conference held in Lexington, Kentucky, in October of 1990. This symposium was supported by several organizations including the National Heart, Lung and Blood Institute and Schering-Plough Corporation. University of Kentucky support came from many different offices, including Research and Graduate Studies, the Chancellor and Dean of the Medical School, University Hospital Admininstration, and the Department of Physiology and Biophysics. Almost two hundred leading scientists from throughout the world met and discussed their ideas and approaches, including many recent technological and methodological advances which have greatly improved our understanding of the respiratory control system. The insights of many of these investigators are shared in this volume.

This meeting provided comprehensive coverage of many of the novel issues and approaches facing future investigation. The chapters in this book bring together a unique blend of investigators studying related issues in widely diverse preparations. Integration of results from different perspectives, ranging from cell membrane properties to functional reflexes and then to coordinated behavior in the human, extends our understanding of respiratory control mechanisms. The use of molecular techniques for addressing physiologic problems such as hypoxia and development is especially exciting. Similarly, reduced preparations such as cell cultures, thick and thin brain slices, and the neonatal isolated brainstem–spinal cord facilitate the study of fundamental properties of respiratory-related neurons. At the organismal level, the reflex connections, electrophysiology, pharmacology, and various modulatory influences are considered. These observations shed new light pertinent to both basic and clinical investigations.

The editors sincerely appreciate the participation of the many experts who attended the meeting and assisted in the preparation of this book. Their input was vital to the success of both endeavors. The efforts of the Session Chairs, Laurie Evans, and the other members of the University of Kentucky Respiratory Group are also gratefully acknowledged.

Dexter F. Speck
Michael S. Dekin
W. Robert Revelette
Donald T. Frazier

PART I

Membrane Properties of Respiratory Neurons

1

An Overview

Michael S. Dekin

A major goal of respiratory neurophysiologists has been to characterize the membrane properties of respiratory neurons and associate these properties with models of the respiratory central pattern generator (respiratory CPG). Much of this effort has been directed towards describing intrinsic cellular mechanisms underlying rhythm generation such as endogenous pacemaker activity and postinhibitory rebound phenomena. More recently we have also begun to appreciate the role of membrane properties in nonrhythm-generating functions such as pattern formation. In this regard, it is now recognized that many respiratory neurons do not act as high fidelity followers of their synaptic inputs. Rather, these neurons possess an impressive repertoire of intrinsic mechanisms for integrating their synaptic inputs (8). These integrative capabilities arise largely as a consequence of the kinetic and neurochemical properties of specific membrane channels found in respiratory neurons. In this brief overview, the experimental strategies used to study membrane channels will be discussed with particular attention given to their strengths and weaknesses. In addition, the types of information gained from such studies will be considered in terms of what they can tell us about the respiratory CPG.

EXPERIMENTAL APPROACHES

Over the past twenty years, it has become apparent that neurons possess many types of membrane channels in addition to the classic sodium and potassium channels responsible for generating the action potential (11). These additional membrane channels include several classes of voltage-dependent potassium (2) and calcium channels (14), as well as channels such as the m-channel (1) which exhibit both chemical and voltage-dependent gating properties. Another important observation is that not all neurons necessarily possess each of the known channel types. A major emphasis of contemporary neurobiology, therefore, has been to determine the unique complement of membrane channels found in specific types of neurons and the integrative capabilities these channels impart. These integrative capabilities define the limits of what specific classes of neurons can and cannot do. A complete understanding of how neuronal circuits such as the respiratory CPG are maintained and modulated will only be realized when such information is available for each type of cell in the network.

In general, membrane channel studies are done using "reduced" *in vitro* preparations so that sophisticated biophysical recording techniques such as voltage clamp can be performed. Mechanical stability for intracellular (or patch) recordings is essential. In addition, these studies require that the particular type of channel being investigated be isolated from other channels in the membrane by utilizing ion substitutions and pharmacological agents. Thus, the reduced preparation must provide not only mechanical stability but also complete control over the extracellular fluid medium. Preparations meeting these criteria include long- and short-term cell cultures, brain slices, and perfused brain preparations. Each comes with a particular set of strengths and weaknesses. For instance, do neurons in culture exhibit the same properties as those in the fully differentiated brain? What are the detrimental effects of cutting neuronal processes during the brain slicing procedure? To what extent does tissue hypoxia compromise the activity of neurons in perfused brain (and brain slice) preparations? In many cases, these criticisms are muted by the fact that similar membrane properties can often be observed in both reduced and whole animal preparations. It is only in the reduced preparation, however, that a quantitative analysis of channel properties can be done.

One criticism which is not easily dismissed is that the loss of synaptic connectivity in reduced preparations, and hence circuit integrity, makes comparisons with intact networks such as the respiratory CPG difficult. The real danger here is that membrane properties might be studied which are not normally expressed by the intact circuit. This is particularly true for studies in cell cultures, and to a lesser extent in brain slices. As will be shown below, assigning a potential function to a given membrane channel without knowing the properties of other channels in the membrane or the synaptic inputs to the cell could easily lead to spurious conclusions. For these reasons, it is always important to interpret data obtained from reduced preparations with caution.

Another major consideration in using reduced preparations such as cell culture or brain slices is verifying that the recorded neurons are actually part of the neuronal network being investigated. For highly organized areas of the brain such as the hippocampus and cerebellum, anatomical localization within the brain slice (or microdissected area for cell culture) is sufficient to ensure that this is the case. For brainstem neurons which make up the respiratory CPG, however, such anatomical delineation is rarely possible. An alternative approach has been to identify unique classes of neurons within respiratory areas of the brain by combining electrophysiological recordings and intracellular labeling with dyes to study cell morphology. Further refinement of the localization process has then been done using tract tracing techniques. This method of identifying putative respiratory neurons has been used in brain slices to successfully study several parts of the respiratory circuit including the dorsal respiratory group (7), the ventral respiratory group (10), and the hypoglossal nucleus (15). It is likely only a matter of time before a similar approach is taken for studying respiratory neurons in cell culture.

TYPES OF INFORMATION NEEDED

Biophysical studies on membrane channels can provide several types of information. Ionic mechanisms, gating properties, inactivation properties, and modulation by neurochemicals are particularly important in describing how a neuronal network functions. Knowledge of the ionic species permeating a membrane channel may suggest functions for the channel in addition to its immediate action on the membrane potential level. For example, activation of calcium channels not only depolarizes the cell but also provides a mechanism for increasing intracellular calcium levels which can then act as a second messenger for specific enzymes and other channels. Specific ionic mechanisms may also suggest pharmacological agents which can be used to alter the channel's activity. The mechanism of channel gating is important for knowing both when and how the channel will be activated. This is especially important in determining if the channel is activated alone or in combination with other types of membrane channels (4, 6). Likewise, the mechanism of inactivating or turning off the channel may place specific constraints on channel activity and even lead to "history"-dependent phenomena which can alter circuit function (5, 6, 8, also see below).

Membrane channel properties (excluding ionic selectivity) are also subject to modulation by endogenous neurotransmitters and neuropeptides. For example, m-channels which are selective for potassium ions are often open at or near resting membrane potentials (1) and have been observed in some respiratory neurons (3). Depolarization causes further opening of these channels. Muscarinic agonists close these channels and this results in a membrane depolarization at resting membrane potentials. In both hippocampal (16) and respiratory neurons (see Champagnat et al., this volume), the neuropeptide somatostatin has been shown to have the opposite effect: that is, it causes further activation of these channels and membrane hyperpolarization. Neurochemical modulation of membrane channels provides a mechanism for altering the integrative capabilities of neurons and by doing so, the ongoing activity of neuronal circuits.

INTERPRETING MEMBRANE PROPERTIES IN THE CONTEXT OF THE WHOLE NEURON

As stated above, a major pitfall in interpreting the role of a particular membrane channel is that the ensemble activity of the neuron must be considered. This ensemble activity arises from both the other types of channels present in the membrane and extrinsic synaptic inputs. This can be illustrated by the following example. Bulbospinal neurons in the dorsal respiratory group (DRG) of the guinea pig possess a large number of different membrane channel types (6, 8). Two of these are the A-channel and a low-voltage-activated (LVA) calcium channel. Activation of A-channels can cause transient membrane hyperpolarization mediated by potassium ions while the LVA calcium channel can both depolarize the membrane potential and contribute to increases in intracellular calcium levels. Together, these channels impart unique integrative capabilities to these neurons (6, 8). In one class of DRG neurons, called type I cells, the voltage dependence of activation of the A-channels and LVA calcium channels is similar; both are turned on by depolarization to membrane potential levels more positive than -60 mV (4). In another class of DRG neurons, called type II, this is not the case. Here the A-channels are activated at membrane potential levels more positive than -50 mV, while the LVA calcium channels are only activated by depolarizations to membrane potential levels more positive than -40 mV (4).

The voltage-dependent gating properties described above will determine when and how the A-channels and calcium channels will be expressed. Normally, DRG neurons receive an alternating pattern of synaptic excitation during inspiration and inhibition during expiration (13). In type I neurons, inspiratory phase depolarization will cause the simultaneous activation of both the outward A-channels and inward calcium channels. Thus, the opposing currents carried by these channels negate their individual effects on membrane potential. Nonetheless, the activation of the LVA calcium channels causes an increase in intracellular calcium and subsequent expression of an outward calcium-activated potassium channel. This calcium-activated potassium channel is responsible for both spike frequency adaptation (6) and a postburst hyperpolarization which may contribute to the initial stages of expiration (12). Thus, the role of the inward calcium current in this cell type appears to be limited to providing a source of intracellular calcium rather than being a mechanism for depolarizing the membrane potential.

In type II neurons, the A-channels will initially be activated alone and the outward current carried by them can compete effectively with the depolarizing drive. As a result, the membrane potential can be kept at a relatively hyperpolarized level, which prevents activation of the calcium channels and causes a long delay (up to several hundred milliseconds) between the onset of depolarization and the beginning of spike activity (5, 6). As the A-channels inactivate, their ability to control the membrane potential will gradually wane, leading to the delayed depolarization of the membrane potential and activation of the LVA calcium channels. Once activated, the inward calcium current will also contribute to the overall depolarizing drive and allow repetitive spike activity to begin. As was the case for type I neurons, the role of these two channel types in controlling the membrane excitability of type II neurons is dependent upon their individual properties as well as their interaction(s).

Finally, both the A-channels and LVA calcium channels display voltage-dependent inactivation during depolarization. Hyperpolarization of the membrane potential level for periods up to several hundred msec is required to remove this inactivation. This property of A-channels and LVA calcium channels makes their expression history dependent. That is, these channels would depend upon expiratory phase inhibition to remove their inactivation so that they can be expressed during subsequent inspiratory phase depolarization. The amount of inactivation removed can be varied by altering the size and duration of the membrane hyperpolarization. As a consequence, the numbers of A-channels and LVA calcium channels expressed during inspiratory phase depolarization can be modulated by the previous expiratory phase inhibition. An example of this history-dependent effect is shown in figure 1.1 for the LVA calcium current in type I neurons activated during a step depolarization to -15 mV. The calcium current in these cells consisted of two components: the LVA current, which completely inactivated with time, and a high-voltage-activated (HVA) current, which did not inactivate. As the pre-depolarization membrane potential level was made more negative, the amplitude of the LVA current increased while the HVA current was not affected. The complete removal of inactivation from the LVA current required pre-depolarization membrane potential levels more negative than -65 mV.

SUMMARY

Our knowledge of the role of membrane channels in determining the activity of individual respiratory neurons has increased greatly over the past few years. In large part, this is due to the development of preparations which are suitable for studying such properties and which also allow putative respiratory neurons to be identified. Problems associated with reduced preparations can be minimized by proper experimental precautions and careful interpretation of the data. When this is done, such preparations can be a powerful tool in describing the membrane properties which generate and maintain the central respiratory rhythm. Equally important, these membrane properties provide a substrate upon which modulation of the central respiratory circuit is played out. The following chapters in this section will provide specific examples of how membrane properties

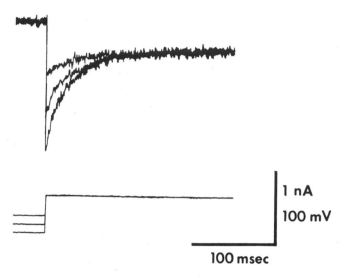

FIG. 1.1 Voltage-dependent removal of inactivation from LVA calcium channels. Upper traces show superimposed calcium currents activated during step depolarizations to -15 mV (inward current shown as a downward deflection). Lower traces are membrane voltage. Pre-depolarization membrane potential levels were -55, -45, and -35 mV.

contribute to sculpturing the repetitive discharge patterns of respiratory neurons and how these discharge patterns can be modulated.

REFERENCES

1. Adams, P.R., D.A. Brown, and A. Constanti. Pharmacological inhibition of the m-current. *J. Physiol.* (London) 332:223-262, 1982.

2. Castle, N.A., D.G. Haylett, and D.H. Jenkinson. Toxins in the characterization of potassium channels. *Trends in Neurosci.* 12:59-66, 1989.

3. Champagnat, J., T. Jacquin, and D. Richter. Voltage dependent currents in neurons of the nuclei of the solitary tract of rat brainstem slices. *Pfluegers Arch.* 406:272-379, 1986.

4. Dekin, M.S. Interaction between the A-current and calcium current in bulbospinal neurons in the ventral part of the nucleus tractus solitarius. *Soc. Neurosci. Abstr.* 14:936, 1988.

5. Dekin, M.S., and P.A. Getting. Firing pattern of neurons in the nucleus tractus solitarius: Modulation by membrane hyperpolarization. *Brain Res.* 324:180-184, 1984.

6. Dekin, M.S., and P.A. Getting. *In vitro* characterization of neurons in the ventral part of the nucleus tractus solitarius. II. Ionic mechanisms responsible for repetitive firing activity. *J. Neurophysiol.* 58:215-229, 1987.

7. Dekin, M.S., S.M. Johnson, and P.A. Getting. *In vitro* characterization of neurons in the ventral part of the nucleus tractus solitarius. I. Identification of neuronal types and repetitive firing properties. *J. Neurophysiol.* 58:195-214, 1987.

8. Dekin, M.S., and G.G. Haddad. Membrane and cellular properties in oscillating networks: implications for respiration. *J. Appl. Physiol.* 69:809-821, 1990.

9. Haddad, G., and P.A. Getting. Repetitive firing properties of neurons in the ventral region of nucleus tractus solitarius. *In*

vitro studies in adult and neonatal rat. *J. Neurophysiol.* 62:1213-1224, 1989.

10. Johnson, S.M., and P.A. Getting. Repetitive firing properties of neurons within the nucleus ambiguus of adult guinea pigs using the *in vitro* slice technique. *Neurosci. Abstr.* 13:825, 1987.

11. Llinas, R. The intrinsic electrophysiological properties of mammalian neurons: insights into central nervous system function. *Science* 242:1654-1664, 1988.

12. Mifflin, S., D. Ballantyne, S.B. Backman, and D.W. Richter. Evidence for a calcium-activated potassium conductance in medullary respiratory neurones. In *Neurogenesis of Central Respiratory Rhythm*, Ed. A.L. Bianchi and M. Denavit-Saubié, 179-181. Lancaster, UK: MTP Press, 1985.

13. Richter, D.W. Generation and maintenance of the respiratory rhythm. *J. Exp. Biol.* 100:93-107, 1982.

14. Tsien, R.W., D. Lipscombe, D.V. Madison, K.R. Bley, and A.P. Fox. Multiple types of neuronal calcium channels and their selective modulation. *Trends in Neurosci.* 11:431-438, 1988.

15. Viana, F., L. Gibbs, and A.J. Berger. Double- and triple-labeling of functionally characterized central neurons projecting to peripheral targets studied *in vitro*. *Neuroscience* 38:829-841, 1990.

16. Watson, T.W.J., and Q.J. Pittman. Pharmacological evidence that somatostatin activates the m-current in hippocampal pyramidal neurons. *Neurosci. Lett.* 91:172-176, 1988.

2

Properties of Brainstem Neurons:
Calcium Currents in Hypoglossal Motoneurons

Albert J. Berger and Felix Viana

The subthreshold and firing behaviors of respiratory-related neurons are governed both by their intrinsic membrane properties and by their synaptic inputs. Recently our interest has turned to investigating intrinsic properties of brainstem respiratory neurons, in particular voltage- and time-dependent conductances that are present in hypoglossal motoneurons. At present little is known about Ca^{++} currents in respiratory motoneurons. We hypothesize that these currents have an important role in determining the subthreshold and firing behaviors of respiratory motoneurons.

Voltage-gated neuronal calcium currents have been categorized in two major ways. The first considers Ca^{++} currents to consist of low-voltage-activated (LVA) and high-voltage-activated (HVA) types of currents (6, 8). The LVA current requires removal of inactivation, by hyperpolarization, and then activation, by depolarization, at membrane potentials somewhat above resting levels. The HVA current is activated at potentials more depolarized than those that activate LVA current. A second categorization scheme considers that there are three types of Ca^{++} channels, the T-, N- and L-channels, each having distinct voltage, kinetic, and pharmacologic properties (6, 8).

In the present study our aim was to determine the types and properties of the Ca^{++} currents present in rat neonatal hypoglossal motoneurons. To do this we used tight-seal whole-cell recordings with patch-type electrodes from visually identified motoneurons in thin medullary slices. We also investigated the role of Ca^{++} currents in the firing behavior of neonatal rat hypoglossal motoneurons recorded intracellularly in conventional slices.

METHODS

Measurements of whole-cell currents were performed using a thin-slice preparation of the medulla. In brief, we removed the brainstem from the skull of decapitated neonatal (3- to 10-day-old) rats, chilled the tissue block in ice-cold Ringer's solution, and then cut thin slices (120–130 μm) of the medulla. Following incubation of 1 h at 35°C, slices were transferred to a specially designed perfusion chamber mounted on a modified Zeiss light microscope. Slices were viewed with differential interference optics, and individual neurons were visualized. The membrane above the

cell was then cleaned of overlying debris using a recently reported method (4). The voltage-clamped hypoglossal motoneurons were studied with tight-seal whole-cell recordings using patch pipettes. In some animals, a fluorescent dye (rhodamine-dextran-lysine) was injected into the tongue to label hypoglossal motoneurons retrogradely (9). Single-labeled motoneurons were observed in the living slice and were cleaned for whole-cell recording. The perfusion fluid and the pipette solution used to block voltage-dependent currents other than Ca^{++} currents have been described previously (2), with the modification that in the present experiments the Ca^{++} was reduced in the perfusion fluid from 10 to 5 mM and Cs^+ (2 mM) was added to this fluid to block the inward rectifier current (I_h) that is present in these neonatal cells (1).

In other experiments using thick medullary slices (400 μm) from neonatal rats, we studied hypoglossal motoneurons in current-clamp mode. The cells were impaled with conventional intracellular microelectrodes. We examined the possible role of Ca^{++} on the subthreshold membrane potential changes as well as its effect on suprathreshold firing behavior.

RESULTS

In voltage-clamp, step depolarizations from a holding potential V_h of approximately −90 mV to a command voltage (V_c) of approximately −55 mV produced a small-amplitude inward current (fig. 2.1A, upper left). This inward current was transient and was fully inactivated by the end of the 500-msec depolarizing voltage step. It is similar to the LVA Ca^{++} current observed in other neuronal systems (2, 3, 5, 6, 8). Further increases in V_c resulted in an inward current of much larger amplitude that consisted of both inactivating and non-inactivating components (fig. 2.1A, upper right) and is similar to the HVA Ca^{++} current that has been observed previously (2, 5, 6, 8). Next, after changing V_h to approximately −60 mV, step depolarizations failed to activate the LVA current but did activate the HVA Ca^{++} current (fig. 2.1A, lower panels). Figure 2.1B shows the I-V relationships for the peak inward current generated by step depolarizations from V_h of −91 and −61 mV. These I-V relationships show that the LVA current requires hyperpolarization in order to be activated by the depolarizing cur-

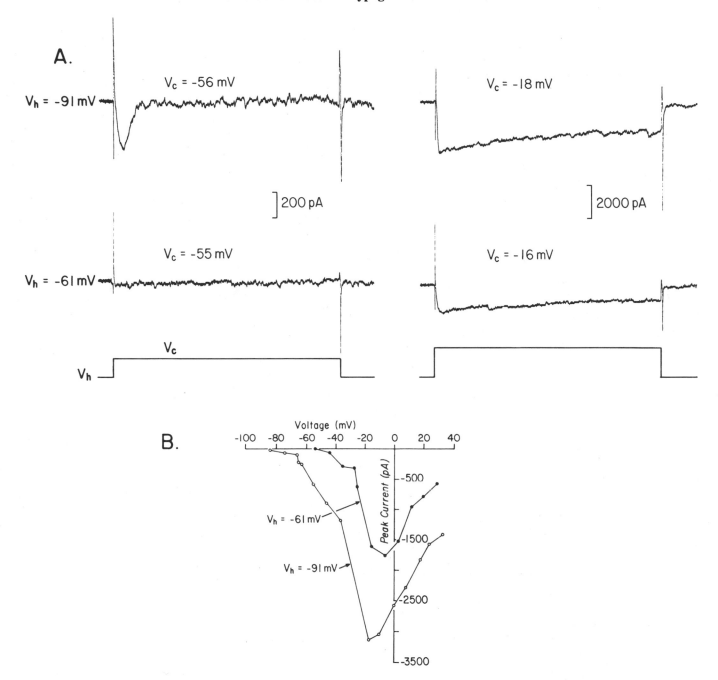

FIG. 2.1 LVA and HVA Ca^{++} currents and their voltage-dependency recorded from a voltage-clamped hypoglossal motoneuron. (A) Whole-cell current recording at two different holding potentials (V_h) in response to two different depolarizing steps (V_c) applied for 500 msec. Depolarization to −56 mV from a V_h of −91 mV resulted in a transient inward current (the LVA current: upper left). Stepping to −18 mV caused a much larger amplitude and long-duration inward current (the HVA current: upper right). Stepping to similar levels from a more depolarized V_h (−61 mV) failed to activate the LVA current but did activate the HVA current (lower traces). (B) The I-V relationships for the peak inward current obtained from the two V_h (−61 mV, filled circles; −91 mV, open circles). Data in A and B are from the same hypoglossal motoneuron, and all data are shown leak-subtracted.

rent steps. A detailed look at the data presented in figure 2.1 reveals a reduction in the HVA current when holding at depolarized compared with hyperpolarized potentials. This may be due to rundown of this current and/or some degree of voltage-dependent inactivation. Both the LVA and HVA currents are carried by Ca^{++} because they are reversibly

abolished or markedly diminished by a nominally Ca^{++}-free bathing medium (fig. 2.2).

The LVA current was investigated in greater detail. First, the time course of removal of inactivation was studied by hyperpolarizing the cell for varying periods and measuring the peak amplitude of the inward current generated after

FIG. 2.2 Effects of removing Ca^{++} from the bathing medium on the LVA and HVA Ca^{++} currents. The perfusion fluid was changed from the control, which contained 5 mM Ca^{++} and 1 mM Mg^{++}, to a solution that was nominally Ca^{++}-free and with 5 mM Mg^{++}; during the wash period the perfusion fluid was returned to its control composition. The lefthand column of traces shows the LVA current produced by applying a hyperpolarizing pulse of 500-msec duration to remove inactivation; in the control and wash records, the transient LVA current is activated when V_h is returned to -45 mV. A nominally Ca^{++}-free solution abolished this LVA current. The righthand column of traces shows the HVA current produced by applying a 500-msec depolarizing pulse from a V_h of -63 mV. A nominally Ca^{++}-free solution markedly reduced this HVA current. In the wash solution, the HVA current returned toward its control value. The traces for the LVA current are single sweeps, whereas the traces for the HVA current are leak-subtracted. LVA and HVA records are from different hypoglossal motoneurons. Both of the 0 Ca^{++} records were taken after 4 min in this solution; the wash records were obtained after bathing the slice for 5 min in the control solution.

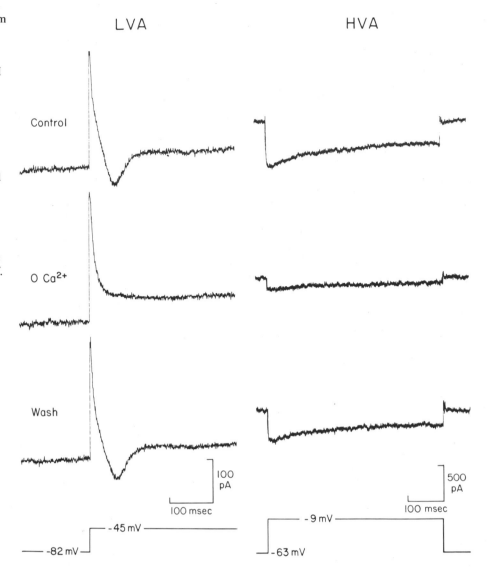

return of the cell to its V_h (fig. 2.3A). We observed that the time course of removal of inactivation fitted a single exponential. The time constant for the single exponential was 481 ± 110 msec (mean $\pm$ SD for n = 8 cells).

Second, inactivation curves were determined by hyperpolarizing a cell to different voltages and measuring the peak amplitude of the inward current generated following return of the cell to its V_h where the LVA current was activated, but at a potential below that which activated the HVA current (fig. 2.3B). The voltage-dependency of inactivation was fitted with a Boltzman relationship. For five cells in which this was done, the voltage for half-inactivation removal was -90.3 ± 2.5 mV, and the slope factor was 5.09 ± 1.06 mV per e-fold change.

We also investigated the possible relevance of LVA and HVA Ca^{++} currents on the subthreshold and firing behaviors of hypoglossal motoneurons. Hypoglossal motoneurons were impaled with microelectrodes while bathing the slice with standard Ringer's solution (containing 2 mM Ca^{++}

and 2 mM Mg^{++})—a solution that did not block ionic currents. These experiments were carried out in current-clamp mode. Figure 2.4A illustrates that injection of 0.5 nA depolarizing current pulses from a resting potential of -70 mV resulted in only a passive-type response of the membrane. Hyperpolarizing prepulses caused a transient depolarization of the membrane (fig. 2.4A, arrow), and, with slightly stronger depolarizing current pulses, this transient depolarization gave rise to a rebound, all-or-none fast action potential. The transient depolarization and rebound response were abolished when the same slice was bathed in a nominally Ca^{++}-free Ringer's solution (fig. 2.4B). These findings suggest that the transient depolarizing response occurring in the presence of a conditioning hyperpolarization is caused mostly by activation of the LVA Ca^{++} current present in these motoneurons.

We investigated next the role of Ca^{++} currents on the action potentials and after-potentials. Figure 2.4C shows that when a slice is bathed in nominally Ca^{++}-free Ring-

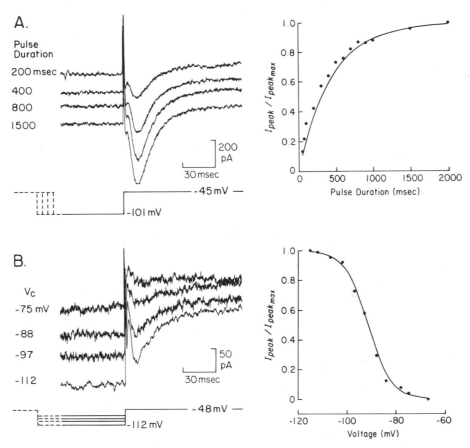

FIG. 2.3 Properties of inactivation of the LVA Ca^{++} current. (A) Time course of removal of inactivation. *Left:* Whole-cell current traces showing return of the membrane potential from −101 mV to −45 mV for four different hyperpolarizing pulse durations. *Right:* The relationship between the normalized transient peak inward current and the hyperpolarizing pulse duration. Filled circles represent total data set from the hypoglossal motoneuron whose current traces are shown in the lefthand panel. The line indicates the exponential fit of the data points obtained by linear regression. (B) Voltage-dependence of inactivation. *Left:* Whole-cell current traces showing return of the membrane potential to a V_h of −48 mV from varying (and indicated) hyperpolarizing levels. The hyperpolarizing pulse duration was 500 msec. *Right:* The relationship between the normalized transient peak inward current and the hyperpolarizing pulse amplitude. Filled circles: Total data set from the hypoglossal motoneuron whose current traces are shown in the lefthand panel. The line indicates the Boltzman equation that was fitted to these data [$I_{peak}/I_{peakmax} = 1/(1 + \exp(V-V_{1/2})/K)$, where $V_{1/2} = −91.4$ mV and $K = 4.82$ mV per e-fold change]. In A and B there is an arbitrary vertical displacement of the current traces one from another for ease in visualizing the transient inward current activated when the voltage was returned to V_h. Records are single sweeps and have not been leak-subtracted. Data in A and B are from different hypoglossal motoneurons.

er's solution, the afterhyperpolarization (AHP) that follows the action potential is markedly reduced. The cell illustrated was kept somewhat depolarized (−62 mV), suggesting that the HVA and not the LVA current contributed exclusively to the Ca^{++} current that was generated. We suggest that during the action potential, activation of the HVA Ca^{++} current causes Ca^{++} to enter the cell and that this is sufficient to activate a Ca^{++}-dependent K$^+$ conductance that is responsible for the AHP. Further, compared with bathing the slice in standard Ringer's solution, a bath of nominally Ca^{++}-free solution had no effect on the shape or duration of a single action potential (fig. 2.4D).

The relevance of Ca^{++} entry into the cell and the effect of the resultant AHP on the repetitive firing behavior of hypoglossal motoneurons is illustrated in figure 2.5. We observed that compared with the control, the steady-state firing frequency was increased when Ca^{++} was absent

from the perfusing solution. This result suggests that Ca^{++} entry through the HVA Ca^{++} channels during an action potential causes activation of a Ca^{++}-dependent K$^+$ conductance, which in turn causes the firing frequency to be reduced.

DISCUSSION

As in the case of other motoneurons, including spinal motoneurons (1) and embryonic chick limb motoneurons (5), neonatal rat hypoglossal motoneurons were found to express both LVA and HVA Ca^{++} currents. The LVA current was activated by depolarization at somewhat above resting levels. Hyperpolarization of hypoglossal motoneurons caused removal of inactivation of the LVA current, and this removal was both time- and voltage-dependent. The HVA current was of a much larger amplitude and was activated

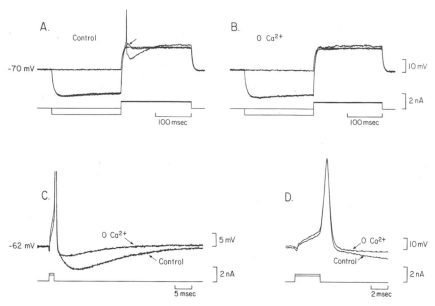

FIG. 2.4 The multiple role of calcium in motoneuronal firing. (A) The response of a neonatal hypoglossal motoneuron to bipolar (hyperpolarizing-depolarizing) current pulses in standard Ringer's solution (2 mM Ca^{++}, 2 mM Mg^{++}). The hyperpolarizing prepulse (200 msec) gives rise to a transient depolarization of the membrane (arrow). A slight increase in the amplitude of the depolarizing pulse results in a rebound action potential (cell resting membrane potential = −70 mV). (B) Same stimulation protocol as in A but in Ringer's solution containing 0 Ca^{++}, 5 mM Mg^{++}, 0.5 mM EGTA (to chelate residual Ca^{++} in extracellular solution). The transient depolarization is now blocked, as is the resulting rebound excitation. (C) The same 0 Ca^{++}/high Mg^{++} solution strongly reduces the afterhyperpolarization that follows a single action potential (resting membrane potential = −62 mV). (D) Lack of effect of the 0 Ca^{++}/high Mg^{++} on the shape and duration of the action potential. All records are from the same motoneuron (A and B were obtained in discontinuous current clamp; C and D in bridge mode). The full size of the spike in A has been reduced by the digitizing procedure. All data are from the same hypoglossal motoneuron. Recordings were made at 32°C.

FIG. 2.5 The role of Ca^{++} in repetitive firing of hypoglossal motoneuron. (A) *Left:* The initial response of a hypoglossal motoneuron to a depolarizing current pulse (1.25 nA). Note the (early) initial doublet followed by a prolonged interspike interval. *Right:* The same pulse as in A (*left*), but in 0 Ca^{++}/high Mg^{++}. Note the decreased interspike interval following the initial doublet. (B) *Left:* The adaptation curve (frequency-time) of motoneuronal firing to the same 1.25 nA(+) current pulse (1 sec duration). *Right:* Removal of Ca^{++} causes a pronounced increase in the steady-state firing. All data are from the same motoneuron as in fig. 2.4. The resting membrane potential = −71 mV.

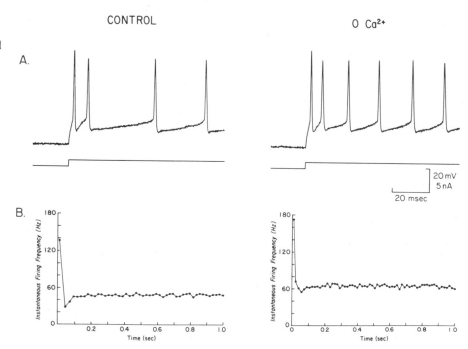

at potentials more depolarized than those that activated the LVA current. Both of these currents have properties similar to those present in other neuronal systems (6, 8).

Of interest is the importance of these two Ca^{++} currents for the behavior of neonatal hypoglossal motoneurons.

A portion of the LVA current is activated in the subthreshold range and therefore may contribute to membrane potential changes in this voltage range. Thus the LVA current can produce a transient depolarization and rebound excitation of hypoglossal motoneurons after its release from hyperpolarizing inputs. This may occur *in vivo* as hypoglossal motoneurons are rhythmically hyperpolarized and depolarized with each respiratory cycle (10). Further, under certain conditions, neonatal hypoglossal motoneurons exhibit a decrementing discharge pattern during inspiration (7). Thus activation of the LVA Ca^{++} current at the start of inspiration may contribute to formation of this type of decrementing burst pattern. The HVA Ca^{++} current may be activated during the action potential, causing a larger influx of Ca^{++}. Although we did not see marked changes in the action potential width following Ca^{++} removal from the perfusion solution (Fig. 2.4*D*), it was evident that removal of Ca^{++} caused a marked reduction in the AHP and also an increase in the firing rate in response to depolarizing current pulses. These results suggest that during a single action potential, the HVA current is activated, causing enough Ca^{++} entry to activate a Ca^{++}-dependent K^+ conductance, and further, that this latter conductance determines the amplitude and duration of the AHP. When K^+ conductances are blocked, as when a slice is perfused with the solution that isolates the Ca^{++} currents, we have observed in current-clamp experiments that long-duration Ca^{++} spikes are generated in response to injection of depolarizing current (not illustrated).

In summary, we have shown that LVA and HVA Ca^{++} currents are present in hypoglossal motoneurons and that these are important in both the sub- and suprathreshold behaviors of this class of brainstem respiratory motoneuron. Of considerable interest is the possibility of modulation of these Ca^{++} currents by neurotransmitters known to be present in the hypoglossal nucleus.

ACKNOWLEDGMENTS

This work was supported by a National Institutes of Health Javits Neuroscience Investigator Award, NS 14857. Special thanks go to Hanna Atkins for editing the manuscript and preparing the illustrations.

REFERENCES

1. Berger, A.J. Recent advances in respiratory neurobiology using *in vitro* methods. *Am. J. Physiol.: Lung Cell. Molec. Physiol.* 3:24-29, 1990.

2. Berger, A.J., and T. Takahashi. Serotonin enhances a low-voltage-activated calcium current in rat spinal motoneurons. *J. Neurosci.* 10:1922-1928, 1990.

3. Carbone, E., and H.D. Lux. Kinetics and selectivity of a low-voltage-activated calcium current in chick and rat sensory neurones. *J. Physiol.* (London) 386:547-570, 1987.

4. Edwards, F.A., A. Konnerth, B. Sakmann, and T. Takahashi. A thin slice preparation for patch clamp recordings from neurones of the mammalian central nervous system. *Pflügers Arch.* 414:600-612, 1989.

5. McCobb, D.P., P.M. Best, and K.G. Beam. Development alters the expression of calcium currents in chick limb motoneurons. *Neuron* 2:1633-1643, 1989.

6. Miller, R.J. Multiple calcium channels and neuronal function. *Science* 235:46-52, 1987.

7. Sica, A.L., A.M. Steel, M.R. Gandhi, and N. Prasad. Factors affecting central inspiratory modulation of hypoglossal motoneuron activity in newborn pigs. *J. Dev. Physiol.* 10:285-295, 1988.

8. Tsien, R.W., D. Lipscombe, D.V. Madison, K.R. Bley, and A.P. Fox. Multiple types of neuronal calcium channels and their selective modulation. *Trends in Neurosci.* 11:431-438, 1988.

9. Viana, F., L. Gibbs, and A.J. Berger. Double- and triple-labeling of functionally characterized central neurons projecting to peripheral targets studied *in vitro*. *Neuroscience* 38:829-841, 1990.

10. Withington-Wray, D.J., S.W. Mifflin, and K.M. Spyer. Intracellular analysis of respiratory modulated hypoglossal motoneurons in the cat. *Neuroscience* 25:1041-1051, 1988.

3

Neuronal Membrane Properties during O_2 Deprivation: *In Vitro* Intracellular Studies

Gabriel Haddad and Chun Jiang

INTRODUCTION

It is well recognized that cellular and membrane properties play an important role in the repetitive firing of neurons in the central nervous system (CNS) of vertebrates as well as invertebrates (9). Although the importance of these membrane properties in respiratory neurogenesis and rhythm maintenance have not been demonstrated fully in *in vivo* conditions, a number of examples in vertebrates have been well documented (3, 4, 5, 10). Nowhere have these examples been more readily available than in adult hippocampal neurons (3), in cerebellar and thalamic neurons (10), and in spinal motoneurons (5). Neural oscillatory activities such as seizures, alternating states of consciousness, and locomotion have been much better understood recently with the use of cellular and molecular approaches (4, 5, 10).

Neuronal membrane properties and their importance in neuronal activity and firing patterns have been generally described under "resting" conditions, whether *in vivo* or *in vitro* (4). However, membrane properties may not be fully expressed and may be totally missed if the membrane potential is not altered (e.g., low and high threshold Ca^{++} currents, A-current) or if intracellular biochemical components or second messenger systems are not modulated (2, 13). We have recently discovered the presence of a K^+ current that is activated by anoxia (and a presumed drop in ATP levels) in hypoglossal motoneurons. We are currently characterizing this K^+ current and channel, its activators, and regulation of its gating and biophysical properties. The purpose of this chapter is to detail some of our experiments which led to the discovery, albeit indirect, of this K^+ current and its function during O_2 deprivation.

METHODS

The brainstem slice preparation was used in most of our experiments. The advantages of this preparation and the general procedure have been described previously (4, 6, 7, 8). In brief, adult rats were lightly anesthetized by methoxyflurane and decapitated. Two to three 350–400 μm-thick transverse slices were obtained between 1 mm rostral to the obex and 0.5 mm caudal to the obex. These slices were placed in a chamber and allowed to equilibrate for 20–30 min. The time between decapitation and placement of the slices in the recording chamber was within 6.0 minutes. Flow of oxygenated Ringer's saline (95% O_2, 5% CO_2) was

2–3 ml/min and slices were kept subfused throughout the experiment. The same gas that oxygenated the saline also flowed over the slices after being warmed and humidified. The Ringer's solution was at pH 7.4 after equilibration with 5% CO_2 and contained the following (in mM): NaCl = 125, KCl = 3, $MgSO_4$ = 1.3, $CaCl_2$ = 2.5, $NaHPO_4$ = 2.5, $NaHCO_3$ = 26, glucose = 10. Brainstem slices remained viable for at least 6–8 hours.

We focused on hypoglossal (HYP) neurons for two reasons: (1) These cells are relatively large in the adult rat and (2) the hypoglossal nucleus is well delineated in the slice preparation. We also studied the density of HYP neurons with retrograde tracing techniques. A cut HYP nerve was soaked in wheat-germ lectin conjugated with horseradish peroxidase (HRP-WGA). Two days after exposure to HRP, animals were sacrificed (using deep pentobarbital anesthesia) and the brain processed for HRP histochemistry using the tetramethylbenzidine (TMB) method (11).

Our protocol had three phases. In the first we determined the properties of neurons before O_2 deprivation. In the second phase we determined these same neuronal properties during 5 min of anoxic exposure. The third was the recovery phase. Anoxia was induced by switching the perfusate to one equilibrated with 95% N_2, 5% CO_2 and by flowing 95% N_2, 5% CO_2 over the slices. Drugs were applied by switching perfusion solutions. All solutions bathed slices for at least 20 minutes before anoxic exposure was attempted. Ion fluxes were measured with ion-selective microelectrodes similar to those described previously (1). For intracellular recordings, double-barreled microelectrodes were employed, in which one barrel was used for measurement of intracellular K^+ activity ($[K^+]i$) and the other for electrical activity (1, 8). DC potential was also measured and was used to correct for extracellular potential shift. For baseline characterization of HYP neurons, single- or double-barreled microelectrodes were used (8). Extracellular K^+ activity ($[K^+]o$) was measured using single-barreled electrodes with tips of about 4 μm. DC potential was also used for correction. The rest of the procedures were the same as those for $[K^+]i$. Calibrations of $[K^+]i$ or $[K^+]o$ were made as previously described (1, 8).

RESULTS AND DISCUSSION

The HYP nucleus contained neurons of shapes and sizes different than other brainstem areas. HYP cells were among the largest cells seen in the brainstem (30–50 μm). The density of HYP neurons within the HYP nucleus was comparatively low.

Following impalement, neurons were hyperpolarized for a few minutes in order to stabilize the recording. Current was removed and once the membrane potential was stable the resting potential was measured and test paradigms started. Adult HYP neurons had a membrane potential of −80 ± 2 mV (mean ± SEM, n = 22). Most adult neurons (>95%) did not fire spontaneously and required relatively large currents to fire, with a rheobase of about 2nA.

In response to hyperpolarizing current pulses, adult HYP neurons displayed a "sag" or inward rectification which was more marked with higher currents. About 40% of the cells displayed a sag of 20% or more from the peak voltage change. Input resistance (R$_N$) averaged 20.9 ± 1.5 Mohms when calculated with the peak voltage change and 14.6 ± 1.4 Mohms when considering the steady state voltage change. Postinhibitory rebound (PIR) was also present in these cells but appeared mainly with large changes in membrane potentials (>20mV) with negative current injections. PIR was also enhanced if resting membrane potential became lower.

HYP neurons showed little spike frequency adaptation (SFA). The SFA index (defined as steady state frequency over peak frequency × 100) in adult HYP neurons was 70 to 90% (n = 10) with most of the decline in firing rate occurring between the first and the second interspike interval. Frequency–current plots revealed that there were generally two slopes. At relatively low currents (<1.3 nA), the firing rate increased more slowly than at higher currents (>1.5 nA) (fig. 3.1).

Additional experiments showed that HYP neurons have tetrodotoxin-sensitive Na channels which are responsible for the rising phase of action potentials (n = 3). When these cells were exposed to tetraethylammonium (TEA, 20 mM), they showed a marked prolongation of action potentials with no repolarization shoulder. CoCl$_2$ (1 mM), a Ca^{++} channel blocker, when used after TEA did not change the trajectory of action potentials. HYP neurons showed no delayed excitation or any major Ca^{++} currents (7).

We conclude from these experiments that adult HYP neurons have cellular properties that are different from those of other brainstem neurons (vagal neurons or cells in the nucleus tractus solitarius) in that these HYP cells are not endowed with major Ca^{++} currents. Since some of these properties (PIR, sag after hyperpolarization, and the absence of A-current) enhance depolarization and excitability and since HYP motoneurons innervate an important upper airway muscle (genioglossus), these properties seemingly would help ensure airway patency before diaphragm contraction in *in vivo* situations.

During anoxia [K$^+$]o measurements were made in 32 adult rat slices. Anoxia induced a 4- to 6-fold increase in K$^+$ activity in the interstitial fluid. With reoxygenation, [K$^+$]o was quickly reduced to or even be-

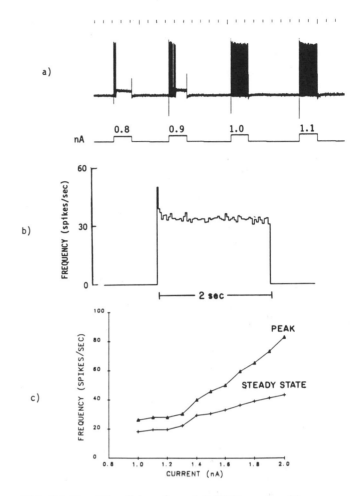

FIG. 3.1 Repetitive firing of an adult HYP neuron with a membrane potential of −78 mV. (A) Response to depolarizing pulses with increasing current intensities. Horizontal scale = 1 sec; vertical scale = 40 mV. (B) Frequency–Time profile. (C) Frequency–current plot for the same HYP neuron.

low baseline levels and gradually came back to baseline in about 6–8 min.

In the slice preparation, our results indicate that the increase in [K$^+$]o is not due to shrinkage of the extracellular compartment. Hence, we raise the question as to whether K$^+$ is leaking from neurons or whether glia, under anoxic conditions, cease to function as K$^+$ sinks and actually leak K$^+$. In order to answer whether K$^+$ leaks from HYP neurons, we measured [K$^+$]i in addition to intracellular potential in all three phases of our protocol in HYP neurons.

[K$^+$]i was measured in ten neurons. During baseline, [K$^+$]i was 98.7 ± 4.7 mM. During anoxia, HYP cells depolarized as we have previously shown (8). Furthermore, there was a major decrease in [K$^+$]i that started 2 min into anoxia. The nadir was quickly reached and averaged about 40% of control values (fig. 3.2). When O$_2$ was reintroduced, [K$^+$]i started to increase and returned back to baseline within 8–10 min.

Since there is evidence from previous studies (8) that the Na-K ATPase pump is inhibited during anoxia (for lack of

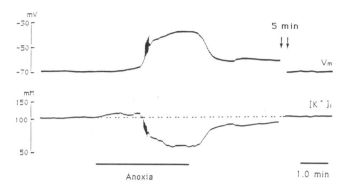

FIG. 3.2 Intracellular recordings of membrane potential (upper trace) and $[K^+]i$ (lower trace) from an adult HYP neuron. At about 1–2 min into anoxia, the neuron started to depolarize and $[K^+]i$ was rapidly reduced. When O_2 was switched back, $[K^+]i$ increased rapidly after a short delay. Ten min later, $[K^+]i$ had recovered to the pre-anoxia levels.

ATP as a substrate), an increase in $[K^+]o$ could result. The question was therefore whether the increase in $[K^+]o$ is solely related to this inhibition or whether there are other mechanisms that are important in K^+ release.

We first used high doses of ouabain (5 mM) to totally block the Na-K pump, then subsequently induced anoxia in the presence of ouabain and measured $[K^+]o$. $[K^+]o$ increased with ouabain but increased *further* with anoxia. This suggested that other mechanisms were active.

Additional experiments showed that TEA and CsCl, but not 4-aminopyridine or apamin, blocked K^+ leakage during anoxia. Even more interesting was our observation that glibenclamide, a specific blocker of ATP-sensitive K^+ channels (2, 12, 13), decreased the release of K^+ by about 60%. In addition, neurons depolarized more during anoxia in the presence of glibenclamide than in its absence.

We conclude, therefore that (1) anoxia produces K^+ leakage from HYP neurons; (2) leakage is a major cause of anoxia-induced K^+ accumulation in the interstitial fluid; (3) the shrinkage in extracellular volume during anoxia does not play a major role in the increase in $[K^+]o$; (4) the increase in $[K^+]o$ during anoxia is probably related to two membrane properties: (*a*) inhibition of the Na-K pump and (*b*) activation of K^+ channels that are generally known to be inactive at rest; and (5) anoxia, by decreasing ATP or by modulating intracellular biochemical events, activates a recently described group of K^+ channels in nerve cells (12).

These channels (or currents) serve to limit depolarization or to hyperpolarize neurons during anoxia, a strategy which would decrease neural activity and energy utilization, thus delaying injury and cell death.

REFERENCES

1. Ammann, D., P. Chao, and W. Simon. Valinomycin-based K^+ selective microelectrodes with low electrical membrane resistance. *Neurosci. Lett.* 74:221-226, 1987.
2. Ashford, F.M. Adenosine 5'-triphosphate-sensitive potassium channels. *Ann. Rev. Neurosci.* 11:97-118, 1988.
3. Brown, T.H., E.W. Kairiss, and C.L. Keenan. Hebbian synapses: Biophysical mechanisms and algorithms. *Ann. Rev. Neurosci.* 13:475-511, 1990.
4. Dekin, M.S., and G.G. Haddad. Membrane and cellular properties in oscillating networks: Implications for respiration. *J. Appl. Physiol.* 69:809-821, 1990.
5. Grillner, S. Neurobiological basis of rhythmic motor acts in vertebrates. *Science* 228:143-149, 1985.
6. Haddad, G.G., and P.A. Getting. Repetitive firing properties of neurons in the ventral region of the Nucleus Tractus Solitarius. *In vitro* studies in adult and neonatal rat. *J. Neurophysiol.* 62:1213-1224, 1989.
7. Haddad, G.G., D.F. Donnelly, and P.A. Getting. Biophysical properties of hypoglossal motoneurons *in vitro*: Intracellular studies in adult and neonatal rats. *J. Appl. Physiol.* 69:1509-1517, 1990.
8. Haddad, G.G., and D.F. Donnelly. O_2 deprivation induces a major depolarization in brainstem neurons in the adult but not in the neonatal rat. *J. Physiol.* (London) 429:411-428, 1990.
9. Llinas, R.R. The intrinsic electrophysiologic properties of mammalian neurons: Insights into central nervous system function. *Science* 242:1654-1663, 1988.
10. McCormick, D.A. Cholinergic and noradrenergic modulation of thalamocortical processing. *Trends in Neurosci.* 12:215-221, 1989.
11. Mesulam, M.M., E. Hegarty, H. Barbas, K.A. Carson, E.C. Gower, A.G. Knapp, M.B. Moss, and E.J. Mufson. Additional factors influencing sensitivity in the Tetramethylbenzidine method for Horseradish Peroxidase neurochemistry. *J. Histochem. Cytochem.* 28:1255-1259, 1980.
12. Mourre, C., Y. Ben-Ari, H. Bernardi, M. Fosset, and M. Lazdunski. Antidiabetic sulfonylurea: Location of binding sites in the brain and effects on the hyperpolarization induced by anoxia in hippocampal slices. *Brain Res.* 486:159-164, 1989.
13. Noma, A. ATP-regulated K^+ channels in cardiac muscle. *Nature* 305:147-148, 1983.

4

New Insights on Synaptic Transmission in the Nucleus Tractus Solitarius

J. Champagnat, P. Branchereau, M. Denavit-Saubié, G. Fortin, T. Jacquin, and P. Schweitzer

Most synaptic interactions in the central nervous system involve more than one messenger molecule. Functional pools of different transmitters can be co-regulated at pre- and postsynaptic sites. At presynaptic sites, neurotransmitters are co-localized and different patterns of afferent input may determine differential release of transmitters. At postsynaptic sites, multiple transmitter actions are integrated at different steps of the chain of events initiated by the agonists' actions on receptive sites, intracellular messenger pathways, and membrane permeabilities. These synaptic influences operating in brainstem structures such as the nucleus tractus solitarius (NTS) probably contribute to central modulation of respiratory patterns.

The NTS is involved in synaptic transmission of vagal and glossopharyngeal sensory primary afferent signals, including those relevant to reflex regulation of respiratory function. The ventrolateral subnucleus of the cat NTS contains the dorsal group of medullary respiratory neurons receiving monosynaptic inputs from pulmonary afferents and the retrofacial respiratory group. Synaptic transmission by fast excitatory (EPSPs) and inhibitory postsynaptic potentials (IPSPs) in the NTS is widely documented *in vitro* and *in vivo* (fig. 4.1). A considerable amount of data is available on the histochemistry of the NTS and neurotransmitters with potential biological and pharmacological interest at this level (see 28). Only a small number of these transmitters, mainly amino acids as discussed by several authors in this volume, are likely to produce fast postsynaptic potentials (PSPs) such as chloride-dependent IPSPs mediated by glycine- or GABA-like transmitters (11, 15, 21, 23) or cationic currents mediated by excitatory amino acid-like transmitters (10, 13, 14, 25). Thus, many putative transmitters identified in the NTS are probably not (or not only) mediators of fast PSPs: this chapter presents studies performed *in vivo* or in brainstem slices during the last few years to understand the function of these transmitters.

Brainstem slices were used because they enable control of medium composition on both sides of the neuronal membrane: on the extracellular side by superfusion of the preparation and application of known concentrations of agonists; on the intracellular side using drugs which cross the plasma membrane. The intracellular cytosolic medium can also be manipulated with the help of whole-cell patch-clamp recordings with relatively large electrode tips: this method

has been recently found applicable to NTS slices (fig. 4.1). Most slice experiments and histochemical observations on the NTS have been performed on rodents. Recent electrophysiological observations on rodent brainstems *in vivo* led to controversial conclusions about the significance of the dorsal respiratory group in these animals (16, 33, see Mc-Crimmon, this volume) and it has been suggested that the population of large inspiratory neurons which have been impaled in the ventrolateral NTS of cats (see 29) may not exist in rats (35). Studies of the dorsal respiratory group in slice preparations thus require a comparative approach on several animal species, including cat brainstem slices which retain ventrolateral NTS neurons with morphological properties comparable to those described in the dorsal respiratory group *in vivo* (4).

Two types of postsynaptic responses are elicited in slices by stimulation of the solitary tract: fast EPSPs and IPSPs generated by increased membrane conductances, and prolonged EPSPs associated with decreased neuronal input conductance and increased background synaptic activity and firing (3, 4). Identification of these two types of synaptic potentials is confirmed by bath applications of exogenous neurotransmitters, which decrease or increase neuronal input resistance in the NTS (fig. 4.2). Synaptic potentials related to a conductance decrease indicate regulation of non-inactivating permeabilities which have to be available before neurotransmitter action. Potentials associated with decreased input conductance can be mediated by several transmitter candidates, all active on potassium conductances: substance P (18), acetylcholine via muscarinic receptors (7), serotonin (18) via 5HT-2 receptors (6), cholecystokinin via CCK-B receptors (2). Other currents controlling firing patterns are also modified by various neurotransmitters. Combination of potassium currents with high and low threshold calcium currents produces a beating pattern of activity in a population of NTS neurons (5, 7). The relative importance of transient potassium currents and low threshold transient calcium currents determines excitability (see Dekin, this volume). Transmitters such as thyrotropin-releasing hormone (9), substance P or serotonin (18), when applied exogenously, modify the balance of calcium and potassium currents and may therefore change firing patterns in the absence of classical PSPs. These effects, however, have not yet been identified following stimulation of endogenous pathways in the NTS.

FIG. 4.1 Gigaohm seal formation and whole-cell recording of EPSC and IPSC in rat ventral NTS from 450 μm thick brainstem slices. *Upper*: approach of the membrane using suction through the 2μm diameter tip of the micropipette (left arrow), current injection (upper trace), and voltage recording (lower trace) to monitor resistance: gigaohms are measured when membrane properly seals to the pipette (cell-attached situation). Further suction (right arrow) breaks the membrane patch at the pipette tip (whole cell recording, membrane potential: −70 mV): action potentials (truncated by the penwriter) are induced by depolarizing current injections. *Lower*: Whole-cell voltage-clamp recording of early postsynaptic currents induced by a single electrical stimulus in the solitary tract (TS, arrow): inward EPSC (downward) is followed by outward IPSP (upward); chloride-free (potassium gluconate-containing) pipette, holding potential −40mV.

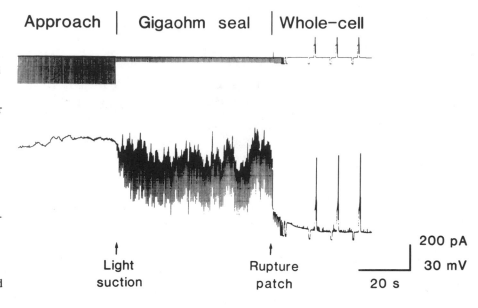

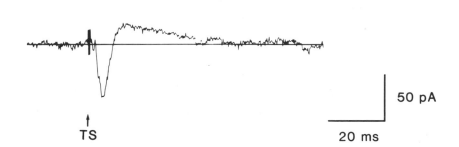

Several sensory inputs to the NTS exhibit periodic discharge of spike trains in relation to the ventilatory or cardiac cycles *in vivo*. The effects of such repetitive trains of stimuli have been studied on slices (4, 8, 24, 34). Comparison with single stimuli demonstrates differential regulation of PSPs by presynaptic patterns. Early PSPs associated with conductance increases are generally depressed by repetitive stimulations, while the background synaptic activity and the PSPs associated with conductance decreases are exaggerated. Responses lasting several minutes were recently obtained after single trains of stimuli. Therefore, periodic repetition of these trains in respiratory afferents has probably two functional consequences in the NTS *in vivo*: transmission of phasic signals and control of tonic excitability in the brainstem. The only transmitter candidates so far available to initiate this tonic control are those which decrease non-inactivating potassium conductances.

Depression of early PSPs during repetitive afferent stimulation might result from failure of action potential propa-

gation in the extensive ramifications of sensory afferents (as discussed in 24), reduction of synaptic release by primary afferent depolarization (see 31), transmitter action on presynaptic calcium currents, or transmitters such as opioids (10) interacting postsynaptically with excitatory transmitters. Other regulatory mechanisms may relate to the important role of excitatory amino acids (EAA) and N-methyl-D-aspartate receptors (NMDA-R). Synaptic excitation by amino acids takes place in the NTS neuronal networks (14, 25). Recently, G. Fortin studied the pharmacology of the first milliseconds of excitatory postsynaptic currents (EPSC) in the NTS and concluded that part of the EAA pool released by primary afferent terminals were active on non-NMDA-R and NMDA-R (3). Involvement of NMDA-R in brainstem networks generating the respiratory off-switch has been established by Foutz et al. (13). Metabolic consequences of excitation by EAA in the brainstem, therefore, deserve discussion. (1) EAAs modify transmembrane ionic gradients and increase extracellular potassium concentration as measured *in vitro* after bath applications

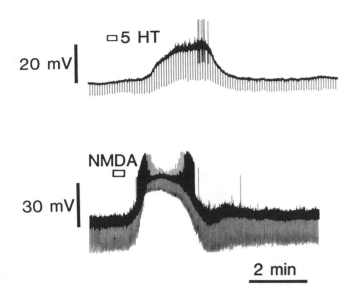

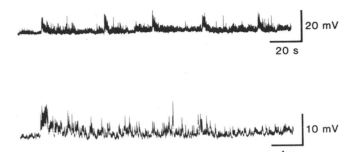

FIG. 4.2 Measurement of membrane potential during bath application of serotonin (5HT, upper trace) and N-methyl-D-aspartate (in the absence of extracellular magnesium; NMDA, lower trace). Neurotransmitter-induced depolarization of NTS neurons may be related to an increase or decrease of the input resistance. Input resistance is monitored by the amplitude of voltage transients (downward deflections of traces) induced by constant 500 ms intracellular current injections (upper: 0.05 nA; lower: 0.1 nA). Neurons have been impaled with a K-acetate-containing electrode. Note that background synaptic activity is increased during the action of 5HT (upper trace) and by removal of extracellular magnesium (compare upper and lower traces); it is decreased by shunting during the action of NMDA. Action potentials (upward) are truncated by the penwriter.

FIG. 4.3 Periodic pattern of "spontaneous" inhibitory synaptic background activities in the rat ventral NTS. Membrane potentials are measured by impalement of the neuron with a KCl-containing micropipette (membrane potential, −70 mV). The two samples were obtained from the same neuron at different time scales. Background activities result from summation of reversed Cl-dependent IPSPs generated within the NTS. In this particular case, each burst of synaptic inhibition exhibits a rapidly increasing–slowly decreasing profile; periodicity (2/min) developed during the time (about 1.5 hour) of a pharmacological study of the neuron by bath application of cholecystokinin analogs; the periodic pattern thereafter persisted until the end of cell recording (about 2 hours). Such periodic patterns are only occasional (i.e., observed in 10% or less of the cases) in NTS neurons in slices.

of agonists or repetitive stimulations of the solitary tract (3, see also 30). (2) EAAs also interact with intracellular pH and the energy-rich phosphorylated metabolites, phosphocreatine and ATP (19): a relationship between amino acid action and mitochondrial respiration has been established pharmacologically in slices (20). It is not known, however, how local ionic or metabolic regulation within the brainstem tissue controls transmission of sensory afferent inputs or generation of respiratory potentials *in vivo*.

In the absence of afferent stimulation, sustained discharge of fast PSPs indicative of spontaneous presynaptic firing can be recorded from most NTS neurons in slices (4). A transient increase of this background synaptic activity is induced by repetitive solitary tract stimulation: the late part of this response is probably initiated by transmitter-induced conductance decreases at presynaptic sites and can be reproduced by bath application of agonists (see the effect of 5HT in fig. 4.2). *In vivo*, a periodic increase of synaptic background activity is recorded in respiratory neurons during the respiratory cycle. Slicing eliminates connections of NTS neurons with different brainstem respiratory areas and with the spinal motor neurons. Spontaneous periodic activities resembling respiratory patterns are, therefore, generally not found in brainstem slices (5) although they can be

occasionally observed in the NTS (12, fig. 4.3) and in the hypoglossal nucleus of brainstem slices from newborns (22, see Smith et al., this volume). The role of endogenous transmitters in the initiation of these periodic patterns *in vitro* remains to be investigated.

Several transmitters appear to reduce membrane permeability *in vitro*. Depolarization by these transmitters leads to an excitatory action which has been described in respiratory neurons *in vivo* by microiontophoretic application of substance P, serotonin, acetylcholine or the tetrapeptide fragment of cholecystokinin; however, effects of these agonists *in vivo* are generally more variable than *in vitro* (1, 26, 27, see 28). Effects were also found highly modifiable *in vitro* when different transmitters were investigated simultaneously. Regulation of potassium permeability in the NTS appears to involve the contribution of several co-released transmitters, several postsynaptic receptive sites, and intracellular messengers.

(1) Potassium permeability of NTS neurons can be either decreased as described above or increased by the same transmitter acting at different receptive sites. Serotonin, via 5HT-1A receptors (6), and cholecystokinin, via CCK-A receptors (2), inhibit discharges by increasing potassium permeability. In these cases, a given transmitter leads to multiple excitatory and inhibitory effects, as previously described using microiontophoresis on respiratory neurons *in vivo*.

(2) Transmitters such as substance P and serotonin are co-localized in the same axon terminals within the NTS and may dramatically change synaptic transmission when released simultaneously. In control situations, serotonin operating on 5HT-2 receptors has an excitatory effect as

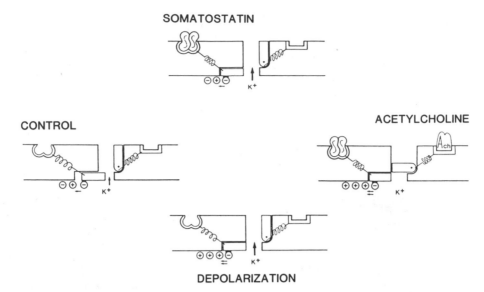

FIG. 4.4 Schematic presentation of interactions between somatostatin, muscarine, and M-current in the NTS (see 17). The potassium current is both voltage- and agonist-gated: (1) it is not detected at membrane potentials more hyperpolarized than -70 mV (*left*), (2) it is increased by membrane depolarization (*lower*), and (3) it is blocked by acetylcholine acting on muscarinic receptors (*right*). Somatostatin approximately doubles conductance underlying the M-current (*upper*) while voltage-dependent properties and sensitivity to acetylcholine are preserved. Regulation by intracellular messengers (46) is not included in this figure. Note that acetylcholine blocks more potassium current in the presence than in the absence of somatostatin, at the same membrane potential. These data provide evidence for a transmitter (somatostatin) with both an inhibitory action on resting excitability and a selective enabling action on excitatory (muscarinic) transmission.

described above. When substance P is released for a prolonged period of time, the excitatory 5HT-2 effect is occluded and the inhibitory 5HT-1A action is revealed (18).

(3) A different type of interaction is illustrated in figure 4.4. It is related to our finding that somatostatin increases the same current previously found sensitive to muscarine. Results suggests that (*a*) somatostatin-containing elements in the NTS play an inhibitory role through the activation of postsynaptic permeability to potassium ions and (*b*) the same ion channel type may be co-regulated by two neurotransmitter candidates, somatostatin and acetylcholine, through a reciprocal control mechanism (17).

(4) Transmitter-gated potassium currents are under the final control of intracellular messengers. Identification of these messengers is required to fully understand synaptic interactions in the NTS. Second messengers involved in the action of somatostatin are probably metabolites of arachidonic acid and different from those mediating the muscarinic effect (32). Intracellular messengers also explain the occlusion of 5HT-2 excitations by substance P because in these experiments two membrane receptors were independently activated by the agonists, while occlusion involved different membrane permeabilities: occlusion thus takes place at an intracellular step located after receptor activation and before channel modifications (18).

Muscarinic agonists and somatostatin were found *in vitro* to control a current comparable to I_M, a voltage and chemically gated potassium current. This is a non-inactivating current which is absent at potentials more hyperpolarized than -70 mV, which activates with a slow time constant upon depolarization by a few millivolts above resting

membrane potential (7). This outward potassium current is inhibitory in function and therefore tends to reduce neuronal activity produced by membrane depolarization. This mechanism probably operates *in vivo* during periodic depolarizations of respiratory neurons: muscarinic excitation of respiratory neurons has been described *in vivo* (27); the few millivolts required for activation of I_M are compatible with the amplitude of respiratory potentials measured *in vivo*. Recently, intracellular injections of cesium (used to block outward potassium currents) into bulbospinal expiratory neurons were found to increase the amplitude of respiratory-related potentials *in vivo* (3). One can propose a new model of respiratory pattern modulation in which neurotransmitters control potassium currents that damp down oscillations of the membrane potential.

CONCLUSION

There is a complex neurobiological substrate for synaptic transmission within the NTS: a plethora of transmitter candidates and a variety of chemically gated conductances. To some extent the complexity of these mechanisms reflects the multiple functions of synapses in the NTS: (1) fast PSPs transmit phasic sensory events, (2) slower synapses acting pre- or postsynaptically tune amplification of responses before propagation outside the NTS, (3) slow synaptic potentials generate on-going background activity and determine tonic activity in brainstem centers, (4) voltage-dependent characteristics of neurotransmission are critical when postsynaptic neurons exhibit periodic respiratory potentials. The number of available transmitter candidates remains larger than expected from the variety of functions, and there are examples of different transmitters having comparable postsynaptic actions. In these cases, functional pools of several transmitters should be considered because synaptic responses may vary considerably when different members of a pool are released simultaneously. Combining *in vitro* and *in vivo* approaches will help our understanding of how multitransmitter systems of the NTS operate in relation to patterns of incoming signals, postsynaptic membrane responsiveness, and intracellular regulation of metabolic pathways.

REFERENCES

1. Böhmer, G., K. Schmid, and M. Baumann. Evidence for a respiration-modulated cholinergic action on the activity of medullary respiration-related neurons in the rabbit: An iontophoretic study. *Pflügers Arch.* 415:72-80, 1989.

2. Branchereau, P., G.A. Böhmer, J. Champagnat, M. Denavit-Saubié, M.P. Morin-Surun, and B.P. Roques. Effets différentiels de la CCK8 sur les sites A et B du noyau du tractus solitaire. *Arch. Int. Physiol. Bioch.* 98:A135, 1990.

3. Champagnat, J., K. Ballanyi, P. Branchereau, M. Denavit-Saubié, G. Fortin, T. Jacquin, D. Richter, and P. Schweitzer. The cardiorespiratory network: Dynamics of cardiorespiratory network interaction. *Euro. J. Neurosci.* Suppl. 3:171, 1990.

4. Champagnat, J., M. Denavit-Saubié, K. Grant, and K.F. Shen. Organization of synaptic transmission in the mammalian solitary complex, studied in vitro. *J. Physiol.* (London), 381:551-573, 1986.

5. Champagnat, J., M. Denavit-Saubié, and G.R. Siggins. Rhythmic neuronal activities in the nucleus of the tractus solitarius isolated *in vitro*. *Brain Res.* 280:155-159, 1983.

6. Champagnat, J., T. Jacquin, and M. Denavit-Saubié. Occlusion of serotonin (5HT-2) excitations by substance P in the nucleus tractus solitarius. *Soc. Neurosci. Abst.* 15:226, 1986.

7. Champagnat, J., T. Jacquin, and D.W. Richter. Voltage-dependent currents in neurones of the solitary tract of rat brain stem slices. *Pflügers Arch.* 406:372-379, 1986.

8. Champagnat, J., K.F. Shen, G.R. Siggins, L.Y. Koda, and M. Denavit-Saubié. Synaptic processing and effects of neurotransmitters in the rat nucleus tractus solitarius *in vitro*. *J. Autonom. Nerv. Sys.* Suppl.:125-131, 1986.

9. Dekin, M.S., G.B. Richerson, and P.A. Getting. Thyrotropin-releasing hormone induces rhythmic bursting in neurons of the nucleus tractus solitarius. *Science* 29:67-69, 1985.

10. Denavit-Saubié, M., J. Champagnat, and W. Zieglgänsberger. Effects of opiates and methionine-enkephalin on pontine and bulbar respiratory neurones of the cat. *Brain Res.* 155:55-67, 1978.

11. Denavit-Saubié, M., A. Foutz, and K. Schmid. Evidence for GABAergic inhibition of medullary respiratory neurones during their active phase in anaesthetized or decerebrated cats. *J. Physiol.* (London) 422:96P, 1990.

12. Du, H.J., L. Chen, and W.H. Xiong. Spontaneous rhythmic bursting activity of rat solitary tract neurons *in vitro* and effect of morphine. *Chin. J. Physiol. Sci.* 5:89-93, 1989.

13. Foutz, A.S., J. Champagnat, and M. Denavit-Saubié. N-methyl-D-aspartate (NMDA) receptors control respiratory off-switch in the cat. *Neurosci. Lett.* 87:221-226, 1988.

14. Guyenet, P.G., T.M. Filtz, and S.R. Donaldson. Role of excitatory amino acids in rat vagal and sympathetic baroreflexes. *Brain Res.* 407:272-284, 1987.

15. Haji, A., J.E. Remmers, C. Connelly, and R. Takeda. Effects of glycine and GABA on bulbar respiratory neurons of cat. *J. Neurophysiol.* 63:955-965, 1990.

16. Hilaire, G., R. Monteau, P. Gauthier, P. Rega, and D. Morin. Functional significance of the dorsal respiratory group in adult and newborn rats: *In vivo* and in vitro studies. *Neurosci. Lett.* 111:133-138, 1990.

17. Jacquin, T., J. Champagnat, S. Madamba, M. Denavit-Saubié, and G.R. Siggins. Somatostatin depresses excitability in neurons of the solitary tract complex through hyperpolarization and augmentation of I_M, a non-inactivating voltage-dependent outward current blocked by muscarinic agonists. *Proc. Natl. Acad. Sci. USA*, 85:948-952, 1988.

18. Jacquin, T., M. Denavit-Saubié, and J. Champagnat. Substance P and serotonin mutually reverse their excitatory effects in the rat nucleus tractus solitarius. *Brain Res.* 502:214-222, 1989.

19. Jacquin, T., G. Fortin, C. Pasquier, B. Gillet, J.C. Béloeil, and J.C. Champagnat. Metabolic acidosis induced by N-methyl-D-aspartate in brain slices of neonatal rat: ^{31}P- and ^{1}H-magnetic resonance spectroscopy. *Neurosci. Lett.* 92:285-290, 1988.

20. Jacquin, T., B. Gillet, G. Fortin, C. Pasquier, J.C. Béloeil, and J. Champagnat. Metabolic action of NMDA in newborn rat brain ex-vivo: ^{31}P magnetic resonance spectroscopy. *Brain Res.* 497:296-304, 1989.

21. Livingston, C.A. and A.J. Berger. I. Immunocytochemical localization of GABA in neurons projecting to the ventrolateral nucleus of the solitary tract. *Brain Res.* 494:143-150, 1989.

22. McLean, H., and J. Remmers. Development of a thick medullary slice preparation for the study of respiratory rhythm generation. *Soc. Neurosci. Abstr.* 14:935, 1988.

23. Mifflin, S.W., K.M. Spyer, and D.J. Withington-Wray. Baroreceptor inputs to the nucleus tractus solitarius in the cat: postsynaptic actions and the influence of respiration. *J. Physiol.* (London) 399:369-387, 1988.

24. Miles, R. Frequency dependence of synaptic transmission in nucleus of the solitary tract *in vitro*. *J. Neurophysiol.* 5:1076-1090, 1986.

25. Miller, B.D., and R.B. Felder. Excitatory amino acid receptors intrinsic to synaptic transmission in nucleus tractus solitarii. *Brain Res.* 456:333-343, 1988.

26. Morin-Surun, M.P., P. De Marchi, J. Champagnat, J.J. Vanderhaeghen, J. Rossier, and M. Denavit-Saubié. Inhibitory effect of cholecystokinin octapeptide on neurons in the nucleus tractus solitarius. *Brain Res.* 265:333-338, 1982.

27. Morin-Surun, M.P., J. Champagnat, M. Denavit-Saubié, and S. Moyanova. The effects of acetylcholine on bulbar respiratory related neurones, consequences of anaesthesia by pentobarbital. *Naunyn Arch. Pharmacol.* 325:205-208, 1984.

28. Moss, I.R., M. Denavit-Saubié, F.L. Eldridge, R.A. Gillis, M. Herkenham, and S. Lahiri. Neuromodulators and transmitters in respiratory control. *Fed. Proc.* 45:2133-2147, 1986.

29. Otake, K., H. Sasaki, K. Ezure, and M. Manabe. Axonal trajectory and terminal distribution of inspiratory neurons of the dorsal respiratory group in the cat's medulla. *J. Comp. Neurol.* 286:218-230, 1989.

30. Richter, D.W., H. Camerer, and U. Sonnhof. Changes in extracellular potassium during the spontaneous activity of medullary respiratory neurons. *Pflügers Arch.* 376:139-149, 1978.

31. Richter, D.W., D. Jordan, D. Ballantyne, M. Meesman, and K.M. Spyer. Presynaptic depolarization in myelinated vagal afferent fibres terminating in the nucleus of the tractus solitarius in the cat. *Pflügers Arch.* 406:12-19, 1986.

32. Schweitzer, P., S. Madamba, and G.R. Siggins. Arachidonic acid metabolites as mediators of somatostatin-induced increase of neuronal M-current. *Nature* 346:464-467, 1990.

33. Saether, K., G. Hilaire, and R. Monteau. Dorsal and ventral respiratory groups of neurons in the medulla of the rat. *Brain Res.* 419:87-96, 1987.

34. Tell, F., L. Fagni, and A. Jean. Neurons of the nucleus tractus solitarius, *in vitro,* generate bursting activities by solitary tract stimulation. *Exp. Brain Res.* 79:436-440, 1990.

35. Zheng, Y., J.C. Barillot, and A.L. Bianchi. Intracellular study of the respiratory neurones in the medulla oblongata of the decerebrated rat. *Euro. J. Neurosci.* Supp. 2:618, 1989.

5

Modulation of Respiratory Patterns during Hypoxia

D.W. Richter, A. Bischoff, K. Anders, M. Bellingham, and U. Windhorst

Mammals react with a diphasic change in respiration when acute systemic hypoxia persists for longer than a few minutes (18, 46). This response starts with an initial increase of respiration which then turns to depression and terminates in apnea when partial oxygen pressure is below a value of 15 torr within the extracellular space of the respiratory network (1, 32, 45). When such severe hypoxia continues, inspiratory muscles are only transiently activated during gasps which are supposed to be organized by structures other than the medullary respiratory network producing the normal respiratory rhythm (40). This observation supports the hypothesis of a differential sensitivity, or a certain hierarchy of vulnerability, of various respiration-related structures in the brain (28).

The basic mechanisms responsible for these hypoxia-induced disturbances of the central respiratory rhythm are as yet unknown. Primary augmentation of respiration has been attributed to stimulation of peripheral chemoreceptors (42) or activation of nervous structures localized rostral to the brainstem which presumably exert an excitatory influence on the bulbar network (11). Several possibilities have been considered as mechanisms producing the secondary depression of ventilation: (1) the reduction of central chemoreceptor activation by chemoreflex-mediated tachypnea (4, 47) or by hypoxia-induced vasodilatation of cerebral vessels and a secondary alkalotic shift in the cerebrospinal fluid at the ventral surface of the medulla; (2) the release of neuromodulators such as adenosine (20, 39, 48) and/or endogenous opioids (16, 41); (3) the imbalance of neurotransmitter release involving excitatory amino acids such as glutamate and aspartate (17, 24), of inhibitory neurotransmitters such as GABA (12, 22, 49), and also of biogenic amines (5, 27), resulting in a net increase in neuronal inhibition due to an alteration of the balance between excitatory and inhibitory neurotransmitter levels, with subsequent membrane hyperpolarization of respiratory neurons.

Favoring the latter possibility, in a recent review Neubauer et al. (28) concluded that the bulbar network of respiratory neurons is relatively undisturbed during hypoxia, and depression of respiration is not due to a metabolic impairment of cellular functions or to failure of synaptic interaction between respiratory neurons. This is in disagreement with evidence for disturbance of the ionic environment within the respiratory network during hypoxia (1, 2, 3, 32, 45; Ballanyi and Richter, unpublished). We therefore tend to oppose the suggestion that the respiratory network is protected better than other nervous structures (28), and we have tested respiratory neurons within the lower brainstem for hypoxia-induced changes in excitability, intrinsic membrane properties, and postsynaptic activity (2, 3).

METHODS

Measurements were performed in cats of either sex (body weight 2.5–4.5 kg) which were anesthetized with sodium pentobarbitone (35–40 mg/kg ip initial dose). Supplementary anesthetic was administered as required (in doses of 4–8 mg, iv). Animals were paralyzed with gallamine triethiodide (10 mg/kg iv initial dose and then 1–2 mg/kg iv hourly) and artificially ventilated by a positive pressure pump with oxygen-enriched air. Ventilatory volume and rate were adjusted to maintain an end-tidal CO_2 level at 3–5%. The O_2 partial pressure of the inspired gas and the end-tidal CO_2 pressure were continuously monitored and blood gas analysis was performed several times during an experiment. Atropine sulphate (0.1–0.2 mg/kg iv) was given to reduce salivation and dexamethasone (0.2 mg/kg) was given im to protect the brain from edema. In some experiments the arterial blood pressure was stabilized by infusing saline solutions containing epinephrine (40 µg/ml).

Femoral arteries were cannulated for monitoring blood pressure and taking blood samples for blood gas analysis. Femoral veins were cannulated for drug injection. In experiments in which effects of ischemia were tested, both common carotid arteries and one vertebral artery were ligated. A cannula was inserted into the trachea below the larynx for artificial ventilation. A wide pneumothorax was established bilaterally to avoid respiratory movements of the thorax and to increase the stability of recordings in the brainstem. Atelectasis of the lungs was prevented by applying positive pressure (1–2 cm H_2O) to the expiratory outflow. Body temperature was maintained between 36 and 38°C by external heating.

Peripheral chemoreceptors were denervated by sectioning the vagal and carotid sinus nerves bilaterally. Phrenic nerves (C5 branches) were exposed on both sides by a dorsal approach and sectioned. The spinal cord was exposed by laminectomy from C2 to C4 for stimulating the reticulospinal tracts of both sides with an array of four bipolar

FIG. 5.1 Response of medullary respiratory activity during complete brainstem ischemia produced by bilateral occlusion of common carotid and vertebral arteries. PN; phrenic nerve activity; LRN; recurrent laryngeal nerve activity recorded from the cervical vagal nerve; index A; moving averages of discharges; BP; arterial blood pressure.

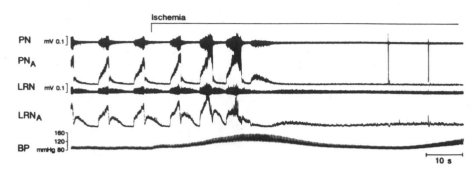

concentric stainless steel electrodes with tip diameters of 100 μm. After placement of these electrodes, the spinal cord was covered with agar dissolved in Ringer's solution. The cat's head was mounted rigidly in a head holder and the spinous processes of T1 and L5 were clamped to a frame. The skull was opened by craniotomy of the occipital bone, and the head was ventroflexed to expose the dorsal surface of the medulla.

Cervical vagal and phrenic nerves were prepared for the recording of their efferent activity. Discharge activity was amplified, bandpass-filtered (0.1–10 kHz) and registered on a chart recorder as the direct discharge or as a moving average of activity. Phrenic activity was taken as an index of the central respiratory rhythm. Glass microelectrodes filled with 4M NaCl (impedance 5–10 MΩ) were used for recording extracellularly the discharges of respiratory neurons of the ventral group. Axons and neurons were recorded intracellularly with micropipettes (30–70 MΩ) filled with 3M KCl. Potentials were recorded with a D.C. electrometer equipped with bridge balance and capacity compensation circuits, amplified and displayed on an oscilloscope. A chart recorder provided permanent records of the membrane potential of respiratory neurons, phrenic nerve discharge, arterial blood pressure, and tracheal pressure. All signals were stored on magnetic tape for off-line analysis.

Experimental protocol: Normocapnic hypoxia was produced by replacing the hyperoxic ventilation gas mixture (80–90% O_2) with a gas mixture of 5 to 10% O_2 in N_2. The ischemic response of respiratory neurons was tested by transiently occluding one intact vertebral artery via a dorsal approach, after both common carotid arteries and one vertebral artery had been ligated previously. During all tests, the O_2 partial pressure of the inspiratory gas and the end-tidal CO_2 pressure was continuously monitored with CO_2- and O_2-meters, and blood gas analysis was performed before, during, and after some tests. This analysis showed that the arterial partial oxygen pressure fell to 20–30 mmHg, which is consistent with the observation that tissue oxygen pressure within the region of ventral respiratory neurons falls nearly to zero levels under comparable conditions (1, 32).

During such severe hypoxia, arterial blood pressure increased transiently to levels of 150–180 mmHg and then

fell. The hypoxia tests were continued until the arterial blood pressure had fallen to 40–60 mmHg. Under these conditions heart beats started to fail regularly.

Suitable stable recording conditions for hypoxia tests and analysis were established in 25 neurons with respiration-related discharges or fluctuations in membrane potential. In these neurons, maximal membrane potentials ranged between −45 and −75 mV during control conditions. The neurons were classified as inspiratory (I), postinspiratory (PI), or stage 2 expiratory (E2) neurons (for identification of neurons see 31).

RESULTS

Initial augmentation of respiration was followed by depression when the oxygen supply of the network within the brainstem was severely reduced for periods lasting longer than 1–2 min. The overall response during ischemia (fig. 5.1) was comparable with the response during systemic hypoxia (fig. 5.2). Initial augmentation of respiratory activity became evident by increased frequency and strength of inspiratory discharge of phrenic and cervical vagal nerves, including efferent recurrent laryngeal fibers, while secondary depression became evident by rapid decrease and cessation of inspiratory discharge. Prolonged postinspiratory after-discharge of phrenic and recurrent laryngeal activity, following the final inspiratory burst, faded slowly and led to silence in both nerves, which we defined as hypoxic apnea. Only very short, irregularly occurring gasplike discharges of declining strength were observed in the neurograms of both nerves when severe hypoxia persisted (fig. 5.1).

The maximal frequency of discharge of action potentials of I, PI, and E2 neurons also increased transiently but then was reduced, with final blockade of action potential generation during prolonged periods of hypoxia (fig. 5.2).

Intracellular recordings from E2 neurons revealed that synaptic interaction between respiratory neurons is disturbed during hypoxia (figs. 5.3 and 5.4). During initial augmentation of respiration, maximal membrane potentials during stage 2 expiration were slightly more depolarized than control levels. This was accompanied by increased synaptic noise (fig. 5.3). The most obvious change, however, was a regularly observed decrease in synaptic inhibi-

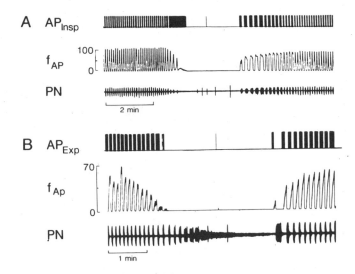

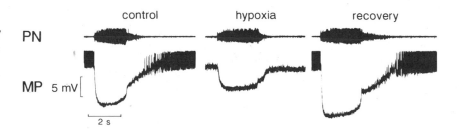

FIG. 5.2 Responses of medullary inspiratory (*A*) and stage 2 expiratory (*B*) neurons to systemic hypoxia starting 20–30 sec after the beginning of the traces. AP_{Insp}; action potential discharge of an inspiratory neuron; AP_{Exp}; action potential discharge of an expiratory neuron; f_{AP}; frequency of action potential discharge in Hz; PN; phrenic nerve activity.

polarization was no longer related to the strength of inspiratory output activity in phrenic and laryngeal nerves. During hypoxia there was rapid membrane hyperpolarization with the onset of inspiration and a sudden depolarization during the start of expiration, presumably because of the loss of PI slowing of membrane depolarization. These changes were accompanied by a shortening of the PI afterdischarge in phrenic nerves. Membrane potential trajectories during control, during hypoxia, and at the beginning of recovery from hypoxia are shown in figure 5.4.

In several hypoxia tests, we saw significant changes in the inhibitory mechanisms acting at the transition from inspiration to stage 2 expiration (fig. 5.5). Phrenic nerve discharge was prolonged and displayed large oscillations in activity during this period, with amplitudes that were comparable with the maximal amplitude of the inspiratory burst. This prolonged activity was clearly distinguishable from the normal inspiratory burst discharge of phrenic nerves and was accompanied by a less prominent membrane hyperpolarization of E2 neurons, which showed os-

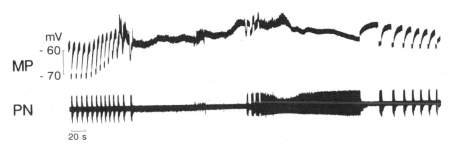

FIG. 5.3 Membrane potential changes during severe systemic hypoxia induced by ventilating the animal with a gas mixture containing 5% oxygen in nitrogen. The membrane potential (MP) of an E2 neuron revealed initial depolarization of maximal membrane potential, which was combined with increased synaptic noise activity. Periodic inspiratory inhibition decreased, although the phrenic nerve (PN) still discharged enhanced inspiratory bursts. The respiratory rhythm disappeared 1–2 min after the the onset of hypoxia. Electrical stimulation of the superior laryngeal nerves evoked reappearance of rhythmic phrenic nerve discharges, which then turned to a tonic discharge. The E2 neuron revealed fairly shallow membrane hyperpolarizations, mirroring this phrenic nerve activity.

FIG. 5.4 Comparison of membrane potential trajectories of a stage 2 expiratory neuron during control, systemic hypoxia, and the first period of recovery from hypoxia. MP; membrane potential; PN; phrenic nerve discharge.

tion during inspiration while phrenic and recurrent laryngeal nerves still showed enhanced inspiratory activity. Finally, inspiratory membrane hyperpolarization of E2 neurons and inspiratory discharge of phrenic nerves disappeared completely.

Disturbances of network functions became evident in changes of cyclic membrane potential changes of single neurons. The amplitude of inspiratory membrane hyper-

cillations of the same frequencies (8–20 Hz), as seen in phrenic nerve activity. These large oscillations of phrenic nerve discharge were followed by a PI after-discharge similar to that of control postinspiration. At the same time, another inhibitory mechanism became active in E2 neurons, producing a further delay of their discharge. The findings reveal that, during hypoxia, the reversible inspiratory off-switch mechanism is affected by disturbance of the inhibitory mechanisms acting during the transition from inspiration to postinspiration.

During apnea, synaptic noise was reduced and the membrane potentials of E2 neurons were held between −45 and −55 mV, which was only slightly more positive than the maximal potential of the control E2 phase. Nevertheless, most E2 neurons failed to discharge action potentials spontaneously. Antidromic excitation of E2 neurons by spinal cord stimulation was possible throughout the period of stable membrane potential, the action potentials revealing only slight inactivation of sodium conductance (not illustrated). During the early stage of hypoxic apnea, electrical stimulation of the superior laryngeal nerves evoked rhythmic phrenic nerve activity, which often turned to a tonic discharge. E2 neurons revealed membrane hyperpolarizations which mirrored this phrenic nerve activity, although hyperpolarization was reduced in amplitude (fig. 5.3).

Hypoxia-induced effects on membrane conductances were verified by measuring the input resistance (R_N) of E2 neurons. The first significant effect was a reduction of the usual decrease in R_N during inspiratory synaptic inhibition, while maximal values of R_N during stage 2 expiration remained rather constant. The relative constancy of maximal membrane potential and maximal R_N, combined with reduced membrane hyperpolarization and diminished decreases in R_N in E2 neurons during inspiration, indicates that the disturbance of synaptic interaction within the network occurs at sites presynaptic to E2 neurons. During apnea, neuronal R_N remained increased for 2–4 min but finally decreased to, or below, the lowest control values (fig. 5.6), indicating activation of membrane conductances of E2 neurons.

DISCUSSION

The results reveal a sequence of disturbance of the respiratory network, summarized in figure 5.7 together with possible mechanisms. In medullary respiratory neurons, hypoxia obviously starts with ATP depletion of the respiratory neurons, resulting in the reduction and blockade of active transport mechanisms and consequent disturbance of ion homeostasis. Various membrane conductances might also be activated. These changes could account for previously observed increases in extracellular potassium and proton concentration and changes in extracellular calcium concentration (1, 29, 32, 35, 45; Ballanyi and Richter, unpublished). This is then followed by reversal and blockade of IPSPs, which is accompanied by enhanced depolarizing postsynaptic activity and the reduction of membrane potentials of respiratory neurons. This blockade of inhibitory synaptic transmission probably occurs presynaptically. The disturbance of inhibitory synaptic transmission (10, 15, 23) and consequent abolition of the postsynaptic voltage effect of inhibitory synaptic potentials on the low-voltage calcium current (33, 34, 36, 37) could result in apnea.

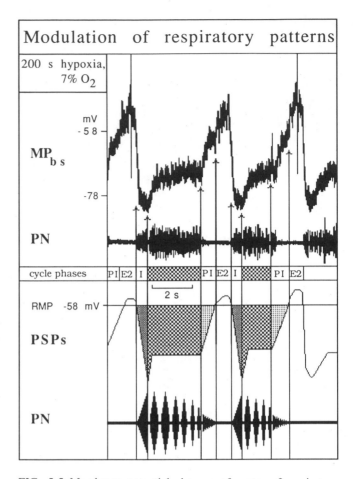

FIG. 5.5 Membrane potential changes of a stage 2 expiratory neuron during hypoxia indicate the existence of complex inhibitory mechanisms acting at the transition from inspiration to postinspiration. The various patterns of synaptic activity are indicated as dotted areas. (For further explanation see text.) MP; membrane potential; PN; phrenic nerve activity; PSP; postsynaptic activity; I; inspiratory phase; PI; postinspiratory phase; E2; stage 2 of expiration.

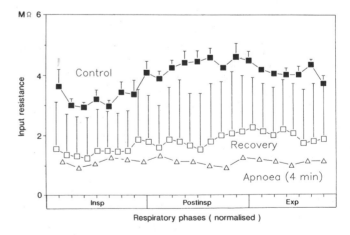

FIG. 5.6 Temporal changes of neuron input resistance before, during, and after systemic hypoxia. The durations of the cycle phases are given in normalized form.

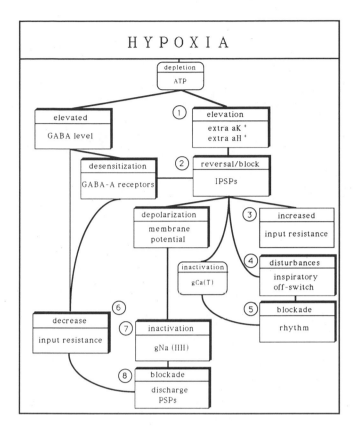

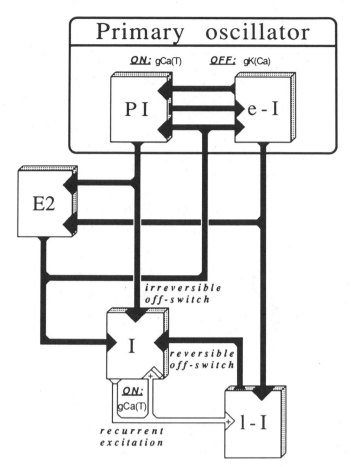

FIG. 5.7 The sequence of disturbances to the respiratory network. The experimentally observed sequence of disturbances is shown in numbered shadowed boxes. Possible mechanisms are given in rounded boxes. gCa(T), low-voltage-activated calcium conductance; gNa(HH), sodium conductance; extra aK$^+$, extracellular activity of potassium; aH$^+$, extracellular activity of hydrogen.

Respiratory apnea is not produced by failure of spike discharge, as antidromic action potentials remain relatively unaffected during this stage. Inactivation of sodium conductances and spike failure occur with a significantly longer delay than apnea and are accompanied by terminal membrane depolarization.

The changes in neuron R_N are complex and are related to the block of receptor-controlled (synaptic) conductances and to the modification of membrane conductances directly or indirectly linked to ATP depletion. The initial increase in neuron R_N, which we relate to the reduction of synaptic interaction, is followed by a pronounced decrease that seems to be related to the effects on membrane conductances and hypoxic damage of the neurons.

The failure of the respiratory rhythm following blockade of synaptic inhibition can be explained by the functional organization of the respiratory network (fig. 5.8; see also 31, 34). This network seems to involve a primary rhythm-generating network consisting of postinspiratory and early-inspiratory neurons. The neurons might be spontaneously active because of intrinsic beating or bursting pacemaker capacities (7, 13, 44) and/or tonic drive from other sources

FIG. 5.8 Schematic illustration of the rhythm- and pattern-generating components of the medullary respiratory network. The illustration is a simplified version of the model proposed by Richter et al. (34).White arrows indicate excitatory connections; black arrows indicate inhibitory connections. Intrinsic membrane properties that determine the function of the rhythm generator and in part also of the inspiratory ramp generator are the low-voltage-activated calcium conductance, gCa(T), and the calcium-dependent potassium conductance, gK(Ca). Other ligand-controlled conductances, such as non-NMDA and NMDA conductances may also be involved, but the functional significance of these is still unknown. PI, postinspiratory neurons; E2, stage 2 of expiratory neurons; I, inspiratory neurons; e-I, early inspiratory neurons; 1-I, late inspiratory neurons.

(21, 36). In this network, the conversion of primary tonic activity into rhythmic oscillations between inspiration and postinspiration seems to be linked to reciprocal inhibition. These oscillations start with rapid onset of activity, triggered by low-voltage calcium conductances which need a preceding membrane hyperpolarization (6). Accommodation of activity follows due to the activation of calcium-and voltage-dependent potassium conductances (8, 9, 25, 26). Finally, phase-switching is produced by disinhibition of one population of neurons and antagonistic synaptic inhibition of the other population (30, 31, 36).

Synaptic inhibition is also necessary in the pattern-generating network in order to stabilize the activation of ramp-I and E2 neurons. The blockade and reversal of IPSPs during hypoxia should, therefore, have a dual effect on the respiratory rhythm: first, the disturbance of phase switching in the pattern-generating network, and second, apnea when inhibition is blocked in the rhythm-generating network. The functional consequence of the reversal or blockade of IPSPs on central rhythm generation is illustrated in figure 5.9. Inhibitory GABAergic interneurons seem to be highly susceptible to hypoxia (14, 38, 43) and hypoxic damage to GABAergic interneurons would explain our observation that some IPSPs were completely blocked during severe hypoxia. As GABAergic inhibition was found to be essential for respiratory rhythm generation (19, 30, 31, 34), such damage could also explain the development of hypoxic apnea. However, hypoxia seems not only to affect presynaptic inhibitory interneurons but also IPSPs in the postsynaptic target neurons receiving inhibitory synaptic inputs. The changes consist of a spontaneous reversal of the IPSP polarity. We consider the disturbances of the Cl^-/HCO_3^- gradients across the membrane of respiratory neurons to play an essential role in such IPSP reversal. Finally, GABA-A receptors seem to be rapidly desensitized by elevated levels of GABA in the extracellular space, decreasing the postsynaptic effects of this neurotransmitter. Since this desensitization is not complete, part of the final decrease in R_N during apnea might thus also be explained by the residual effect of elevated GABA level.

We thus conclude that hypoxia-induced changes of IPSPs lead to respiratory failure because of the disturbance of phase switching and blockade of the activity trigger mediated by low-voltage calcium conductances. As apnea is preceded by disturbances of the inspiratory off-switch mechanisms, we propose that the different inhibitory mechanisms acting during the transition from inspiration to postinspiration are most susceptible to hypoxia and produce the primary disturbances of respiration during hypoxia. The assumption that disturbance of inhibition is the reason for arrhythmia within the respiratory network would fit the observation that reappearance of rhythmic respiratory activity during recovery from hypoxia always is introduced by inhibition which is either inspiratory or postinspiratory.

Our results have shown that the hypothesis that depression of respiration is due to increased membrane hyperpolarization of respiratory neurons, originating from a net increase in neuronal inhibition due to an alteration of the balance of excitatory and inhibitory neurotransmitter levels toward inhibition (28), is wrong. The bulbar network of respiratory neurons is directly disturbed, and depression is due to metabolic impairment or failure of synaptic interaction between respiratory neurons.

ACKNOWLEDGMENT

This work was supported by the SFB 330.

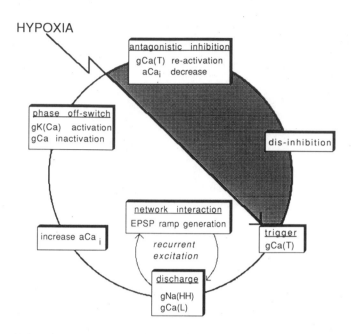

FIG. 5.9 Schematic illustration of the mechanisms (clockwise) necessary for phase switching within the respiratory network and the effect of hypoxia-induced blockade of synaptic inhibition. gCa(T), low-voltage-activated calcium conductance; aCa$_i$, activity of intracellular calcium; gNa(HH), sodium conductances; gCa(L), long-lasting non-inactivating channel; gK(Ca), calcium-dependent potassium conductance; gCa, calcium conductance. (For further explanation see text.)

REFERENCES

1. Acker, H., and D. Richter. Changes in potassium activity and oxygen tension in the extracellular space of inspiratory neurones within the NTS of cats. In *Neurogenesis of central respiratory rhythm,* ed. A.L. Bianchi and M. Denavit-Saubié, 183-186. Lancaster, U.K.: MTP Press, 1985.

2. Anders, K., and D.W. Richter. Hypoxia response of the medullary respiratory network of cats. *Pflügers Arch.* 411:R113, 1988.

3. Anders, K., and D.W. Richter. Hypoxic apnoea in the anaesthetized cat. *J. Physiol.* 417:119P, 1989.

4. Berkenbosch, A., C.N. Olivier, J. De Goede, and J.H.G.M. Van Beek. Carbon dioxide tension in the CSGF- and depression of ventilation by brain stem hypoxia. In *Modelling and Control of Breathing,* ed. B.J. Whipp and D.M. Wiberg, 107-114. New York: Elsevier Biomedical, 1983.

5. Brown, R.M., S.R. Snider, and A. Carlsson. Changes in biogenic amine synthesis and turnover induced by hypoxia and/or foot shock stress, II. The central nervous system. *J. Neurol. Trans.* 35:293-305, 1974.

6. Carbone, E., and H.D. Lux. Kinetics and selectivity of a low-voltage activated calcium current in chick and rat sensory neurones. *J. Physiol.* 386:547-570, 1987.

7. Champagnat, J., M. Denavit-Saubié, and G.R. Siggins. Rhythmic neuronal activities in the nucleus of the tractus solitarius isolated *in vitro. Brain Res.* 280:155-159, 1983.

8. Champagnat, J., T. Jacquin, and D.W. Richter. Voltage-dependent currents in neurones of the nuclei of the solitary tract of rat brainstem slices. *Pflügers Arch.* 406:372-379, 1986.

9. Champagnat, J., K. Ballanyi, P. Brancherau, M. Denavit-Saubié, G. Fortin, T. Jacquin, D.W. Richter, and P. Schweitzer. Dynamics of cardio-respiratory network interaction. *Euro. J. Neurosci.* Suppl. 3:171, 1990.

10. Eccles, R.M., Y. Loyning, and T. Oshima. Effects of hypoxia on the monosynaptic reflex pathway in the cat spinal cord. *J. Neurophysiol.* 29:315-332, 1966.

11. Eldridge, F.L., P. Gill-Kumar, and D.E. Millhorn. Input-output relationships of central neural circuits involved in respiration in cats. *J. Physiol.* 311:81-95, 1981.

12. Erecinska, M., D. Nelson, D.F. Wilson, and I.A. Silver. Neurotransmitter amino acids in the CNS. I. Regional changes in amino acid levels in rat brain during ischemia and reperfusion. *Brain Res.* 304:9-22, 1984.

13. Feldman, J.L., and J.C. Smith. Cellular mechanisms underlying modulation of breathing pattern in mammals. *Ann. NY Acad. Sci.* 563:114-130, 1989.

14. Francis, A. and W. Pulsinelli. The response of GABAergic and cholinergic neurons to transient cerebral ischemia. *Brain Res.* 243:271-278, 1982.

15. Fujiwara, N., H. Higashi, K. Shimoji, and M. Yoshimura. Effects of hypoxia on rat hippocampal neurones *in vitro*. *J. Physiol.* 384:131-151, 1987.

16. Grunstein, M.M., T.A. Hazinski, and H.A. Schlueter. Respiratory control during hypoxia in newborn rabbits: Implied action of endorphins. *J. Appl. Physiol.* 51:122-130, 1981.

17. Hagberg, H., A. Lehmann, M. Sandberg, B. Nystrom, I. Jacobson, and A. Hamberger. Ischemia-induced shift of inhibitory and excitatory amino acids from intra- to extracellular compartments. *J. Cerebral Blood Flow and Metabolism* 5:413-419, 1985.

18. Haddad, G.G., and R.B. Mellins. Hypoxia and respiratory control in early life. *Ann. Rev. Physiol.* 46:629-643, 1984.

19. Haji, A., J.E. Remmers, C. Connelly, and R. Takeda. Effects of glycine and GABA on bulbar respiratory neurons of cat. *J. Neurophysiol.* 63:955-965, 1990.

20. Hedner, T., J. Hedner, P. Wessberg, J. Jonason. Regulation of breathing in the rat: Indications for a role of central adenosine mechanisms. *Neurosci. Lett.* 33:147-151, 1982.

21. Hugelin, A., and M.I. Cohen. The reticular activating system and respiratory regulation in the cat. *Ann. NY Acad. Sci.* 109:586-603, 1963.

22. Iverson, K., T. Hedner, and P. Lundborg. GABA concentrations and turn-over in neonatal rat brain during asphyxia and recovery. *Acta Physiol. Scand.* 118:91-94, 1983.

23. Kass, I.S., and P. Lipton. Mechanisms involved in irreversible anoxic damage to the *in vitro* hippocampal slice. *J. Physiol.* 332:459-472, 1982.

24. Meldrum, B.S. Excitatory amino acids and anoxic/ischaemic brain damage. *Trends in Neurosci.* 1988:47-48, 1985.

25. Mifflin, S.W., D. Ballantyne, S.B. Backman, and D.W. Richter. Evidence for a calcium activated potassium conductance in medullary respiratory neurones. In *Neurogenesis of central respiratory rhythm*, ed. A.L. Bianchi and M. Denavit-Saubié, 179-182. Lancaster, U.K.: MTP Press, 1985.

26. Mifflin, S.W., and D.W. Richter. Effects of QX-314 on medullary respiratory neurones. *Brain Res.* 420:22-31, 1987.

27. Millhorn, D.E., F.L. Eldridge, and T.G. Waldrop. Prolonged stimulation of respiration by endogenous central serotonin. *Resp. Physiol.* 42:171-188, 1980.

28. Neubauer, J.A., J.E. Melton, and H.H. Edelman. Modulation of respiration during brain hypoxia. *J. Appl. Physiol.* 68:441-449, 1990.

29. Nolan, W.F., P.C. Houck, J.L. Thomas, and D.G. Davies. Ventral medullary extracellular fluid pH and blood flow during hypoxia. *Am. J. Physiol.* 242:R195-R198, 1982.

30. Pack, A.I., and D.W. Richter. Modelling cardio-respiratory activities. *Euro. J. Neurosci.* Suppl. 3:172, 1990.

31. Richter, D.W. Generation and maintenance of the respiratory rhythm. *J. Exp. Biol.* 100:93-107, 1982.

32. Richter, D.W., and H. Acker. Respiratory neuron behavior during medullary hypoxia. In *Chemoreceptors and reflexes in breathing: Cellular and molecular aspects,* ed. S. Lahiri, 267-274. New York: Oxford University Press, 1989.

33. Richter, D.W., D. Ballantyne, and S.W. Mifflin. Interaction between postsynaptic activities and membrane properties in medullary respiratory neurones. In *Neurogenesis of central respiratory rhythm*, ed. A.L. Bianchi and M. Denavit-Saubié, 172-178. Lancaster, U.K.: MTP press, 1985.

34. Richter, D.W., D. Ballantyne, and J.E. Remmers. How is the respiratory rhythm generated? A model. *News in Physiol. Sci.* 1:109-112, 1986.

35. Richter, D.W., H. Camerer, and U. Sonnhof. Changes in extracellular potassium during spontaneous activity of medullary respiratory neurons. *Pflügers Arch.* 376:139-149, 1978.

36. Richter, D.W., J. Champagnat, and S. Mifflin. Membrane properties involved in respiratory rhythm generation. In *Neurobiology of the Control of Breathing,* ed. C. von Euler and H. Lagercrantz, 141-147. New York: Raven Press, 1986.

37. Richter, D.W., J. Champagnat, and S. Mifflin. Membrane properties of medullary respiratory neurones of the cat. In *Respiratory muscles and their neuromotor control,* ed. G.C. Sieck, S.C. Gandevia, and W.E. Cameron, 9-15. New York: Alan R. Liss, 1987.

38. Romjin, H.J. Preferential loss of GABAergic neurons in hypoxia-exposed neocortex slab cultures is attenuated by the NMDA receptor blocker D-2-amino-7-phosphoheptanoate. *Brain Res.* 501:100-104, 1989.

39. Runold, M., H. Lagercrantz, N.R. Prabhakar, and B.B. Fredholm. Role of adenosine in hypoxic ventilatory depression. *J. Appl. Physiol.* 67:541-546, 1989.

40. St. John, W.M. Neurogenesis, control and functional significance of gasping. *J. Appl. Physiol.* 68:1305-1315, 1990.

41. Schaeffer, J.I., and G.G. Haddad. Ventilatory response to moderate and severe hypoxia in adult dogs: Role of endorphins. *J. Appl. Physiol.* 65:1383-1388, 1988.

42. Schwieler, G.H. Respiratory regulation during postnatal development in cats and rabbits and some of its morphological substrate. *Acta Physiol. Scand.* Suppl. 304:1-123, 1968.

43. Sloper, J.J., P. Johnson, and T.P.S. Powell. Selective degeneration of interneurons in the motor cortex of infant monkeys following controlled hypoxia: A possible cause of epilepsy. *Brain Res.* 198:204-209, 1980.

44. Suzue, T. Respiratory rhythm generation in the *in vitro* brain stem-spinal cord preparation of the neonatal rat. *J. Physiol.* 354:173-183, 1984.

45. Trippenbach, T., D.W. Richter, and H. Acker. Hypoxia and ion activities within the brain stem of newborn rabbits. *J. Appl. Physiol.* 68:2494-2503, 1990.

46. Weil, J.V., and C.W. Zwillich. Assessment of ventilatory response to hypoxia: Methods and interpretation. *Chest* 70, Suppl.:124-128, 1976.

47. Weiskopf, R.B., and R.A. Gabiel. Depression of ventilation during hypoxia in man. *J. Appl. Physiol.* 39:911-915, 1975.

48. Winn, H.R., R. Rubio, and R.M. Berne. Brain adenosine concentration during hypoxia in rats. *Am. J. Physiol.* 241:H235-H242, 1981.

49. Wood, J.D., W.J. Watson, and A.J. Drucker. The effect of hypoxia on brain gamma-aminobutyric acid levels. *J. Neurochem.* 15:603-608, 1968.

II

In Vitro Studies of Respiratory Control

6

An Overview

Gordon S. Mitchell

In vitro experimental preparations have proven to be invaluable in many areas of contemporary neuroscience, allowing insights into the form and function of neural systems that were elusive with more traditional approaches (e.g., 31). Among the more powerful advantages of *in vitro* preparations are the following: (1) direct access to neurons of interest, allowing direct visualization with modern microscopic techniques; (2) mechanical stability, thereby improving the stability of intracellular recordings with conventional or whole-cell patch techniques; and (3) improved control of the environment surrounding the neurons.

By 1931 an *in vitro* preparation had already been applied to respiratory neurobiology (1), permitting the fundamental question of the minimal anatomical substrate necessary for rhythm generation to be addressed. Adrian and Buytendijk (1) used cotton wick electrodes to demonstrate that an isolated (*in vitro*) goldfish medulla generates electrical field oscillations corresponding to respiratory rhythm. Only a handful of studies concerning respiratory neurobiology utilized *in vitro* preparations in the subsequent fifty years. In the past decade, however, there has been a remarkable resurgence of interest in the application of *in vitro* experimental techniques to studies of respiratory control (for review see 2).

In vitro preparations used in studies on respiratory control include brain slices (5), isolated and perfused brains (24), intact superfused brainstem–spinal cord preparations from neonatal rats (22, 28, 30) or adult poikilothermic vertebrates (7), and dissociated/cultured neurons from the CNS (20) or carotid body (3, 16). Each preparation has distinct advantages and drawbacks for studies of the neuronal network subserving respiratory control.

The chapters in this section utilize *in vitro* brainstem–spinal cord preparations, either from neonatal rats or larval amphibians (tadpoles). The overriding advantage of these relatively intact preparations is that they preserve sufficient neuronal circuitry to produce the behavior of interest: respiratory output. As such, these preparations allow investigations into fundamental processes such as rhythm generation, burst pattern formation, and central integration of modulatory inputs. On the other hand, there are factors limiting the experiments that may be performed using such preparations, or that raise concerns over the applicability of the results obtained to intact animals. Thus, I will discuss the implications of these papers and some of the experimental advantages/limitations of *in vitro* brainstem–spinal cord preparations in general.

RHYTHM GENERATION

Identifying the site and mechanism of respiratory rhythm generation is a fundamental biological issue. Until recently, most hypotheses concerning this process centered on neural network models that relied on extensive mutual inhibition. However, two papers in this symposium utilized the brainstem–spinal cord preparation from neonatal rats to provide exciting evidence that respiratory rhythm generation results from conditional pacemaker neurons. Smith and colleagues utilized precision microsectioning of the medulla to demonstrate that a limited region of the ventrolateral medulla termed the "pre-Bötzinger region" is necessary for continued rhythmic output in both cervical and cranial motoneurons. Furthermore, slice preparations from this region contain rhythm-generating neurons that oscillate conditionally; the incidence and frequency of oscillations is dependent on membrane potential. Homma and colleagues also provide compelling evidence for a population of cells located more rostrally in the ventrolateral medulla that discharge prior to respiratory activity in the cervical roots. These cells have been termed "pre-I" neurons, and are also considered to have intrinsic pacemaker activity. Both groups suggest that the pacemaker cells are embedded in a neuronal network providing for a rich array of synaptic interactions. The major difference between these studies concerns the location of putative pacemaker cells, an apparent conflict that awaits resolution.

Pack and colleagues have utilized a comparative approach to ventilatory control, providing evidence that there are many similarities between elements of the control system in air-breathing fish or amphibia and mammals. One approach was to exploit the advantages of a brainstem–spinal cord preparation from larval bullfrogs. By using GABA receptor antagonists or chloride-free media to investigate the role of synaptic inhibition in rhythm generation, they demonstrated that these bimodal breathers utilize distinct mechanisms of rhythm generation for gill versus pulmonary ventilation. The gill rhythm generator appears to rely on synaptic inhibition and differs both temporally and functionally from the pulmonary rhythm generator, which more likely results from pacemaker activity since it does not require inhibitory synaptic interactions.

It has been suggested that the branchiomeric rhythm generator in fish is the phylogenetic precursor of an upper airway rhythm generator in mammals (27). Could it be that there remain multiple rhythm generators in mammals and that these rhythm generators correspond to the "pre-

Bötzinger" (pulmonary) and "pre-I" (upper airway) regions? The invertebrate literature on neural networks has many examples of anatomical networks that function in a variety of (circuit) modes (cf. 10). Similarly, the neural network subserving ventilatory control in mammals may have several functional modes, possibly subserving diverse functions such as sighing, gasping, emesis, and respiration. It is not necessary to postulate discrete neural networks for each (see below).

BURST PATTERN FORMATION

An equally, if not more, demanding task for the respiratory control system is to shape the spatiotemporal pattern of motor output to the various muscles engaged in the act of breathing. Once again, *in vitro* brainstem–spinal cord preparations can be useful in studies of this process. For example, Liu and colleagues studied synaptic inputs and intrinsic membrane properties governing the excitability of phrenic motoneurons in the neonatal rat preparation. By determining the major descending synaptic drive to phrenic motoneurons, and the dominant neurotransmitters mediating this drive, they provide novel insights into the determinants of inspiratory motor output to the diaphragm and establish the basis for studies on modulation of these drives by other transmitter systems. For example, serotonin injected into the phrenic nucleus of rabbits amplifies descending inputs, greatly enhancing the resulting phrenic output within a breath (26). There remains much to be discovered concerning the processes of burst pattern formation and the spatiotemporal distribution of inspiratory and expiratory drives to various motoneuron pools.

CENTRAL INTEGRATION OF MODULATORY INPUTS

Recent advances in understanding the operation of neural networks have led to the emergence of two general concepts (11): (1) the operation of neural networks depends on the interplay of multiple, nonlinear, and dynamical processes at several levels of organization and (2) modulation of these properties can fundamentally alter network function. The significance of modulation in defining network behavior in a qualitative versus quantitative manner is often underestimated by mammalian neurophysiologists. By changing the functional connectivity and synaptic strength via modulation and/or neuroplasticity, the potential exists to change the fundamental computation of a neural network, imparting the ability to achieve multiple functions in the same neural network or to adapt network function so that it remains appropriate in the face of changing system conditions (10, 12). For example, conditional pacemaker cells (see above) imply qualitative behavioral changes (i.e., oscillations) as a result of modulatory inputs that elicit depolarizing currents.

Hilaire and colleagues investigated modulation of the respiratory rhythm generator by projections from pontine noradrenergic area A5. Using a variety of techniques in the neonatal rat preparation, they showed that norepinephrine tonically inhibits rhythm generation, possibly causing hyperpolarizing currents in conditional pacemaker cells of the rostral ventrolateral medulla. Similar results were reported by Homma and colleagues, and both groups suggest that these effects are mediated by $\alpha2$ adrenergic receptors; however, it is notable that disparate results were obtained when using the well-known $\alpha2$ receptor agonist clonidine. Homma and colleagues report that clonidine was effective at mediating this behavior, whereas it was ineffective in the hands of Hilaire and colleagues. Although the reasons for this difference are not clear, it may relate to different experimental conditions despite superficially similar experimental preparations (see below).

There are virtually limitless modulatory inputs that must be considered before a full understanding of respiratory control is realized. Examples include synaptic inputs from sensory feedback, modulatory neurotransmitter systems such as the cholinergic or monoaminergic systems, hormonal status, "state," and so on (for review see 18). Many but not all of these factors can be addressed effectively with *in vitro* preparations.

EXPERIMENTAL LIMITATIONS

The size of any nonperfused *in vitro* preparation from mammalian tissues is a serious limitation since substantial gradients for oxygen and carbon dioxide may alter tissue and limit its viability. For example, the outermost layers of an *in vitro* brainstem are expected to be severely hyperoxic, possibly resulting in hyperoxic toxicity. On the other hand, interior tissues are predicted to be severely hypoxic, or even anoxic, leading to accumulation of acid metabolites (21). As a result, alterations may occur in neurotransmitter systems such as monoamines that are sensitive to oxygen levels or pH (4). Simple model calculations (e.g., 23) suggest that mammalian brain tissue will be totally anoxic at depths greater than 400 μm, even in a bathing medium equilibrated with 95% oxygen. Unstirred boundary layers would make the problem of anoxia worse. Thus, experimenters have resorted to using animals that are small and tolerate hypoxia well (e.g., neonatal rat pups) and to lowering the medium temperature to decrease oxygen consumption. Even at lower temperature, however, substantial oxygen gradients most likely exist unless the interior tissues have died and no longer consume oxygen.

Reducing the temperature of any *in vitro* mammalian tissue may have consequences beyond the desired effect of reducing metabolic rate and prolonging the "viability" of the preparation. For example, reductions in temperature reduce membrane fluidity, thereby altering the function of membrane-bound proteins, including receptors and ion channels. Decreased temperature decreases channel conductance but increases the channel opening time at mouse neuromuscular junctions (8). Similar effects may underlie qualitative behavioral changes in neuronal function when temperature is decreased. Temperature reductions convert certain chemoreceptors from regular to bursting discharge patterns at otherwise constant conditions (6). Temperature effects on the neuromuscular junction and chemoreceptors occur between 25 and 27°C, a temperature range commonly used for *in vitro* studies.

It is also relevant to ask what the most appropriate pH would be at a lower temperature. Most experimenters use a default gas mixture of 95% O_2 and 5% CO_2 to establish a pH of 7.4. However, since imidazole groups have a temperature-dependent pK in the physiological pH range, the charge state of proteins will change with temperature at constant pH (cf. 19). Alteration in the charge state of proteins may alter their conformation or biological reactivity, preventing normal function. Since many neuronal receptor types and ion channels have an abundance of histidine residues (and therefore imidazole groups) (19), membrane conductances, membrane potential, and neuronal function may be affected by an imbalance between the pH and pK. Would it be wise to adjust PCO_2 and pH so that charge state is preserved? To do so requires only that pH be increased approximately 0.015 pH units/°C decrease by lowering the CO_2. Interactions between temperature and pH may also influence the effectiveness of pharmacological agents. Could it be that clonidine (an imidazoline with a pK in the physiological pH range) was inactive in the study of Hilaire and colleagues due to a different pH/temperature relationship affecting the drug or its associated receptor?

There are numerous other concerns that may limit the applicability of information derived from *in vitro* preparations to intact, behaving animals. For example, critical anatomical structures, trophic factors, or transmitters may be missing from the bathing medium, thereby preventing expression of important behaviors (e.g., 25, 13, 14) or manifesting inappropriate behaviors. Examples include the neuronal excitability changes elicited when normal CSF levels of glutamate (10–50 μM) are restored in the bath (25) or the plateau potentials in motoneurons that are expressed only in the presence of serotonin (13, 14).

SIGNIFICANCE OF A COMPARATIVE APPROACH

In vitro preparations from poikilothermic vertebrates have been successfully utilized in many areas of neurophysiology, including preparations from lampreys (11), frogs (29), and turtles (15), among others. Similar preparations offer powerful advantages in the study of respiratory control; for example, the turtle brainstem–spinal cord preparation has been observed to produce rhythmic respiratory output for as long as five days *in vitro* (7). The brain structures of poikilothermic vertebrates are smaller than comparably sized mammals (even in adults); metabolic rates are typically lower than mammalian tissues at the same temperature, although this may not always be the case (17); the tissues are

adapted to a wide range of body temperatures, thus allowing further decrease in metabolic rate; and, many poikilothermic vertebrates are remarkably tolerant of hypoxia and even anoxia due to their capacity to utilize alternate metabolic pathways (cf. 17). Simple calculations based on the model of Piiper and Scheid (23) suggest that it may be wise to expose an *in vitro* frog brainstem–spinal cord at room temperature to oxygen levels no higher than 30%. By lowering the external oxygen tension, hyperoxic toxicity may be avoided without risk of tissue anoxia at the center of the preparation.

Although parallels with adult mammals are not assured, valuable insights into the function of neural networks subserving respiratory control are the likely result of *in vitro* studies on poikilothermic vertebrates, providing insight into mammalian ventilatory control either by similarity or by contrast. Comparative studies on motor control indicate that there are often many neural solutions to the same problem and that apparently similar neural networks sometimes serve radically different functions (10). The system may also undergo transformation rather than reduction as control system elements are removed or constrained (9). Thus, excessive focus on too few experimental systems may give rise to models and hypotheses that are too narrow in scope to be widely applicable to vertebrates or even mammalian species.

CONCLUSIONS

In vitro preparations offer major experimental advantages in studies on the neural network subserving respiratory control at the molecular, cellular, and network levels (2, 31). Such reductionist approaches have already proven to be highly beneficial, laying the foundation for understanding the integrated control system. However, synthesis and integrative thought must follow in order to discover the emergent properties of neural networks. Advances in modeling nonlinear systems offer much promise in this regard (12), although it is essential to retain the greatest degree of biological revelance possible in these models so that meaningful and testable hypotheses emerge (10). Only by studies of the system at multiple levels of organization are we likely to gain a full appreciation of the respiratory control system and its behavior in awake, behaving animals.

REFERENCES

1. Adrian, E.D., and F.J.J. Buytendijk. Potential changes in the isolated brain stem of the goldfish. *J. Physiol.* (London) 71:121-135, 1931.

2. Berger, A.J. Recent advances in respiratory neurobiology using *in vitro* methods. *Am. J. Physiol.* 259:L24-L29, 1990.

3. Biscoe, T.J., and M.R. Duchen. Electrophysiological responses of dissociated type I cells of the rabbit carotid body to cyanide. *J. Physiol.* (London) 413:447-468, 1989.

4. Davis, J.N., A. Carlsson, V. MacMillan, and B.K. Siesjo. Brain tryptophan hydroxylation: Dependence on arterial oxygen tension. *Science* 182:72-76, 1973.

5. Dekin, M.S., and P.A. Getting. Firing pattern of neurons in the nucleus tractus solitarius: Modulation by membrane hyperpolarization. *Brain Res.* 324:180-184, 1984.

6. Douse, M.A., and G.S. Mitchell. Temperature effects on CO_2-sensitive intrapulmonary chemoreceptors in the lizard, *Tupinambis nigropunctatus. Resp. Physiol.* 72:327-342, 1988.

7. Douse, M.A., and G.S. Mitchell. Episodic respiratory related discharge in turtle cranial motoneurons: *in vivo* and *in vitro* studies. *Brain Res.* 536:297-300, 1990.

8. Dreyer, F., K.D. Muller, K. Peper, and R. Sterz. The M. omohyoideus of the mouse as a convenient mammalian muscle preparation: A study of junctional and extrajunctional acetylcholine receptors by noise analysis and cooperativity. *Pflügers Arch.* 367:115-122, 1976.

9. Feldman, J.L., J.C. Smith, H.H. Ellenberger, C.A. Connelly, G.Liu, J.J. Greer, A.D. Lindsay, and M.R. Otto. Neurogenesis of respiratory rhythm and pattern: Emerging concepts. *Am. J. Physiol.* 259:R879-R886, 1990.

10. Getting, P.A. Emerging principles governing the operation of neural networks. *Ann. Rev. Neurosci.* 12:185-204, 1989.

11. Grillner, S., P. Wallen, N. Dale, L. Brodin, J. Buchanan and R. Hill. Transmitters, membrane properties and network circuitry in the control of locomotion in the lamprey. *Trends in Neurosci.* 10:34-42, 1987.

12. Hopfield, J.J., and D.W. Tank. Computing with neural circuits: A model. *Science* 233:625-633, 1986.

13. Hounsgaard, J., H. Hultborn, B. Jespersen, and 0. Kiehn. Intrinsic membrane properties causing a bistable behaviour of α-motoneurones. *Exp. Brain Res.* 55:391-394, 1984.

14. Hounsgaard, J., and O. Kiehn. Ca^{++} dependent bistability induced by serotonin in spinal motoneurons. *Exp. Brain Res.* 57:422-425, 1985.

15. Larson-Prior, L.J., D.R. McCrimmon, and N.T. Slater. Slow excitatory amino acid receptor–mediated synaptic transmission in turtle cerebellar purkinje cells. *J. Neurophysiol.* 63:637-650, 1990.

16. Lopez-Barneo, J., J.R. Lopez-Lopez, J. Urena, and C. Gonzalez. Chemotransduction in the carotid body: K^+ current modulated by PO_2 in type I chemoreceptor cells. *Science* 241:580-582, 1988.

17. Lutz, P.L. Mechanisms for anoxic survival in the vertebrate brain. *Ann. Rev. Physiol.* (In press), 1991.

18. Mitchell, G.S., M.A. Douse and K.T. Foley. Receptor interactions in modulating ventilatory activity. *Am. J. Physiol.* 259:R911-R920, 1990.

19. Nattie, E.E. The alphastat hypothesis in respiratory control and acid-base balance. *J. Appl. Physiol.* 69:1201-1207, 1990.

20. Neubauer, J.A., W. Chou, S.F. Gonsalves, A.M. Martin, H.M. Geller, and N.H. Edelman. Chemosensitivity of medullary neurons in tissue explant cultures. *FASEB J.* 2:A1295, 1988.

21. Okada, Y., K. Muckenhoff, and P. Scheid. Tissue pH in the isolated brainstem of the neonatal rat. *Proceedings of the International Conference Modulation of Respiratory Pattern: Peripheral and Central Mechanisms.* 67, 1990.

22. Onimaru, H., A. Arata, and I. Homma. Localization of respiratory rhythm-generating neurons in the medulla of brainstem–spinal cord preparations from newborn rats. *Neurosci. Lett.* 78: 151-155, 1987.

23. Piiper, J., and P. Scheid. Cross sectional PO_2 distributions in a Krogh cylinder and solid cylinder models. *Resp. Physiol.* 64:241-251, 1987.

24. Richerson, G.B., and P.A. Getting. Maintenance of complex neural function during perfusion of the mammalian brain. *Brain Res.* 409:128-132, 1987.

25. Sah, P., S. Hestrin, and R.A. Nicoll. Tonic activation of NMDA receptors by ambient glutamate enhances excitability of neurons. *Science* 246:815-818, 1989.

26. Schmid, K., G. Böhmer, and S. Merkelbach. Serotonergic control of phrenic motoneuronal activity at the level of the spinal cord of the rabbit. *Neurosci. Lett.* 116:204-209, 1990.

27. Smatresk, N. Chemoreceptor modulation of endogenous respiratory rhythms in vertebrates. *Am. J. Physiol.* 259:R887-R897, 1990.

28. Smith, J.C., J.L. Feldman, and B.J. Schmidt. Neural mechanisms generating locomotion studied in mammalian brainstem spinal cord *in vitro. FASEB J.* 2:2283-2288, 1988.

29. Sykova, E., and L. Vyklicky. Isolated spinal cord of the frog: An *in vitro* model for the study of neuronal mechanisms of pain. *Physiol. Bohemoslov.* 28:227-229, 1979.

30. Suzue, T. Respiratory rhythm generation in the *in vitro* brain stem-spinal cord preparation of the neonatal rat. *J. Physiol.* (London) 354:173-183, 1984.

31. Walton, K., J. Feldman, P. Getting, L. Renaud, and R. Llinas. New directions in mammalian CNS *in vitro:* Beyond the slice. *Soc. Neurosci. Abst.* 13:1430, 1987.

7

Novel Approaches to the Study of Cellular Mechanisms Generating Respiratory Rhythm *in Vitro*

**Jeffrey C. Smith, John J. Greer, Klaus Ballanyi,
Jack L. Feldman, and Diethelm W. Richter**

The neuronal mechanisms underlying respiratory rhythm-generation in the mammalian nervous system are unknown. Although there has been substantial progress in identifying cellular and synaptic properties of medullary respiratory neurons (11), the cellular mechanisms responsible for rhythm generation have not been elucidated. This is largely because the rhythm-generating neurons in the medulla have not been identified, due in part to technical limitations of experimental approaches applied to this problem in the nervous system *in vivo*.

Isolated preparations of the mammalian brainstem that preserve respiratory network and cellular function *in vitro* allow the application of a broader range of neurobiological techniques and provide the opportunity to identify neuronal mechanisms of rhythmogenesis. Recently, by exploiting the unique properties of *in vitro* neonatal rat brainstem–spinal cord preparations, for example, it has been established that neuron populations distributed in the ventral medulla are sufficient for respiratory rhythm- and motor pattern–generation (15, 16), and the involvement of various synaptic mechanisms in rhythmogenesis has been investigated (4, 6). The *in vitro* systems provide conditions that allow the application of most current biophysical techniques, including patch-clamp techniques (1, 2, 8), for the analysis of cellular properties. Indeed, once the rhythm-generating cells are identified, a major challenge will be to apply voltage-clamp recording techniques for the analysis of neuronal membrane currents to distinguish contributions to the rhythm-generation process of intrinsic membrane properties and synaptic interactions. Conditionally bursting pacemaker neurons have recently been hypothesized to be involved in rhythm generation *in vitro* (4, 19, 20). If this turns out to be the case, voltage-clamp techniques will play a particularly important role in identifying the intrinsic membrane channels and currents responsible for oscillatory properties of the rhythm-generating cells.

In this paper, we describe recently developed *in vitro* methods for both locating and isolating regions of the mammalian medulla containing rhythm-generating neurons, and for applying whole-cell patch-clamp recording techniques to study the biophysical properties of respiratory cells in these regions. These techniques represent a powerful set of new approaches for the identification and analysis of cellular mechanisms of rhythm generation in the mammalian nervous system.

METHODS AND RESULTS

The method for locating medullary regions containing rhythm-generating neurons involves simultaneous recording of respiratory motoneuron activity and precision microsectioning of the medulla of isolated neonatal rat brainstem–spinal cord preparations *in vitro* (16, 20). We have previously established that neurons generating the rhythm *in vitro* are located in the ventral medulla (15, 16). Furthermore, the spontaneously active respiratory neuron populations in the ventral medulla *in vitro* are distributed in longitudinal columns in the ventrolateral reticular formation (18), analogous to cell distributions in the ventrolateral medulla of the adult mammal. The method is therefore designed to determine the locus of rhythm-generating neurons along these ventral cell columns. The medulla is serially microsectioned in the transverse plane with a vibratome, and simultaneous recordings are made of the spontaneous discharge of respiratory motoneuron populations remaining in the neuraxis before and after each section. This procedure allows systematic analysis of perturbations of the respiratory rhythm as cell populations at successive levels of the ventrolateral reticular formation are removed.

The neonatal brainstem–spinal cords are isolated from 1- to 4-day-old Sprague Dawley rats as previously described (13, 18). Details of the brainstem–spinal cord preparation, techniques for nerve recording and data acquisition, and detailed descriptions of the spatiotemporal patterns of motor and medullary neuron activity *in vitro* have been presented elsewhere (18). The neuraxis is pinned down on a rigid, paraffin-coated block, and the block is mounted in the specimen vise in the bath of the vibratome (Technical Products International, VT 1000) with the neuraxis oriented vertically. The medulla is sectioned serially in 50 or 75 μm–thick sections starting from either the pontine-medullary junction in medulla–spinal cord preparations, or from the caudal medulla in isolated medulla preparations. With this section thickness we achieve a high spatial resolution for defining the involvement of cell populations in local regions of the medullary reticular formation. The slicing is continuously observed through a dissecting microscope, and each slice is immediately collected and fixed in 10% formalin solution and subsequently stained for histological identification of reticular formation regions contained within the slice. Motoneuron discharge is recorded bilaterally from cranial and/or spinal ventral roots containing axons of spontaneously active respiratory motoneurons (18). In experiments where the medulla is serially sectioned along the neuraxis in the rostral to caudal direction, recordings are made simultaneously from cranial nerves (IX, X, or XII) and C4 or C5 spinal ventral roots (containing phrenic motoneuron axons). Rhythmic motoneuron discharge is recorded bilaterally from glossopharyngeal nerves in experiments where the isolated medulla is sectioned in the caudal to rostral direction.

Neuroanatomical reconstructions and analysis of perturbations of respiratory rhythm after microsectioning at various medullary levels are presented elsewhere (20). The fundamental result is that successive microsections could be removed from the medulla without significant perturbation of the steady-state rhythm until a unique, limited region of the medulla was reached in which sectioning induced instabilities in the rhythm and eliminated rhythmic motor output. This region is located at the level of the reticular formation, immediately caudal to the retrofacial nucleus and Bötzinger Complex, at the transition zone between the respiratory cell populations of the ventral respiratory group and Bötzinger Complex; we have therefore named this region the pre–Bötzinger Complex (17, 20). In this region, serial sectioning over 150–200 μm (rostral to caudal direction) typically resulted in a progressive reduction in steady-state discharge frequency, an increase in cycle-to-cycle variation in the period, and eventually complete cessation of the rhythmic motor output of all respiratory motoneuron populations, indicating that neurons critical for rhythm generation are distributed throughout this approximately 200 μm–thick medullary region. The elimination of spinal respiratory motoneuron discharge with rostral to caudal sectioning at this level cannot be accounted for by removal of inspiratory bulbospinal neurons, since these premotoneuron populations are concentrated more caudally in the medulla, with highest cell density near the level of the obex (3, 20). Indeed, in these experiments we are exploiting this spatial distribution of pre-motoneurons, which allows us to section serially through much of the rostral medulla without impinging on pre-motor cells transmitting inspiratory drive inputs to the spinal motoneuron populations. We conclude that the pre-Bötzinger Complex contains interneurons involved in rhythm generation.

Microsectioning and recording procedures can be used to obtain isolated medullary slices, containing the pre-Bötzinger Complex, that generate respiratory oscillations (17, 20). These techniques provide the opportunity to probe the oscillatory properties of active respiratory neurons in this region. To obtain these slices, the medulla was sectioned serially from the rostral medulla in medulla–spinal cord preparations to within 150 μm of the rostral boundary of the pre-Bötzinger Complex, and slices of varying thicknesses (200 μm up to 600 μm), containing this and more caudal medullary regions, were cut. Simultaneous recordings of spinal and cranial motoneuron activity were made to confirm that the medulla generated spontaneous oscillations before cutting the slice and for comparisons of the oscillatory period in slice and *en bloc* preparations. The slices were transferred to a recording chamber and bathed in the standard physiological solution (18) during recording experiments. The rostral part of the hypoglossal motor nucleus is contained within these slices, and recordings of hypoglossal motoneuron discharge as well as recordings from neurons within the ventrolateral reticular formation were used for analysis of the patterns of rhythmic neuron activity in the slices.

Slices (≥350 μm thick) containing the pre-Bötzinger Complex generated rhythmic motor discharge bilaterally on hypoglossal roots (fig. 7.1), indicating that they contained not only rhythm-generating neurons, but also local premotoneuronal circuitry for motor output generation. Rhythmically active respiratory neurons in these slices (fig. 7.1) were concentrated in the pre-Bötzinger Complex and more caudally in flanking regions of the ventrolateral reticular formation. In general, slices greater than 500 μm thick generated spontaneous motor output under standard conditions, although the period of spontaneous oscillations and the amplitude of the hypoglossal motoneuron population discharge was typically lower than in the brainstem–spinal cord prior to cutting the slice. The oscillation frequency and discharge amplitude could be increased to those of the *en bloc* medulla–spinal cord preparation by increasing neuronal excitability in the slice (e.g., by elevating the extracellular potassium concentration to 9–10 mM). The thinner slices generated rhythmic motoneuronal discharge when the level of cell excitation was elevated. The reduction in neuronal excitation in the slices is possibly due to changes in the cellular ionic environment with washout of the extracellular space, or removal of excitatory synaptic connections, when the slices are cut. The temporal pattern of motoneuron discharge and synaptic potentials/currents of medullary respiratory neurons generated by all of the slices under the conditions of elevated neuronal excitation closely corresponded to those generated in the *en bloc* brainstem–spinal cord preparation (fig. 7.1). The thinnest slices (350 μm) that generated oscillatory activity contained primarily the pre-Bötzinger Complex in the ventrolateral reticular formation, confirming that rhythm-generating neurons are located at this level of the reticular formation.

There are technical limitations of conventional single-electrode intracellular recording techniques, particularly for obtaining stable, long-term current- and voltage-clamp recordings from small interneurons in the neonatal medullary reticular formation. These limitations can be potentially overcome by whole-cell patch-clamp recording techniques (1, 2, 8). To assess the applicability of these techniques for recording from spontaneously active respiratory neurons in the slice and *en bloc* medulla preparations, we used procedures for blind patch clamping similar to those described by Blanton et al. (1) for whole-cell

FIG. 7.1 Whole-cell current-clamp (*A,
B*) and voltage-clamp (*C*) recordings illustrating typical membrane potentials
and synaptic currents of medullary neurons obtained with the blind whole-cell
patch-clamp technique. Recordings were
obtained from neurons with inspiratory
phase discharge in 500 μm–thick isolated
slice containing the pre-Bötzinger Complex in *A* and in *en bloc* brainstem–spinal
cord preparation in *B* and *C*. The neurons
were located in the ventrolateral reticular
formation. Simultaneous recordings of
hypoglossal (XII) root discharge in the
slice and C_4 phrenic motor discharge in
the *en bloc* preparations are shown. The
bottom traces in *B* and *C* show membrane
potentials and synaptic currents, respectively, on a faster time base. The holding
potential for the voltage clamp in *C* was
−70 mV. The neurons exhibit 15 to 20
mV–depolarizing synaptic drive potentials under current clamp, and 400–700
pA peak synaptic currents under voltage
clamp during the inspiratory phase. Temporal patterns of motoneuron discharge,
neuronal spiking, and synaptic drive po-
tentials/currents in the isolated slice
closely correspond to patterns generated
in the *en bloc* preparation. Electrode resistance = 5 MΩ, series resistance (Rs)
= 30 MΩ, membrane capacitance C_M =
16 pF, and membrane resistance (R_M) =
450 MΩ for neuron in *A*; Rs = 26 MΩ,
C_M = 14 pF, R_M = 500 MΩ for neuron
in *B* and *C*.

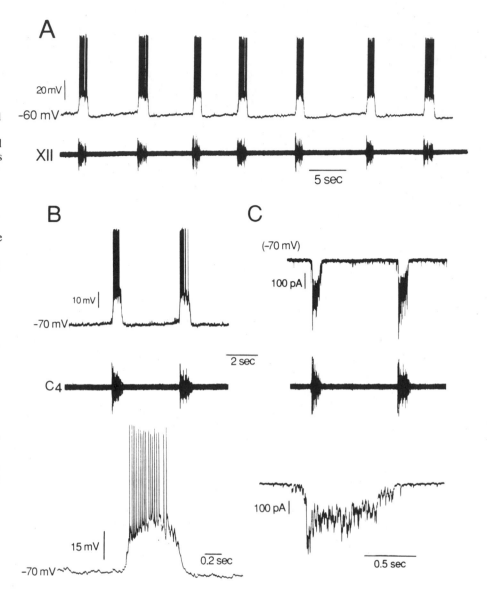

recording in reptilian and mammalian cortical slices. These
techniques were modified for use in the *en bloc* medulla–
spinal cord preparations. The respiratory neurons are sufficiently deep within the medulla (typically 100–300 μm
below the cut surface of slices; 200–500 μm below the ventral surface in the *en bloc* preparations) that the cell somas
cannot be directly visualized during the process of obtaining a whole-cell recording, in contrast to procedures used
for whole-cell patch-clamp recording in thin slice preparations (2, 22). Furthermore, the neuron composition of the
medullary reticular formation is heterogeneous, with nonrespiratory neurons distributed in regions containing respiratory cells. In order to improve the yield of respiratory
neurons, particularly in *en bloc* preparations, we first located spontaneously active respiratory cells by mapping
field potentials to establish the depth of cell somas and determine a point of entry through the medullary surface for
the patch electrodes. In slice preparations where the retic-

ular formation could be viewed and cytoarchitectonic regions (e.g., nucleus ambiguus) distinguished, satisfactory
yields could often be obtained without initially mapping extracellular potentials.

To obtain whole-cell recordings, continuous positive
pressure (160–200 mmHg) was applied to the back of the
pipette from a constant pressure source to keep the pipette
tip clean and maintain tip patency, as indicated by continuous measurement of the pipette resistance under voltage-
clamp conditions. Gigaohm seals (3–10 GΩ) could be
routinely formed on respiratory neurons by application of
slight negative pressure to the pipette. In some cases, the
respiratory cells could be identified prior to seal formation
by recording currents during the rhythmic discharge of action potentials with the pipette tip apposed to the somal
membrane. Whole-cell recordings were obtained after rup-
turing the membrane patch attached to the pipette by applying slight negative pressure to the pipette. For neuronal

recording under standard conditions, the electrodes were filled with solution containing (mM): D–gluconic acid (potassium salt) 120; $CaCl_2$, 1; NaCl, 1; HEPES, 10; BAPTA (tetrapotassium salt), 11; $MgCl_2$, 1; NaATP (pH = 7.4), 0.5.

Stable, long-term (1–3 hr) whole-cell current- and voltage- clamp recordings of rhythmic membrane potentials and currents could be routinely obtained from a number of classes of inspiratory and expiratory neurons previously shown to be spontaneously active in the pre-Bötzinger and adjacent reticular formation regions *in vitro* (18). Figure 7.1 illustrates typical recordings of spike discharge patterns and synaptic drive potentials and currents of neurons with inspiratory phase discharge. These cells exhibited large amplitude (10–20 mV, 600–900 msec duration) rhythmic synaptic drive potentials under current-clamp and excitatory postsynaptic currents (0.3–0.7 nA) under voltage-clamp conditions. Expiratory neurons (not shown) exhibited 10–15 mV membrane potential hyperpolarizations during the inspiratory phase, demonstrating the presence of inhibitory synaptic interactions. Membrane resistances and capacitances of respiratory neurons, measured from currents induced by potential pulses (1–10 mV), under voltage-clamp with greater than 75% series resistance compensation, ranged from 0.3 to 1 GΩ, and from 10 to 25 pF, respectively.

DISCUSSION

We have briefly described methods for locating medullary regions containing neurons involved in rhythm generation, methods for isolating these regions in viable medullary slices that generate respiratory oscillations, and techniques for routinely obtaining current- and voltage-clamp recordings from respiratory neurons in these regions for analysis of cellular and synaptic mechanisms. These techniques represent a powerful set of new approaches for analysis of cellular mechanisms of rhythm generation in the mammalian nervous system. The medullary slice preparations contain not only rhythm-generating neurons but an active local network and therefore also provide the opportunity to analyze synaptic mechanisms involved in rhythmic drive transmission in an isolated, functional respiratory circuit *in vitro*.

The application of blind whole-cell patch-clamp recording techniques, which our results demonstrate is feasible in the isolated slice and *en bloc* brainstem–spinal cord preparations, should rapidly lead to elucidation of cellular and synaptic mechanisms involved in rhythm generation. These methods represent an important advance for analysis of cellular properties underlying respiratory pattern generation. Although we have previously established that conventional single-electrode intracellular recording techniques (including voltage-clamp techniques) can be applied for the analysis of membrane properties of spinal motoneurons in the

in vitro brainstem–spinal cord preparation (7, 14), medullary interneurons in the neonatal brainstem are small, and even stable single-electrode current-clamp recording from medullary cells (18) has proven technically difficult. The whole-cell patch-clamp techniques circumvent the limitations of conventional single-electrode recording techniques applied to small medullary cells. These techniques can also be exploited to obtain information on a number of other cellular properties, as demonstrated for other neurons (see discussions in 1, 2, and 8), including the following: (1) single-channel properties in addition to the macroscopic membrane properties; (2) morphological properties and axonal projections by simultaneous cell staining by intracellular filling from dye-containing recording pipettes; and (3) involvement of cytoplasmic signaling and other intracellular biochemical processes regulating membrane excitability.

The results obtained with the microsectioning method indicate that neurons in the reticular formation at the level of the pre-Bötzinger Complex are essential for rhythm generation in the *in vitro* neonatal rat brainstem (16, 17, 20). The isolated slices containing primarily this region generate respiratory oscillations, confirming that the region contains rhythm generating cells. Perturbations of neuronal excitability in the pre-Bötzinger Complex in these slices and *en bloc* preparations cause profound perturbations of rhythm (5, 20). The microsectioning results indicate that no other medullary region is essential for rhythmogenesis, and therefore do not support the recent proposal (9, 10) that neuron populations located more rostrally in the ventrolateral reticular formation constitute the primary rhythm generator. Removal of these more rostral medullary regions causes no perturbations of the spontaneous rhythm; moreover, these regions were not contained within the rhythmically active medullary slices. The properties of the rhythm-generating neurons and their precise spatial distribution in the reticular formation at the level of the pre-Bötzinger Complex remain to be established. A number of classes of respiratory neurons have been identified in this region, including cells that have neuronal spike discharge starting before the generation of inspiratory phase motoneuron activity (12, 18). Furthermore, by applying the whole-cell patch-clamp recording techniques, we have identified neurons with voltage-dependent oscillatory properties in the pre-Bötzinger Complex in the isolated slice preparations (19, 20, 21), consistent with the hypothesis that a population of synchronized conditionally bursting pacemaker neurons generates rhythm (see discussion in 4). It is possible that rhythm-generating neurons are not strictly confined to the pre-Bötzinger Complex, but are also distributed caudally and rostrally in immediately flanking regions of the reticular formation, since (particularly) more caudal reticular formation regions were also contained within the thicker slices that generated rhythmic neuronal activity. Regardless of the complete spatial distribution, the results suggest that there are rhythm-generating cells in the pre-Bötzinger Complex. This region has not been previously identified as a site for rhythm generation, and properties of neurons within this region should now be analyzed further both *in vitro* and *in vivo*.

ACKNOWLEDGMENTS

This work was supported by NIH HL40959, HL02204, DFG Ba 1095/1–1, and a fellowship from the Alexander von Humboldt Foundation.

REFERENCES

1. Blanton, M.G., J.J. Lo Turco, and A. Kriegstein. Whole cell recording from neurons in slices of reptilian and mammalian cerebral cortex. *J. Neurosci. Methods* 30:203-210, 1989.

2. Edwards, F.A., A. Konnerth, B. Sakmann, and T. Takahashi. A thin slice preparation for patch clamp recordings from neurons of the mammalian central nervous system. *Pflügers Arch.* 414:600-612, 1989.

3. Ellenberger, H., and J.L. Feldman. Subnuclear organization of the lateral tegmental field of the rat I: Nucleus ambiguus and ventral respiratory group. *J. Comp. Neurol.* 294:202-211, 1990.

4. Feldman, J.L. and J.C. Smith. Cellular mechanisms underlying modulation of breathing pattern in mammals. *Ann. NY Acad. Sci.* 563:114-130, 1989.

5. Funk, G., J.C. Smith, and J.L. Feldman. Respiratory oscillations in medullary slices: Critical role of excitatory amino acids. *Soc. Neurosci. Abs.* 17:1580, 1991.

6. Greer, J.J., J.C. Smith, and J.L. Feldman. Role of excitatory amino acids in the generation and transmission of respiratory drive in neonatal rat. *J. Physiol.* (London) 437:727-749, 1991.

7. Liu, G., J.L. Feldman, and J.C. Smith. Excitatory amino acid–mediated transmission of inspiratory drive to phrenic motoneurons. *J. Neurophysiol.* 64:423-437, 1990.

8. Marty, A., and E. Neher. Tight-seal whole-cell recording. In *Single Channel Recording*, ed. B. Sakmann and E. Neher, 107-122, New York: Plenum Press, 1983.

9. Onimaru, H., A. Arata, and I. Homma. Localization of respiratory rhythm-generating neurons in the medulla of brainstem–spinal cord preparations from newborn rats. *Neurosci. Lett.* 78:151-155, 1987.

10. Onimaru, H., A. Arata, and I. Homma. Primary respiratory rhythm generator in the medulla of brainstem–spinal cord preparation from newborn rat. *Brain Res.* 445:314-324, 1988.

11. Richter, D.W., D. Ballantyne, and J.E. Remmers. How is respiratory rhythm generated? A model. *News in Physiol. Sci.* 1:109-112, 1986.

12. Schwarzacher, S.W., J.C. Smith, and D.W. Richter. Respiratory neurones in the pre–Bötzinger region of cats. *Pflügers Arch.* (Suppl. 1) 418:R17, 1991.

13. Smith, J.C., and J.L. Feldman. *In vitro* brainstem–spinal cord preparations for study of motor systems for mammalian respiration and locomotion. *J. Neurosci. Methods* (Special Issue: *Novel Approaches to the Study of Motor Systems*) 21:321-333, 1987.

14. Smith, J.C., G. Liu, and J.L. Feldman. Intracellular recording from phrenic motoneurons receiving respiratory drive *in vitro*. *Neurosci. Lett.* 88:27-32, 1988.

15. Smith, J.C., and J.L. Feldman. Discharge patterns of medullary respiratory neurons in mammalian brainstem *in vitro*. *Soc. Neurosci. Abstr.* 14:1060, 1988.

16. Smith, J.C., J.J. Greer, and J.L. Feldman. Identification of limited region of the medulla that may contain neuron populations generating respiratory rhythm *in vitro*. *Soc. Neurosci. Abstr.* 15: 505, 1989.

17. Smith, J.C., J.J. Greer, and J.L. Feldman. Medullary slices that generate respiratory oscillations *in vitro*. *Soc. Neurosci. Abstr.* 16:1130, 1990.

18. Smith, J.C., J.J. Greer, G. Liu, and J.L. Feldman. Neural mechanisms generating respiratory pattern in mammalian brainstem–spinal cord *in vitro*. I. Spatiotemporal patterns of motor and medullary neuron activity. *J. Neurophysiol.* 64:1149-1169, 1990.

19. Smith, J.C., K. Ballanyi, D.W. Richter, and J.L. Feldman. Conditionally bursting pacemaker neurons in a limited region of the medulla involved in respiratory rhythm generation *in vitro*. *FASEB J.* 5:A734, 1991.

20. Smith, J.C., H. Ellenberger, K. Ballanyi, D.W. Richter, and J.L. Feldman. Pre-Bötzinger Complex: A brainstem region that may generate respiratory rhythm in mammals. *Science* 254:726-729, 1991.

21. Smith, J.C., K. Ballanyi, D.W. Richter, and J.L. Feldman. Oscillatory properties of neurons in an isolated respiratory circuit *in vitro* analyzed by whole-cell patch-clamp techniques. *Soc. Neurosci. Abstr.* 17:1580, 1991.

22. Takahashi, T. and A.J. Berger. Serotonin enhances a low-voltage-activated calcium current in rat spinal motoneurons. *J. Neurosci.* 10:1922-1928, 1990.

8

Respiratory Rhythm Generation in the Ventral Medulla

Ikuo Homma, Akiko Arata, and Hiroshi Onimaru

Respiratory output is shaped by neurons in the dorsal and ventral respiratory groups (DRG and VRG) of the medulla. Although the shape and the amplitude of the inspiratory output are greatly altered by microlesion (19, 20) or by focal cooling (3) of these areas, respiratory rhythm remains. The exact locus and types of neurons constituting the respiratory rhythm generator are unknown. Several recent reports (4, 7) have suggested that structures localized ventral to the VRG are critical in the generation of rhythm and patterns of respiratory activity.

In 1984, Suzue (21) used a brainstem–spinal cord preparation isolated from newborn rats to show respiratory activity *in vitro*. This preparation presents a great advantage in recording central nervous activities isolated from peripheral inputs (6, 10, 18). Using this preparation, we have examined the source of rhythm generation and the location of respiratory neurons in the ventral medulla.

METHODS

The brainstem and spinal cord of 0- to 5-day old Wistar rats were isolated under deep ether anesthesia. The preparation was placed in a small chamber and perfused continuously with modified Krebs solution (mM): NaCl, 124; KCl, 5.0; KH_2PO_4, 1.2; $CaCl_2$, 2.4; $MgSO_4$, 1.3; $NaHCO_3$, 26; glucose, 30; equilibrated with 95% O_2 and 5% CO_2; at 25–26°C, pH 7.4.

Respiratory activity corresponding to inspiration was recorded from the spinal C4 or C5 ventral roots through a glass capillary suction electrode. The respiratory rhythm persisted after removing the pons by transection between the VIth cranial nerve roots and the lower border of the trapezoid body. C4 or C5 respiratory rhythmic bursts could be recorded even after removing the dorsal half of the medulla (2). The ventral medulla thus includes neuronal structures necessary to inspiratory pattern generation as well as rhythm generation. This was also confirmed recently in isolated newborn rabbit preparations (figs. 8.2, 8.3).

RESULTS AND DISCUSSION

Various types of neuronal firing related to rhythmic C4 or C5 activities were recorded in the rostral ventrolateral medulla (RVL) of rat preparations at the levels of the IXth or Xth cranial nerve root and 50–250 μm deep from the ventral surface (2, 12). These respiratory-related units were classified into three types: type 1 exhibited activity that preceded inspiration (Pre-I), type 2 fired during inspiration, and type 3 fired tonically but was inhibited during inspiration. Type 1 and type 2 neurons had subtypes showing more or less tonic activity (fig. 8.1).

In rabbit preparations, several types of respiratory-related neuronal activity could be recorded from the RVL (fig. 8.2). Although some of these discharge patterns were similar to the firing patterns of Pre-I neurons of the rat, detailed properties of these neurons have not yet been examined (see fig. 8.3).

In newborn rat preparations, respiratory rhythm is produced primarily by Pre-I neurons. This is suggested by the following results: (1) Single shock stimulation of the RVL induced Pre-I activity and reset the phase of the respiratory rhythm (12, 13); (2) electrolytic lesion in the RVL slowed or stopped the rhythmic activity (12); (3) Pre-I activity was not always followed by C4 activity, although spontaneous C4 activity was preceded by Pre-I activity without exception (11); (4) after electrolytic lesion of the caudal ventrolateral medulla at the level of the medial roots of the XII cranial nerve, C4 activity disappeared, but Pre-I activities remained (13); (5) electric stimulation applied to the vagus nerve inhibited C4 inspiratory activity, but rhythmic Pre-I activity remained (11); (6) Pre-I-like rhythmic bursts were also recorded from the RVL of the ventral half of blocks of the rostral medulla (11); and (7) intracellular membrane potential analyses of inspiratory neurons revealed excitatory synaptic connections from Pre-I neurons to inspiratory neurons (unpublished observation). These results strongly suggest that the primary rhythm generator, which is separate from the neural mechanism of inspiratory pattern generation, is located in the RVL and that Pre-I neurons are the primary rhythm generator neurons. However, characterization of Pre-I neurons remains to be determined, and the population of Pre-I neurons may be found to be heterogeneous.

About half of the Pre-I neurons retained their rhythmic burst activity after chemical synaptic transmission was blocked in low Ca^{++}, high Mg^{++} solution (15). These Pre-I neurons are believed to possess intrinsic bursting pacemaker properties. The intrinsic Pre-I rhythm in low Ca^{++}, high Mg^{++} solution was inhibited by the α2-agonist, clonidine (1), and enhanced by the adenylate cyclase activator, forskolin (unpublished observation). A role for cAMP in the rhythm generation is thus suggested. The

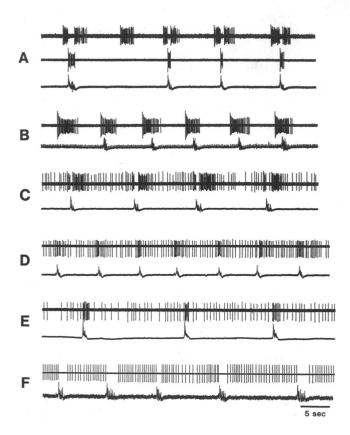

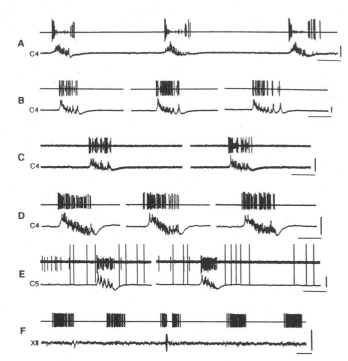

FIG. 8.1 Firing pattern of several respiration-related neurons in the ventral medulla of the newborn rat preparation together with C4 (or C5) inspiratory activity (lower trace in each record). (*A*) Typical Pre-I and inspiratory (I) neurons. (*B*) Pre-I neuron whose firing is not inhibited during I phase. (*C*) Tonic Pre-I neuron that fires virtually continuously, but whose activity increases just before and after the I phase. (*D*) Tonic Pre-I neuron whose firing is only weakly depressed during I phase. (*E*) Tonic I neuron that fires virtually continuously, but whose activity increases during the I phase. (*F*) Tonically firing neuron that is inhibited during I phase.

FIG. 8.2 Firing patterns of several respiration-related neurons recorded from the RVL of medulla isolated from a 0-day-old rabbit together with C4, C5 or XII inspiratory activity (lower trace in each record). (*A, B*) Preparations with medulla intact. (*C*) Preparation in which the dorsal half of the medulla was removed. (*D–F*) Preparations with intact medulla, perfused with modified Krebs solution from a small glass capillary inserted into the basal artery. This arterial perfusion is necessary to maintain neuronal activity for more than 1 hr. Calibration: 0.1mV and 2 sec.

intrinsic pacemaker mechanism should be studied in detail by analyzing the intracellular membrane potentials of Pre-I neurons.

Pre-I neuronal firing was usually inhibited during inspiration and was biphasic in nature (Fig. 8.1*A*). This inhibition disappeared after perfusions of bicuculline, picrotoxin, or strychnine, or during reduction of Cl$^-$ concentration (17). Figure 8.4 shows that the inhibition of activity during inspiration disappeared after microiontophoretic application of bicuculline to a Pre-I neuron. The results suggest that the Pre-I neurons receive Cl-dependent GABA- (or glycine-) like synaptic inhibition during inspiration. Such inhibition, however, was not required to produce the rhythmic Pre-I bursts.

A role for excitatory amino acid (EAA) receptors in respiratory rhythm generation in the brainstem was recently suggested (5). We examined the effects of some EAA antagonists on Pre-I and inspiratory neuron activity (16). Kynurenic acid (KYN, 0.1–0.5 mM, 5–10 min perfusion

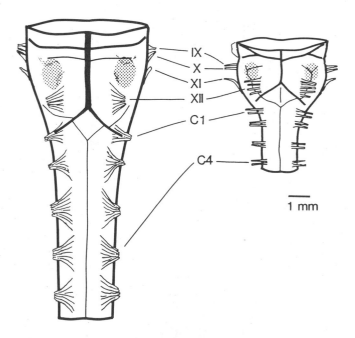

FIG. 8.3 Ventral view of brainstem–spinal cord preparation from newborn rabbit (*left*) and newborn rat (*right*). IX–XII, cranial nerves. C1–C4 cervical ventral nerves. Unit activities of neurons in the rostral ventrolateral medulla were recorded extracellularly by glass microelectrodes from within the shaded area.

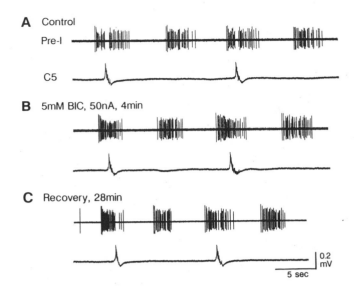

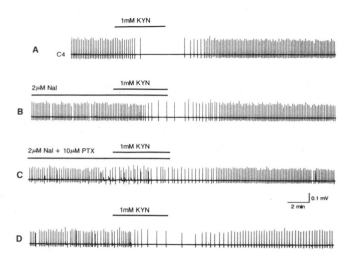

FIG. 8.4 Effects of iontophoretic application of bicuculline (BIC) on Pre-I neuron activity. (A) Pre-I and C5 activity in the control. (B) Activity after application of bicuculline ejected by 50 nA DC current (4 min) through drug electrode filled with 5 mM bicuculline and cemented 30 μm back from tip of recording electrode. Note disappearance of inhibition of Pre-I firing during inspiration. (C) Activity 28 min after ejection was stopped.

FIG. 8.5 Reduction of kynurenic acid (KYN) –induced inhibition of rhythmic C4 activity by pretreatment with antagonists of inhibitory transmitter. (A) Disruption of the rhythm by brainstem perfusion with 1 mM KYN. (B) Effects of KYN after 13 min of pretreatment with 2 μM naloxone (Nal). (C) Effects of KYN after 23-min pretreatment with 2 μM naloxone plus 10 μM pictrotoxin (PTX). Note KYN inhibition of breathing is diminished. (D) Effects of KYN 27 min after perfusate was returned to standard solution. All records are from the same preparation.

reduced the intraburst firing frequency and the burst duration of Pre I neurons. Right and left Pre-I firing tended to be desynchronized, so C4 bursts were intermittent, and the C4 burst rate was thus reduced with no significant reduction of amplitude or duration. 2-amino-5-phosphonovaleric acid (2-APV, 50–100 μM) and 6-cyano-7-nitroquinoxaline-2, 3,-dione (CNQX, 0.2–1 μM) produced effects similar to those of KYN. At higher doses (0.5–1 mM), KYN strongly reduced the rate of Pre-I bursts. The inhibitory effect of brainstem perfusion with 1 mM KYN was antagonized considerably with 2 μM naloxone plus 10 μM picrotoxin (fig. 8.5). These results suggest that EAA transmitters are involved in the synchronization between Pre-I neurons and in burst generation, which can thus be regulated by balancing excitatory and inhibitory synaptic inputs.

Although the properties of the inspiratory pattern generator (IPG) are less understood and the precise location of the IPG is unknown at present, it is presumed to be located in the ventrolateral medulla, more caudal than the RVL (14). Perfusion (20–30 min) of the brainstem with 1 mM KYN reduced the amplitude and duration of spontaneous or stimulus-induced C4 bursts (unpublished observation). Thus EAA may be involved in inspiratory pattern generation in the medulla.

It is thought that stimulation of the vagus inhibits C4 inspiratory activity, probably via inhibition of IPG, since Pre-I firing was not depressed in most cases (11). Inhibition of inspiratory activity by lung inflation is reported to be via GABA (and/or glycine) receptors (9). On the other hand, GABA (0.2 mM) or glycine (0.5 mM) perfusion (10–30

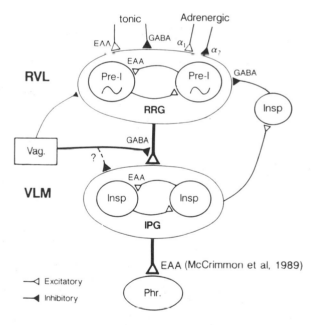

FIG. 8.6 Neuronal groups and possible synaptic interactions involved in the generation of rhythmic respiratory activity. RRG, respiratory rhythm generator; IPG, inspiratory pattern generator; Phr., phrenic motoneurons; Vag., vagal afferents. Pre-I, Pre-I neurons; Insp, inspiratory neurons. RVL, rostral ventrolateral medulla; VLM, ventrolateral medulla. EAA, excitatory amino acid transmitter; GABA, GABA- and/or glycine-like Cl⁻-dependent synaptic inhibition. The RRG is composed of Pre-I neurons in the RVL, some of which possess intrinsic pacemaker properties. The RRG produces the primary rhythm of respiration and triggers IPG. McCrimmon et al. (8) have suggested that excitatory synaptic impulses are transmitted via EAA receptors from bulbospinal inspiratory neurons to phrenic motoneurons.

min) did not depress the amplitude of spontaneous or stimulus-induced C4 activity, whereas the burst rate was extremely reduced (17). This implies that the IPG has fewer GABA or glycine receptors than the RRG. Therefore, vagal afferents might act at presynaptic sites of excitatory input to the IPG.

CONCLUSION

In brainstem–spinal cord preparations isolated from newborn rats, respiratory rhythm is probably generated primarily by a neuronal network composed of excitatory synapses among, mainly, Pre-I intrinsic pacemaker cells in the rostral ventrolateral medulla. Figure 8.6 shows neuronal groups and possible (simplified) synaptic interactions involved in the generation of rhythmic respiratory activity.

REFERENCES

1. Arata, A., H. Onimaru, and I. Homma. A possible role of adrenaline on respiratory rhythm generation in the medulla of newborn rat *in vitro. Neurosci. Res.* Suppl. 11:S22, 1990.

2. Arata, A., H. Onimaru, and I. Homma. Respiration-related neurons in the ventral medulla of newborn rats *in vitro. Brain Res. Bull.* 24:599-604, 1990.

3. Budzinska, K., C. von Euler, F.F. Kao, T. Pantaleo, and Y. Yamamoto. Effects of graded focal cold block in the solitary and para-ambigual regions of the medulla in the cat. *Acta Physiol. Scand.* 124:317-328, 1985.

4. Budzinska, K., C. von Euler, F.F. Kao, T. Pantaleo, and Y. Yamamoto. Effects of graded focal cold block in rostral areas of the medulla. *Acta. Physiol. Scand.* 124:329-340, 1985.

5. Feldman, J.L., and J.C. Smith. Cellular mechanisms underlying modulation of breathing pattern in mammals. In *Ann. NY Acad. Sci.* vol. 563, *Modulation of defined vertebrate neural circuits,* ed. M. Davis, B.L. Jacobs, and R.I. Schoenfeld, New York: NY Acad Sci, 114-130, 1989.

6. Harada, Y., M. Kuno, and Y.Z. Wang. Differential effects of carbon dioxide and pH on central chemoreceptors in the rat *in vitro. J. Physiol.* (London) 368:679-693, 1985.

7. Homma, I., A. Isobe, M. Iwase, A. Kanamaru, and M. Sibuya. Two different types of apnea induced by focal cold block of ventral medulla in rabbits. *Neurosci. Lett.* 87:41-45, 1988.

8. McCrimmon, D.R., J.C. Smith, and J.L. Feldman. Involvement of excitatory amino acids in neurotransmission of inspiratory drive to spinal respiratory motoneurons. *J. Neurosci.* 9:1910-1921, 1989.

9. Murakoshi, T., and M. Otsuka. Respiratory reflexes in an isolated brainstem-lung preparation of the newborn rat: Possible involvement of γ-aminobutyric acid and glycine. *Neurosci. Lett.* 62:63-68, 1985.

10. Murakoshi, T., T. Suzue, and S. Tamai. A pharmacological study on respiratory rhythm in the isolated brainstem–spinal cord preparation of the newborn rat. *Br. J. Pharmacol.* 86:95-104, 1985.

11. Onimaru, H., and I. Homma. Respiratory rhythm generator neurons in medulla of brainstem–spinal cord preparation from newborn rat. *Brain Res.* 403:380-384, 1987.

12. Onimaru, H., A. Arata, and I. Homma. Localization of respiratory rhythm–generating neurons in the medulla of brainstem–spinal cord preparations from newborn rats. *Neurosci. Lett.* 78:151-155, 1987.

13. Onimaru, H., A. Arata, and I. Homma. Primary respiratory rhythm generator in the medulla of brainstem–spinal cord preparation from newborn rat. *Brain. Res.* 445:314-324, 1988.

14. Onimaru, H., A. Arata, and I. Homma. Electrophysiological properties and localization of inspiratory pattern generator in medulla isolated from newborn rats. *Jpn. J. Physiol.* 39:249, 1989.

15. Onimaru, H., A. Arata, and I. Homma. Firing properties of respiratory rhythm generating neurons in the absence of synaptic transmission in rat medulla *in vitro. Exp. Brain Res.* 76:530-536, 1989.

16. Onimaru, H., A. Arata, and I. Homma. The role of excitatory amino acid (EAA) transmitter in the generation of respiratory rhythm in medulla isolated from newborn rat. *Jpn. J. Physiol.* 40:s55, 1990.

17. Onimaru, H., A. Arata, and I. Homma. Inhibitory synaptic inputs to respiratory rhythm generator in medulla isolated from newborn rats. *Pflügers Arch.* 417:425-432, 1990.

18. Smith, J.C., and J.L. Feldman. *In vitro* brainstem–spinal cord preparations for study of motor systems for mammalian respiration and locomotion. *J. Neurosci. Methods* 21:321-333, 1987.

19. Speck, D.F., and J.L. Feldman. The effects of microstimulation and microlesions in the ventral and dorsal respiratory groups in medulla of cat. *J. Neurosci.* 2:744-757, 1982.

20. Speck, D.F., and E.R. Beck. Respiratory rhythmicity after extensive lesions of the dorsal and ventral respiratory groups in the decerebrate cat. *Brain Res.* 482:387-392, 1989.

21. Suzue, T. Respiratory rhythm generation in the *in vitro* brainstem–spinal cord preparation of the neonatal rat. *J. Physiol.* (London) 354:173-183, 1984.

9

Noradrenergic Modulation of the Medullary Respiratory Rhythm Generator by the Pontine A5 Area

G. Hilaire, R. Monteau, S. Errchidi, D. Morin, and J.M. Cottet-Emard

Cardiovascular and respiratory regulation are based on intermingled mechanisms which interact peripherally and/or centrally. Therefore, it is often difficult to define the functional entirety of the central structures implicated in these regulations (11). Previous reports demonstrated that the pontine A5 area is involved in cardiovascular regulation (7). To define whether the A5 area also participates in respiratory regulation, *in vitro* experiments were performed in the isolated brainstem–spinal cord preparation of newborn rats, which retains a respiratory activity after the elimination of all peripheral mechanisms. Results suggested that A5 may exert a tonic inhibitory modulation of the medullary respiratory rhythm generator via a release of endogenous noradrenaline (NA). Some of these results have already been published (5, 9).

METHODS

Experiments were performed in the brainstem–spinal cord preparation of newborn rats as described elsewhere (9, 12, 17, 20). Electrical activities of cervical ventral roots were recorded with suction electrodes. Drugs dissolved in the bathing medium were applied by superfusion or ejected locally with multi-barreled electrodes (pressure pulse, volume injected 5 nl). Electrical stimulation (0.2 msec, 50–100 μA) or lesions (DC current, 2–5 sec, 0.5–1 mA) were administered with either a tungsten microelectrode or the saline-filled central channel of a multibarreled micropipette. Changes in minute respiratory frequency (RF) resulting from drug application, stimulation, or lesion were expressed as percentages of control values defined during a 5 min period prior to the test. Histological controls of sites of stimulation and lesion were performed routinely. Results were given as the mean $\pm$ S.E.M. and changes considered as significant at P values of less than 0.05.

RESULTS

The respiratory frequency (RF), assessed from the rhythmical discharges recorded in cervical ventral roots, was low in ponto-medullary preparations (around 5/min) with restricted variations ($<10\%$). Elimination of the pons by transection (medullary preparations) elicited a sustained increase in RF, which stabilized at twice the control values (10–12/min, fig. 9.1*A*). Electrical stimulation performed in

the pons localized RF inhibitory sites in the vicinity of the A5 area (fig. 9.1*B*) where bilateral electrocoagulation increased RF as transections did.

Bathing the ponto-medullary preparations with medium containing NA antagonists (yohimbine, piperoxane, idazoxan) to block NA receptors doubled RF in 6–9 min and suppressed the effects of A5 electrical stimulation (fig. 9.1*C*). Local application of NA in the A5 sites, assumed to inhibit A5 neurons, increased RF immediately. Glutamate ejection, assumed to excite A5 neurons, delayed onset of inspiration, whereas saline ejection had no effect. Applying medium containing NA or adrenaline (25–100 μM) on medullary preparations decreased RF in a dose-dependent manner (fig. 9.2). These decreases were blocked by NA antagonists and potentiated by inhibition of NA degradation by monoamine oxidase (pargyline). These results suggest a tonic noradrenergic inhibitory drive on the medullary respiratory rhythm generator originating from A5.

In medullary preparations, NA-induced decreases in RF were blocked by α-2 antagonists (yohimbine, piperoxane, and idazoxan) but not by α-1 antagonists (prazosin). Applying medium containing 6-fluoro-NA (α-1 agonist) or isoproterenol (β agonist) did not decrease RF. Therefore, α-2 receptors are likely to be involved in the decrease of RF evoked by NA bathing. However, well-known α-2 agonists had no effect (clonidine, guanfacine) or limited effects (α-CH$_3$-NA), whereas phenylephrine, which is mainly an α-1 and to a lesser degree an α-2 agonist, decreased RF (fig. 9.2).

When the pons was bathed with drugs known to block NA biosynthesis (α-CH$_3$-tyrosine), RF was significantly increased in agreement with a withdrawal of a pontine NA inhibitory effect. In contrast, applying a NA precursor (tyrosine) decreased RF. This effect was potentiated by pargyline (IMAO) and blocked by α-2 antagonist pretreatment. All these RF changes may be due to NA newly synthesized from tyrosine, demonstrating that NA biosynthesis continues under these *in vitro* conditions.

In the absence of any exogenous NA, bathing the ponto-medullary preparations with drugs known to potentiate NA effects (such as pargyline, which inhibits NA degradation, or desipramine, which inhibits its reuptake) decreased RF. Since both the decreases in RF with NA agonists and the increases in RF due to NA antagonists did not appear after elimination of the pons by transection, a

FIG. 9.1 Noradrenergic inhibition from A5 area on the medullary respiratory rhythm generator. *Left*: Schematic drawing showing, at the top, the brainstem with entry points of the stimulating electrode (black points) and the level of transection (double-headed arrow) and, at the bottom, a slice with the effective area of the pons (hatched area). *Right*: Traces of the inspiratory discharge of a cervical ventral root were recorded; beneath each trace is the integrated activity. (*A*) Transection at the ponto-medullary level (horizontal bar) immediately increased the respiratory frequency (RF); (*B*) in another preparation, electrical stimulation (black bar, 10 Hz, 30 µA, 0.3 msec) performed with a tungsten electrode lowered 300 µm below the surface (black points) delayed inspiration; (*C*) after idazoxan bathing (200 µM, 9 min), the RF was doubled and electrical stimulation no longer inhibited inspiration.

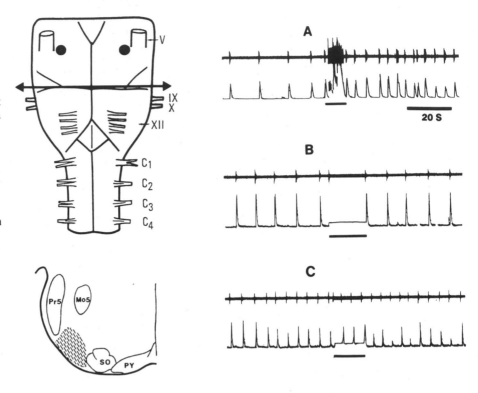

tonic release of NA by the pontine A5 area may be reasonably postulated. On-going HPLC experiments confirm release of endogenous NA by the brainstem in the bathing medium (200 pg/hr).

In order to localize the receptors involved in modulating RF, lesion, local application of drugs, and stimulation experiments were performed within the medulla. Bilateral lesions were made about 300 µm below the surface with a tungsten microelectrode. Extensive lesions of the dorsal medulla in the vicinity of the nucleus tractus solitarius (NTS) did not disturb respiratory activity and did not suppress NA-induced decreases in RF. However, lesions made in the ventral medulla could affect NA responses. In the rostral ventrolateral medulla (RVLM, black area in fig. 9.3), respiratory arrest was evoked with a recovery in 7–10 minutes after a unilateral lesion. A second lesion at the symmetrical contralateral site stopped respiration definitively in all but three cases in which recovery was observed in 10 min. Thereafter, NA did not decrease RF in the three cases. Prior to lesioning, stimulation of the RVLM (single shock) during expiration on-switched inspiration prematurely (fig. 9.3A). In more medial sites, electrical stimulation had no effect and lesions did not induce respiratory arrest. However, NA applied after lesioning frequently elicited increases in RF (hatched area in fig. 9.3).

Applying NA in the RVLM significantly decreased RF during 6–7 min (<1 min latency, fig. 9.3B), whereas clonidine or saline ejection were not effective. At the same site, electrical stimulation initiated inspiration prematurely (fig. 9.3A) whereas lesions stopped respiration (fig. 9.3C). In more medial sites, NA ejections were less effective, of

longer latency (2–3 min) and electrical stimulation was without effect. NA ejections performed deeper (about 700 µm, i.e., at the level of the ventral respiratory group) were only occasionally effective. In the most rostral ventrolateral location, sites were encountered where NA ejection increased RF. These results suggest that the NA depressive effect was not directly on the ventral respiratory group (VRG), but was relayed by some structures located in the RVLM.

DISCUSSION

Lesion, stimulation, and pharmacological experiments demonstrate that (1) NA biosynthesis mechanisms remain functioning under *in vitro* conditions and (2) tonic release of NA from the noradrenergic A5 area depresses the activity of the medullary respiratory rhythm generator. At the medullary level, data from lesioning, stimulation, and local application of drugs suggest that the A5 region does not modulate the respiratory neurons of the VRG directly but rather through neurons sensitive to NA that are located in the RVLM. It remains difficult to identify these neurons more precisely. Close to the RVLM, the C1 nucleus (10) contains NA neurons which are involved in cardiovascular regulation. Since these neurons are sensitive to NA (15), they may relay A5 effects to the respiratory neurons of the VRG. The C1 nucleus, however, is not a homogenous aggregate of adrenergic neurons as it contains non-adrenergic cells also (10). These non-adrenergic neurons may exhibit pacemaker properties (18, 19) and could be sympathoexcitatory cells firing with respiratory modulation (8). Interest-

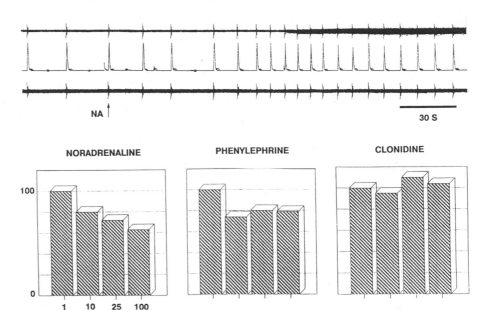

FIG. 9.2 Adrenergic drugs and respiratory frequency (RF). *Top*: Inspiratory activity was recorded in two cervical ventral roots; the center trace is the integrated activity of the bottom trace. Normal medium was replaced at the arrow by medium containing noradrenaline (NA, 100 μM); note the decrease in RF. *Bottom*: Dose-response histograms showing the mean effect on RF (n = 5, expressed as percent of control in ordinate) of bathing the preparation with adrenergic agonists at different concentrations (in abscissa, concentration in μM).

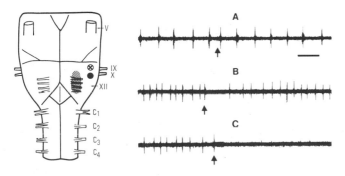

FIG. 9.3 Medullary targets of A5. (*A*) Electrical stimulation via the central barrel of a multibarreled micropipette inserted in the rostral ventrolateral medulla, 300 μm below the surface (black area on the diagram), prematurely on-switched inspiration (at arrow). (*B*) Ejection of noradrenaline (NA, at arrow) lowered the respiratory (RF) immediately (saline had no effect). (*C*) Electrocoagulation (at arrow) stopped breathing. *Left*: Schematic drawing of the analyzed sites; black area, see *A, B* and *C*; hatched area, NA ejection decreased weakly RF with a 2–3 min latency, stimulation and lesion had no effect; crossed area, NA ejection increased RF. Time scale: horizontal bar, 15 sec in *A* and 30 sec in *B* and *C*.

ingly, respiratory neurons have been recorded in the same loci in the *in vitro* brainstem preparation of newborn rats and might be pacemakers of the respiratory rhythm (13, 14). Indeed, the effects of RVLM stimulations or lesions argue for a critical role of the RVLM in respiratory neurogenesis. Whatever the function of these neurons, it is likely that they are under A5 modulation.

Under *in vivo* experimental conditions, changes in cardiovascular variables induce modifications of respiratory related parameters (pulmonary gas exchange, afferents from the baroreceptors and chemoreceptors, etc.), which in turn regulate the activity of the respiratory centers that modify respiration. Similarly, changes in respiration may

elicit cardiovascular adjustments. These interactions complicate the understanding of both regulations (11). It is often difficult to define whether neurons are primarily cardiovascular or respiratory (8); although they form two separate columns in the ventral medulla there is some overlap, which may give rise to central interactions (4). Under *in vitro* conditions all the peripheral effects were eliminated, and the results were consistent with the possibility that central structures involved in cardiorespiratory regulation (both A5 and C1 nuclei) might also be implicated in respiratory modulation, arguing for the existence of central interactions between respiratory and cardiovascular "centers."

Since A5 modulation and NA respiratory effects were blocked by α-2 but not α-1 antagonists, it is likely that α-2 receptors are involved in the A5 modulation of the medullary respiratory rhythm generator. However, well-known α-2 agonists such as clonidine and guanfacine did not elicit NA mimetic effects, and α-CH$_3$-NA (a potent α-2 agonist) was only weakly effective. This raises two questions: (1) Was the α-2 agonist potency of these drugs overestimated? (2) Are the adrenoceptors mature at birth?

Clonidine is an antihypertensive agent, imidazoline in structure, and classified as a potent and selective α-2 agonist (21). Its central site of action has been demonstrated to be the nucleus reticularis lateralis, where local application evoked hypotension (3). Surprisingly, local application in the same site of α-CH$_3$-NA, another α-2 agonist but catecholaminergic in structure, was ineffective (1, 2). It has been suggested that the vasodepressor effects of clonidine are mediated via imidazole but not α-2 adrenergic receptors (16) and that the α-2 potency of clonidine may be questioned.

In neurons of the dorsal motor nucleus of the vagus, α-2 responses did not clearly appear until 8–14 days of age, whereas α-1 receptors were already functioning at birth, revealing immaturity of adrenoceptors and developmentally different onset of α-1 and α-2 adrenergic responses (6). If so, at the differentiation of α-1/α-2 adrenoceptors, various neurovegetative changes may occur, since NA influences gastric motility, cardiovascular and respiratory functions, raphe structures, and others. Any dysfunction in adrenoceptor maturation would lead to multiple difficulties which might be correlated with the various symptoms reported during Sudden Infant Death Syndrome.

ACKNOWLEDGMENTS

This work was supported by CNRS (URA 0205), INSERM (886006) and "Naître et Vivre" Foundation.

REFERENCES

1. Bousquet, P., J. Feldman, R. Bloch, and J. Schwartz. The nucleus reticularis: A region highly sensitive to clonidine. *Euro. J. Pharm.* 69:389-392, 1981.

2. Bousquet, P., J. Feldman, and J. Schwartz. Central cardiovascular effects of α adrenergic drugs: Differences between catecholamines and imidazoline. *J. Pharm. Exp. Therap.* 230:232-236, 1984.

3. Bousquet, P., and J. Feldman. The blood pressure effects of alpha-adrenoreceptor antagonists injected in the medullary site of action of clonidine: The nucleus reticularis lateralis. *Life Sciences* 40:1045-1052, 1986.

4. Ellenberger, H.H., W.Z. Zhan, and J.L. Feldman. Anatomical relationship between respiratory and catecholamine neurons in ventrolateral medulla of rat. *Soc. Neurosci. Abstr.* 13:809, 1987.

5. Errchidi, S., G. Hilaire, and R. Monteau. Permanent release of noradrenaline modulates respiratory frequency in the newborn rat: An *in vitro* study. *J. Physiol.* 429:492-510, 1990.

6. Fukuda, A., J. Nabekura, C. Ito, C. Plata-Salaman, and Y.L. Oomura. Developmentally different onset of α-1 and α-2 adrenergic responses in the neonatal rat dorsal motor nucleus of the vagus *in vitro*. *Brain Res.* 493:357-361, 1989.

7. Guyenet, P. Baroceptor mediated inhibition of A5 noradrenergic neurons. *Brain Res.* 303:31-40, 1984.

8. Haselton, J.R., and P. Guyenet. Central respiratory modulation of medullary sympathoexcitatory neurons in rat. *Am. J. Physiol.* 356:R739-750, 1989.

9. Hilaire, G., R. Monteau, and S. Errchidi. Possible modulation of the medullary respiratory rhythm generator by the noradrenergic A5 area: An *in vitro* study in the newborn rat. *Brain Res.* 485:325-332, 1989.

10. Hökfelt, T., O. Johansson, and M. Goldstein. Central catecholaminergic neurons as revealed by immunohistochemistry with special reference to adrenaline neurons. In *Classical transmitter in the CNS,* Part 2, ed. A. Bjorklund and T. Hökfelt, 157-276. Amsterdam: Elsevier, 1984.

11. Koepchen, H.P. Respiratory and cardiovascular "centres:" functional entirety or separate structures? In *Central Neurone Environment,* ed. M.E. Schlafke, H.P. Koepchen and W.R. See, 221-235, Berlin: Springer, 1983.

12. Murakoshi, T., T. Suzue, and S. Tamai. A pharmacological study on respiratory rhythm in the isolated brainstem−spinal cord preparation of the newborn rat. *Br. J. Pharmacol.* 86:95-104, 1985.

13. Onimaru, H., A. Arata, and I. Homma. Localization of respiratory rhythm generating neurons in the medulla of brainstem−spinal cord preparations from newborn rat. *Neurosci. Lett.* 78:151-155, 1987.

14. Onimaru, H., and I. Homma. Respiratory rhythm generator neurons in medulla of brainstem-spinal cord preparation from newborn rat. *Brain Res.* 403:380-384, 1987.

15. Reis, D.J., A.R. Granata, T.H. Joh, C.A. Ross, D.A. Ruggiero, and D.H. Park. Brainstem catecholamine mechanisms in tonic and reflex control of blood pressure. *Hypertension* 6:7-15, 1984.

16. Reis, D.J., P. Ernsberger, R. Giuliano, R. Willette, and A.R. Granata. The vasodepressor response to clonidine is mediated by imidazole and not α-2 adrenergic receptors in the rostral ventrolateral medulla. *Soc. Neurosci. Abstr.* 13:227, 1987.

17. Smith, J.C., and J. Feldman. *In vitro* brainstem−spinal cord preparation for study of motor systems for mammalian respiration and locomotion. *J. Neurosci. Methods.* 21:321-333, 1987.

18. Sun, M.K., J.T. Hackett, and P. Guyenet. Sympathoexcitatory neurons of rostral ventrolateral medulla exhibit pacemaker properties in the presence of a glutamate-receptor antagonist. *Brain Res.* 438:23-40, 1988.

19. Sun, M.K., B.S. Young, J.T. Hackett, and P. Guyenet. Reticulospinal pacemaker neurons of the rat rostral ventrolateral medulla with putative sympathoexcitatory function: An intracellular study *in vitro*. *Brain Res.* 442:229-239, 1988.

20. Suzue, T. Respiratory rhythm generation in the *in vitro* brainstem−spinal cord preparation of neonatal rat. *J. Physiol.* 93:173-183, 1984.

21. U'Prichard, D.C. Direct binding studies of α-adrenoceptors. In *Adrenoceptors and catecholamine action,* Part A, ed. G. Kunos, 131-179. Rochester, N.Y.: J. Wiley and Sons, 1981.

10

Bulbospinal Transmission of Respiratory Drive to Phrenic Motoneurons

Guosong Liu and Jack L. Feldman

The continuous and reliable transmission of respiratory drive to spinal cord motoneurons controlling the muscles of the respiratory pump is a basic condition for life in mammals. This respiratory rhythm is generated in the brainstem and is transmitted to spinal motoneurons via bulbospinal neurons. Understanding the mechanism controlling the excitability of spinal cord respiratory motoneurons is fundamental to the understanding of neural control of respiration.

Neuronal excitability is determined dynamically by synaptic input and intrinsic membrane properties. To study synaptic input to a neuron, the factors that control the generation and transmission of synaptic current must be determined. This requires identification of presynaptic transmitters, pre- and post-synaptic receptors, and location of the active synapse(s), and the electrotonic attenuation of current during the transfer from synaptic site to the soma. Intrinsic membrane properties, a function of various voltage- or non-voltage-dependent channels in the membrane, control the transformation of synaptic currents into membrane potential, and therefore the excitability of neurons. In this paper we briefly summarize our recent work on bulbospinal transmission of respiratory drive to phrenic motoneurons using intracellular recording (6), single electrode voltage-clamp (6), and whole-cell patch-clamp (5) techniques in the brainstem–spinal cord preparation *in vitro*.

METHODS

Experiments were performed in an *in vitro* preparation of the neonatal rat brainstem–spinal cord. Details of the preparation, the surgical procedure, intracellular recording, single sharp electrode voltage-clamp techniques, and data acquisition have been reported elsewhere (6). Here, we briefly describe the procedures for obtaining whole-cell patch-clamp recordings. Standard intracellular recording was used to locate the phrenic motoneuron pool. To keep patch electrodes clean and avoid the attachment to axons or nonrespiratory neurons, continuous positive pressure was applied to the patch electrode until it arrived at the desired depth. Since the leak of electrolyte (K^+ or Cs^+ and tetraethylammonium) from the patch electrode will perturb neuronal activity, a positive pressure was chosen that kept the patch electrode clean, yet did not disrupt synaptic transmission. The current noise level was monitored continuously when the patch electrode was advanced towards the mo-

toneuron pool. Since the noise level mainly reflects the electrode resistance before seal formation, it can be used as an index of attachment of the patch electrode to the cell membrane, with a decrease in noise level signifying that the electrode tip was approaching the membrane. At this time, slight suction leads to formation of Gigaohm seals (2–10 GΩ). Further suction will rupture the membrane and provide access to the cell interior for whole-cell recording. The junction potential due to the different constituents between the patch electrode solution and the extracellular solution was measured for different intracellular solutions and corrected. Series resistance and whole-cell capacitance were determined by an on-line computer program. These values were used for optimizing series resistance compensation.

RESULTS

To better understand the synaptic transmission of inspiratory drive, both synaptic potentials and currents were studied (fig. 10.1A). In all brainstem–spinal cord preparations there were spontaneously generated rhythmic membrane depolarizations and associated spiking of phrenic motoneurons during the inspiratory phase of the respiratory cycle. The envelope of the spontaneous inspiratory drive potential in a (spiking) phrenic motoneuron had a rapid onset (50 msec) to a peak followed by a plateau/declining phase that lasted 400–700 msec. The peak potential was 10–20 mV above baseline potential. Superimposed on the slow envelope of drive were faster depolarizing potentials, and the initiation of action potentials always seemed to occur with these fast potentials. When the membrane potential of a phrenic motoneuron was clamped at end-expiratory potentials (-60 to -75 mV), the peak amplitude of the synaptic current during inspiration was 1.5 to 3.5 nA. The envelope of the inspiratory postsynaptic current had a similar shape and duration to the synaptic potential. Power spectral analysis of the synaptic drive current and potential revealed that these fast components have a characteristic frequency of 20 Hz. Given the strikingly similar fast depolarizing potentials and inward currents, we presume that they represent similar synaptic events.

To obtain optimal recordings of membrane current, we modified whole-cell patch-clamp techniques for use in the intact brainstem–spinal cord preparation *in vitro*. Unitary

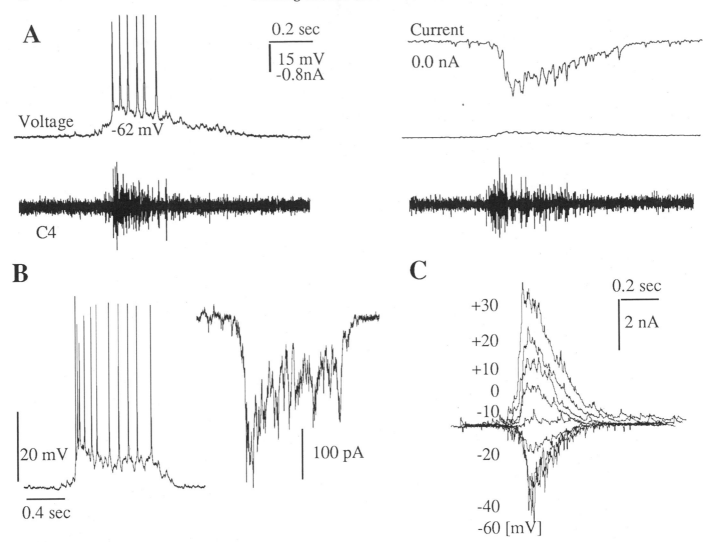

FIG. 10.1 Characteristics of descending inspiratory drive potentials and currents. (*A*) *Left*: A representative intracellular recording of a phrenic motoneuron with a 15 mV depolarization drive potential during the inspiratory phase of the respiratory cycle and a −62 mV potential during the expiratory phase. The lower trace is the C4 root activity recorded simultaneously. *Right*: Inspiratory drive current during voltage-clamp with a peak inward current of −1.4 nA with similar shape and duration as the drive potential. Drive current can be arbitrarily separated into two components, a basic envelope of drive current and fast components superimposed on the envelope. The middle trace is of the voltage during voltage-clamp (6). (*B*) Whole-cell patch-clamp recording from a phrenic motoneuron receiving inspiratory drive. *Left*: Inspiratory drive potential recorded in current-clamp mode. *Right*: Inspiratory drive current recorded in voltage-clamp mode. Note that individual EPSCs can be resolved in the data record. (*C*) Voltage-dependence of inspiratory drive current. Each current trace represents the current at the voltage indicated. The reversal potential was near −10 mV.

excitatory postsynaptic currents (EPSCs) and inhibitory postsynaptic currents (IPSCs) are easily seen because of the high current resolution of patch-clamp technology. Most respiratory neurons recorded with whole cell patch-clamp techniques received strong excitatory drive during inspiration, as illustrated in Fig. 1B. The shape and time course of the drive potentials or currents obtained under the patch-clamp recording were similar to those obtained under the sharp electrode intracellular recording. However, the resolution of voltage-clamp recording is much higher under patch-clamp conditions, such that unitary EPSCs, which

composed the inspiratory drive currents, can be observed. We analyzed the time course of these EPSCs to obtain some information on the properties of channels activated by the endogenous neurotransmitter, which is likely to be an excitatory amino acid (EAA) (6, 7). The rising time of these EPSCs ranged from 0.45 to 1.3 ms with a mean of 0.86 ms. There seemed to be two types of EPSCs, distinguished by their decay time course. One type of decay time course was best fitted by an exponential curve with a single time constant (about 2.5 msec). The other was best fitted by a two time-constant exponential curve. The slow time constant of the decay phase ranged from 2.73 to 9.16 msec with a mean value of 5.18 msec (n = 18). The mean fast time constant was 1.14 msec (n = 6).

To study the type(s) of receptor(s) activated by the endogenous release of neurotransmitter and the ionic mechanisms underlying generation of synaptic current, it is necessary to determine the voltage-dependence and reversal potential of the synaptic current. Studies from cultured neurons (2) have demonstrated the existence of two EPSC components, a slow one mediated by N-methyl-D-aspartate (NMDA) receptors and a fast one mediated by non-NMDA receptors; the reversal potentials of both components are near 0 mV. Slow EPSCs show a strong voltage-dependence. We were interested in whether the same voltage-dependence and reversal potential exists for the inspiratory drive current.

Phrenic motoneuron membrane potential was clamped at voltage levels from −60 to +30 mV. The voltage-dependence of drive current is shown in figure 10.1C. The drive current had a rapid onset and slow decay phase superimposed with fast events (30 msec). The shape of the drive current changed at holding potentials more positive than −20 mV. The amplitude of the drive current at the decay phase (100 msec after the peak) was plotted against holding potential. The current was highly voltage-dependent with a region of negative slope at membrane potentials near −40 mV. The peak current, defined as the maximum net drive current (measured from the steady-state value), is symmetrical in the range of −40 to +30 mV with a reversal potential of −13 mV. These results are consistent with our previous observation that EAA is the major neurotransmitter mediating inspiratory drive (6). These results also revealed that some of the channels activated by the inspiratory drive were both voltage- and ligand-gated. These channels may be those coupled with activation of NMDA receptors.

Our previous finding (7) suggests that EAAs are involved in the bulbospinal transmission of inspiratory drive. To establish the presence of EAA receptors on phrenic motoneuronal membranes and provide information on the available receptor subtypes for action of the endogenously released transmitter, we tested the effects of agonists of the major EAA receptor subtypes on phrenic motoneurons after blocking synaptic transmission (produced by axonal action potentials) by bath application of tetrodotoxin (TTX). We found that phrenic motoneurons have three types of EAA receptors: quisqualate, kainate, and NMDA. To identify the types of receptors mediating endogenous inspiratory drive, the effects of various EAA antagonists on the inspiratory drive potentials or currents were studied. Bath application of 2 μM 6-cyano-7-nitroquinoxaline-2,3-dione (CNQX), a specific non-NMDA receptor antagonist (4), reversibly abolished the spontaneous C4 motor output. Local application of 100 μM CNQX reduced the amplitude of descending inspiratory drive current (fig. 10.2A). On the other hand, local application of 1mM (+)-5-methyl-10,11-dihydro-5H-dibenzo [a,d] cyclohepten-5,10-iminemaleate (MK-801, a

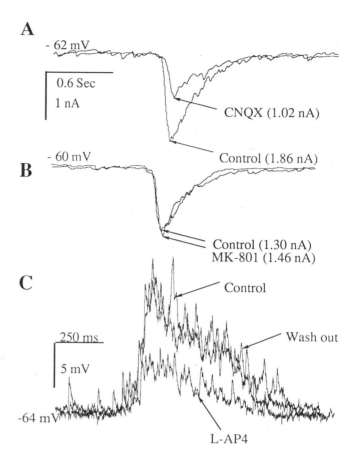

FIG. 10.2 Receptors mediating inspiratory drive. (A) Effect of local application of 100 μM CNQX on the inspiratory drive current (holding potential, −62 mV). (B) Local application of an NMDA receptor antagonist (MK-801) did not affect the inspiratory drive current. (C) Effects of local application of 1 mM AP4 on inspiratory drive potential (6).

specific noncompetitive NMDA receptor antagonist) did not alter the inspiratory drive current detected at −60 mV holding potential (Fig. 10.2B), although there was a 10–15% reduction of the C4 motoneuron population activity. These results suggest that non-NMDA receptors are the primary receptors mediating inspiratory drive transmission.

DL-2-amino-4-phosphonobutyric acid (AP4) is another potent functional antagonist of inspiratory drive (7). To further understand how AP4 affects bulbospinal synaptic transmission, the effects of AP4 on the inspiratory drive potential were studied. Local application of AP4 blocked the motoneuron discharge and reduced the drive potential amplitude within 10–30 sec (fig. 10.2C). This effect of AP4 was not accompanied by any change of the membrane I/V relationship. Moreover, application of this concentration of AP4 did not block the depolarization induced by exogenous application of either quisqualate, kainate, or glutamate. These results demonstrate that AP4 does not block any known postsynaptic EAA receptors on phrenic motoneurons and suggest that AP4 blocks transmission of

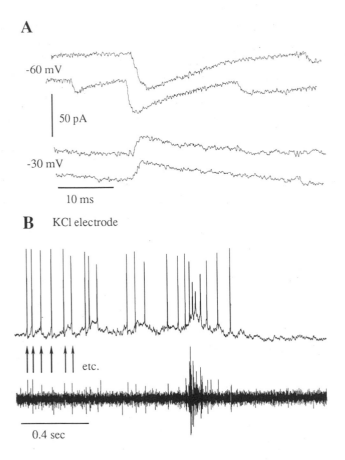

A

-60 mV

50 pA

-30 mV

10 ms

B   KCl electrode

↑ ↑ ↑↑ ↑↑↑   etc.

0.4 sec

FIG. 10.3 Inhibitory synaptic current recorded during expiration. (*A*) Spontaneous IPSCs in a phrenic motoneuron at two membrane holding potentials. The reversal potential of these currents is 40 mV, due to an increase of intracellular Cl⁻ concentration in the experimental conditions. (*B*) The drive potential recorded with a KCl electrode. The potentials prior to inspiration occurred only when a KCl clectrode was used for intracellular recording. In addition, those potentials did not appear until the microelectrode penetrated a neuron for a few minutes. The early depolarizations (arrows) are Cl⁻ dependent reversed inhibitory potentials.

inspiratory drive by acting at presynaptic terminals of bulbospinal neurons (1, 6).

Phrenic motoneurons also receive Cl⁻-dependent inhibitory synaptic inputs during the expiratory period. These inhibitory synaptic currents are easily seen under whole-cell patch-clamp recording. Figure 10.3*A* shows the properties of these spontaneous IPSCs. Both mean rise time (1.1 msec) and decay time constant (7.8 msec) of IPSCs always seemed slower than that of EPSCs. The reversal potential of these IPSCs was −40 mV.[1] The voltage-dependence of this synaptic conductance remains to be analyzed. Interestingly, phrenic motoneurons in some preparations received powerful inhibitory inputs just before and

concurrent with excitatory input during inspiration. As shown in figure 10.3*B*, inhibitory synaptic potentials were sometimes superimposed on the excitatory synaptic potentials at the beginning of the inspiratory phase. The neurotransmitter involved in this inhibitory synaptic transmission remains to be determined.

CONCLUSION

In summary, the goal of this work is to understand the mechanisms for control of excitability of phrenic motoneurons. Although many studies have been done to investigate the motoneuron recruitment by afferent input (3), little is known on the role of descending input in the control of motoneuron excitability. The study of descending synaptic drive to phrenic motoneurons provides the information on how the excitability of motoneurons is controlled by descending input. Our results suggest that the pattern of descending synaptic input plays an important role in the control of motoneuron firing pattern, because the initiation of action potentials always seemed to occur with those fast synaptic events superimposed on a ramp of drive potential. We also identified the various types of transmitters and postsynaptic receptors mediating these synaptic inputs. Determination of the main types of transmitters and receptors which mediate descending inspiratory and expiratory input to phrenic motoneurons will help us understand the generation of inspiratory drive and provide the basis for studying the modulation of these drives by other transmitters, such as serotonin or norepinephrine.

Finally, understanding the mechanisms underlying transmission of respiratory drive to motoneurons is of considerable importance in defining the mechanisms responsible for respiratory homeostasis and for pathologies where ventilatory failure results from the inability to generate the appropriate motor output. Moreover, the mechanisms involved in neurotransmission of drive potential from pre-motor neurons to motoneurons may be common to other motor systems, even to all central nervous system synapses using EAAs as fast neurotransmitters.

ACKNOWLEDGMENT

This work was supported by NIH Grant NS-24742.

REFERENCES

1. Feldman, J.L., and J.C. Smith. Cellular mechanisms underlying modulation of breathing pattern in mammals. *Ann. NY Acad. Sci.* 563:114-130, 1989.

2. Forsythe, I.D., and G.L. Westbrook. Slow excitatory postsynaptic currents mediated by N-methyl-D-aspartate receptors on cultured mouse central neurons. *J. Physiol.* 396:515-533, 1988.

3. Henneman, E., and L.M. Mendell. Functional organization of motoneuron pool and its inputs. In *Handbook of Physiology.* Section 1, vol. 2, ed. V.B. Brooks, 423-507. Bethesda, Md.: American Physiological Society, 1981.

[1]This value is consistent with a Cl⁻-mediated conductance since the intracellular Cl⁻ concentration (19 mM in patch pipette solution) was higher than normal (8 mM) after dialysis of the intracellular environment by patch electrode (estimated E_{Cl} 50 mV for $[Cl]_o:[Cl]_i = [133]:[9]$)

4. Honoré, T., S.N. Davies, J. Drejer, E.J. Fletcher, P. Jacobson, D. Lodge, and F.E. Nielson. Quinoxalinediones: Potent competitive non-NMDA glutamate receptor antagonists. *Science* 241:701-703, 1988.

5. Liu, G., and J.L. Feldman. Whole-cell patch-clamp recording of endogenous synaptic currents in mammalian motoneurons in intact brainstem–spinal cord. *Soc. Neurosci. Abstr.* 16:1184, 1990.

6. Liu, G., J.L. Feldman, and J.C. Smith. Excitatory amino acid mediated transmission of inspiratory drive to phrenic motoneurons. *J. Neurophysiol.* 64:423-436, 1990.

7. McCrimmon, D.R., J.C. Smith, and J.L. Feldman. Involvement of excitatory amino acids in neurotransmission of inspiratory drive to spinal respiratory motoneurons. *J. Neurosci.* 9:1910-1921, 1989.

11
Comparative Approach to Neural Control of Respiration

Allan I. Pack, Raymond J. Galante, Robert E. Walker,
Leszek K. Kubin, and Alfred P. Fishman

Most studies to elucidate the neural basis of respiratory rhythmogenesis have been done in mammals. Less investigation has been done in nonmammalian species. Although studies in *Aplysia* (5), mollusk (41), lamprey (21, 22, 35, 36, 42), and teleost fish (1, 2) have provided certain interesting insights, they have shed little light on the evolution of the respiratory pattern generator. A comparative approach to neural systems can provide important insights (for discussion of this approach, see 4) by relating evolutionary changes in behavior to the neural basis of the behavior. With evolution there have been major changes in the mechanical act of respiration (for summary, see 31). The alteration in the mechanical aspects of the behavior of this neural control system have been well characterized. Little, however, is known about the evolution of the underlying neural systems. In this contribution we describe the beginnings of this type of approach to the respiratory pattern generator.

A logical starting point for this inquiry is to study the neural basis of respiration in the first air-breathing species. Thus, we have concentrated initially on the dipnoan lungfish, which appear early in the evolution of air breathing (33). These lungfish have both gills and lungs. There are three genera: *Protopterus* (African), *Lepidosiren* (South American) and *Neoceratodus* (Australian). There are important differences between them. In particular, the gills of *Neoceratodus fosteri* are sufficient to support gas exchange (14), whereas in the others gills are too rudimentary and air breathing is obligatory (19, 20). The precise relationship of lungfish and tetrapods remains a subject of debate (for summary see 25). One theory argues that they are sister groups (13, 34), while others argue that this is not the case (38). Similarities in the cardiorespiratory systems of modern lungfish and amphibia would therefore be a consequence of convergent evolution (38).

The dipnoan lungfish employ a buccal force pump mechanism to ventilate their lungs (3, 26). The action of this pumping mechanism has been studied by pressure recording (8, 26), electromyography of the action of the buccal muscles (26), and by cine-fluoroscopy (3). Some studies suggest that when lungfish initiate a lung breath, they first expire gas from their lungs. Thereafter, fresh air enters the buccal cavity and is forced into the lungs through an actively opened glottis by the rhythmic contraction of the buccal muscles. It takes a series of contractions to ventilate the lung. Alternatively, however, it has been described that

lungfish first aspirate air into the buccal cavity with the glottis closed (26) preceding expiration from the lung. With expiration, there is mixing of fresh air and lung gas in the buccal cavity. Subsequently, this mixed gas is pumped into the lung by the rhythmic contraction of the buccal musculature (26). A similar buccal force pump mechanism is also employed by amphibia (7, 43).

The lungs in the lungfish are paired, hollow sacs which extend along the dorsal portion of the abdominal cavity. Proximally the two sacs come together to form a common anterior chamber which is connected by a short pneumatic duct to the glottic sphincter of the pharynx (see ref. 9, fig. 1). Trabeculae from the inner walls extend into the central cavity of the lungs. Within these trabeculae and in the tissue surrounding the lungs, there is smooth muscle (17, 30). The lungs are innervated by pulmonary branches of the vagus nerve.

The lungs of these fish contain both slowly adapting and rapidly adapting receptors. This has been demonstrated by our laboratory using both *in vivo* and *in vitro* recording techniques (9). Some slowly adapting receptors were active at resting lung volume. They showed a sigmoid pattern of response to step inflations of the lungs. Inflation of the lungs to pressures above 10 cm H_2O produced little further increase in their activity. Other receptors were not active at resting lung volume and showed varying recruitment thresholds. The slowly adapting receptors also showed a dynamic sensitivity, that is, their firing was determined by both the degree and rate of lung inflation (9). This aspect of their response is similar to that described for mammalian stretch receptors (28). In addition, as described in mammals (37), increasing CO_2 concentration in the lungs caused a decrement in receptor firing (9).

The transduction properties of the rapidly adapting receptors were also similar to those described in mammals (27). Seven of the ten receptors, which we studied, showed firing both during inflation of the lung segment and briefly during deflation. During dynamic inflations of the lungs, the activity of these rapidly adapting receptors was strongly influenced by the rate of lung inflation and to a much lesser extent by the degree of inflation.

These studies confirm that, at this early stage of the development of air breathing, there were highly developed mechanoreceptors in the lungs. The information that they provide to the brainstem about mechanical events in the lungs is similar to that provided by receptors in the mammalian lung. In these studies we did not examine for the presence or response of C-fiber afferents.

As indicated above, the information provided by pulmonary mechanoreceptors in the lungfish is similar to that in mammals. This raises the question as to the role of this information in control of respiratory timing intervals. In a separate series of studies (29), we studied the role of lung inflation in the control of interbreath interval. We utilized two preparations: in one we instrumented the lungfish to measure and control intrapulmonary pressure and to measure opercular pressure; in the other, we created a flow-through lung preparation, in addition to measuring intrapulmonary and opercular pressure. Gas of known composition was passed continuously through the lungs while the glottis was occluded by a balloon catheter. This preparation served to maintain blood gas tensions constant (for further details see ref. 29, fig. 1).

In both preparations, inflation of the lungs with air prolonged the interval between lung breaths. As described previously (18), hypoxia also decreased the interval between lung breaths. At the three levels of oxygen studied (5%, 10%, 18%), increased intrapulmonary pressure prolonged the interval between lung breaths. At higher levels of oxygen, increased intrapulmonary pressure produced more marked prolongation of interbreath interval, as in mammals (45).

These studies also demonstrated a time dependence of the effect of lung inflation on interbreath interval. Pulses of inflation applied early in the interbreath interval, produced less prolongation of that interval than did pulses of inflation applied later in the interval (29). This time dependence is similar to the effects of inflation on the control of expiratory duration in cats (23). Thus these studies demonstrate that there is a reflex in the lungfish similar to the Hering-Breuer expiratory promoting reflex in mammals. Many of the features of this reflex are similar between the different species.

If a Hering-Breuer expiratory promoting reflex is present, is there also an inspiratory-terminating reflex? To address this question, we have conducted another series of studies. We examined the effect of lung inflation on the duration of action of the buccal force pump. Lungfish were instrumented to record intrapulmonary and opercular pressure. The glottis of the fish was occluded by an inflated balloon. At the start of a lung breath, the lungs were inflated to a preset level of pressure. Five different types of tests were performed: no inflation (glottis occluded) and inflations to 2.5, 5.0, 7.5, and 10.0 cm H_2O.

Inflation of the lungs shortened the duration of action of the buccal force pump. There was a large difference in breath duration between the no inflation test and that at 2.5 cm H_2O (see fig. 11.1). Breath duration was determined from the buccal pressure trace (not shown). Further increases in inflation pressure produced little further shortening of breath duration. The shape of the relationship between inflation pressure and breath duration is curvilinear and similar to the relationship between tidal volume and inspiratory duration in mammals (6, 16). This shortening effect of lung inflation on the duration of action of the buccal force pump was not related to changes in blood gas tensions. Inflations with air, 100% oxygen, or 100% nitrogen produce similar shortening of the duration of action of the buccal force pump.

Although mechanoreceptor feedback from the lung had a profound effect on the timing mechanisms for lung ventilation, it had no effect on gill ventilation in the lungfish. Inflation of the lung in the interval between lung breaths produced no alteration in the frequency of gill ventilation (29). This result is in contrast to those in the larval form of amphibia (tadpole) where lung inflation slows the frequency of gill ventilation (44). Such slowing after the lung breaths reduces the loss of oxygen through the gills from the now oxygenated blood. Although lung inflation did not slow gill ventilation in the lungfish, gill ventilation did slow after a lung breath. This interaction is controlled by a central program since it occurs even though intrapulmonary pressure is held constant. With intrapulmonary pressure constant there is an interval following a lung breath in which there is no gill ventilation, after which gill ventilation increases to a new steady state.

Based on these data (29), it seems likely that in the lungfish there are separate circuits for control of pulmonary and gill ventilation. The former receives afferent information from pulmonary mechanoreceptors and is powerfully affected by hypoxia. In contrast, the circuits for generation of gill ventilation are unaffected by input from pulmonary mechanoreceptors (29) and are less affected by hypoxia (18). Although not directly tested by us, it would seem likely that the pattern generator for gill ventilation is influenced from mechanoreceptors on the gill arches, since mechanical agitation of water changes the frequency of gill ventilation (20). The slowing of gill ventilation following a lung breath is likely to be mediated by a direct inhibitory connection from the lung pattern generator to that for the gills (see fig. 9 schematic in ref. 12).

The studies outlined above indicate that there are both vagally mediated expiratory promoting reflexes and inspiratory terminating reflexes in the lungfish, and they seem to operate on similar principles as the corresponding reflexes in mammals. This similarity extends to the quantitative nature of the interrelationships. Thus we conclude that respiratory timing control similar to that in mammals was already developed in the lungfish. This adds weight to the hypothesis of Feldman and colleagues that the circuits for respiratory timing control and those for shaping the respiratory burst are separate although interacting neural systems (10, 11, 39). We would argue that both the pulmonary mechanoreceptor system and the respiratory timing control system were already developed in these early air breathing fish. With evolution, the major changes that have taken

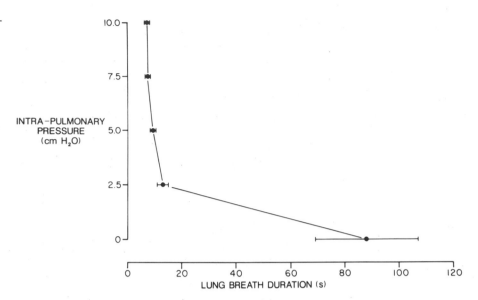

FIG. 11.1 Relationship between the duration of action of the buccal force pump and the intrapulmonary pressure in a single lungfish. The results (mean ± SD) are shown for six to eight tests in which the lung was not inflated (zero pressure) or inflated to pressures of 2.5, 5.0, 7.5, or 10.0 cm H_2O. Breath duration, the dependent variable, is plotted on the x-axis to allow comparison with the V_T/T_I plot in mammals.

place are in the circuits for shaping the respiratory burst, as the mechanical act of breathing has changed from the buccal force pump in air-breathing fish and amphibia to suctional breathing based on contraction of the diaphragm and chest wall musculature. This raises the question as to what happened to the circuits for the branchiomeric ventilatory system. One hypothesis, put forward by Richardson (32), is that the high-frequency oscillations recorded in phrenic nerve output and in the upper airway muscles are the remnant of this neural system.

If the timing mechanisms are present, then can one gain insight into the mechanisms of respiratory rhythmogenesis by studying early air breathing species? Recently a powerful approach to such studies has been the use of *in vitro* neonatal preparations in which rhythmogenesis is maintained (40). We have applied a similar approach to these early air breathing species and have developed a preparation using the isolated brainstem of the larval form (tadpole) of amphibia (*Rana catesbeiana*). This preparation consists of the isolated brainstem of the tadpole, which is placed in a small organ bath and is superfused by an oxygenated physiological solution. The preparation shows rhythmic neural output for several hours when maintained in this state. The neural output, which can be recorded from the motoneuron pools of the vagus and facial nerve, has a pattern that resembles the pattern of changes in buccal pressure that have been measured in freely swimming tadpoles (see fig. 11.2; 44).

To establish that the patterns of neural activities that we are recording are related to pulmonary and gill ventilation, we recorded both neural activity and mechanical events in tadpoles. These studies were done *in vivo* after we had transected the brain through the diencephalon. Multiunit activity from the facial motor nucleus was recorded simultaneously with recordings of either buccal pressure or in-

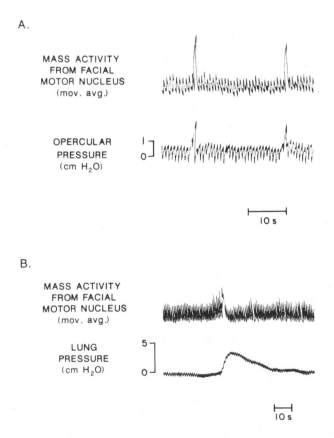

FIG. 11.2 (*A*) Simultaneous recording of the moving average of neuronal activity from the 7th motor nucleus and the opercular pressure. (*B*) Simultaneous recording of the moving average of neural activity from the same nucleus and the intrapulmonary pressure. (For further details see text.)

trapulmonary pressure. The pressure recordings from the buccal cavity showed oscillations that corresponded to neural activity (see fig. 11.2A). The small pressure oscillations correspond to those for gill ventilation, while the larger oscillations were likely to be associated with pulmonary ventilation (44). That the larger of the neural activities was related to pulmonary ventilation was confirmed by measuring intrapulmonary pressure (see fig. 11.2B). Following the largest neural activity, there is an increase in intrapulmonary pressure, which declines in the interbreath interval. Associated with the increase in pulmonary pressure there is a decline in the amplitude of gill ventilation (see fig. 11.2B). This presumably reflects the effects of feedback from pulmonary mechanoreceptors, as alluded to earlier (44). These results indicate that the patterns we are recording *in vitro* represent those for pulmonary and gill ventilation.

The *in vitro* preparation allowed us to manipulate the chemical environment of the pattern generators for gill and pulmonary ventilation. This approach has been extensively used in other systems, for example, studying swimming in isolated lamprey spinal cord (15), gill ventilation in lamprey (36), and respiration in the neonatal rat (10). We have first examined the effects of increasing concentrations of the inhibitory transmitter gamma-amino butyric acid (GABA) on gill and pulmonary ventilation. Studies were done by superfusing the brainstem with concentrations of this neurotransmitter (0–20 mM). The results in a single tadpole are shown in figure 11.3. At low concentrations of GABA (2.5 mM) there is a reduction in the amplitude of the neural output associated with gill ventilation and a slowing of this rhythm. The neural activity associated with lung ventilation is less affected. At higher concentrations of GABA (7.5 mM) the frequency of lung respiration is also slowed and finally at even higher concentrations (10 mM) both rhythms are completely abolished.

These data indicate that GABA can affect the timing circuits for both pulmonary and gill ventilation. There is, however, a differential effect on the different neural systems. Gill ventilation is affected at relatively low concentrations, whereas it takes higher concentrations to alter pulmonary ventilation. This supports our argument that there are separate neural circuits. The pattern generator for gill ventilation may be either more superficially located in the tissue and/or have a higher sensitivity to GABA.

The role of inhibitory transmitters in rhythmogenesis can be assessed by removing chloride from the bathing medium (10, 15, 36). Both GABA and glycine receptors are coupled to chloride channels (24). Thus, when activated there is an inward flux of chloride ion which hyperpolarizes the neuron. If chloride is depleted, the action of these transmitters is effectively blocked. This strategy has revealed the role of inhibitory connections in other pattern generators (10, 15, 36). Network oscillators, which depend on mutually

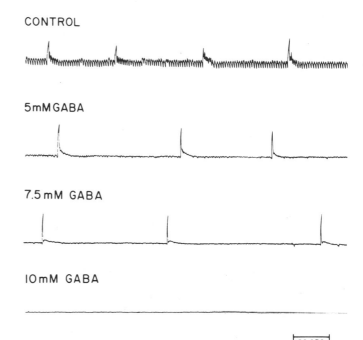

FIG. 11.3 Effect of increasing concentrations of gamma-aminobutyric acid (GABA) on the recorded moving average of neural activity from the 7th motor nucleus of an isolated *in vitro* brainstem of a tadpole. The top recording shows control conditions. The effect of increasing concentrations of GABA are shown below. At low concentrations of GABA (2.5 mM) gill ventilation is slowed and suppressed. Higher concentrations of GABA (10 mM) block both gill and pulmonary ventilation.

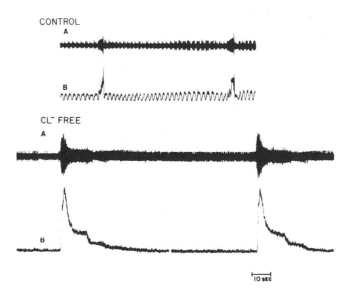

FIG. 11.4 Effect of replacement of chloride ion on the pattern of neural activity (*A*) and the integrated neural activity (*B*). The top two recordings show control conditions and the bottom two traces show the effect during a chloride-free state. With the removal of chloride, gill ventilation stops while pulmonary ventilation continues, albeit with increased amplitude and duration of the neural burst.

TABLE 11.1. Effect of Chloride Ion Replacement on
Respiratory Rhythm[1]

	Control	Chloride Free
Lung breath duration (sec)	3.5 ± 0.9	35.3 ± 9.8
Lung breath frequency (burst/min)	54.9 ± 18.0	39.9 ± 13.7

[1] Results are given for control conditions, and after chloride was
replaced by gluconate (chloride free).

[2] Each value is the average ± SD of data in seven tadpoles.

inhibitory connections between neurons should stop oscillating in the absence of chloride. In contrast, pacemaker-
driven oscillations should continue in the absence of
chloride. Respiratory rhythm in the neonatal rat is maintained without chloride being present (10).

In our studies in tadpoles we have used gluconate to re-
place chloride. Replacement of chloride ion produced a
profound change in respiratory rhythm (see fig. 11.4). Neural activity associated with lung ventilation continued,
while that for gill ventilation disappeared. In the interval
between lung breaths tonic firing of neurons increased. The
duration of the bursts of neuronal activity associated with
lung ventilation increased. There was, on average, little
change in the frequency of lung ventilation. In the seven
tadpoles studied to date, the changes in respiratory timing
are given in table 11.1.

Since gill ventilation stops, these data imply that in tadpoles this rhythm is based on a network oscillator. In contrast, pulmonary ventilation depends on a system involving
some form of pacemaker cell or inhibitory interactions that
are not dependent on chloride ions.

CONCLUSION

In this chapter we have reviewed studies on control of respiratory timing in an early air-breathing species, the lungfish. The data indicate that there is significant similarity
between control of respiratory timing in this fish and in
mammals. This leads us to hypothesize that the circuits for
respiratory timing control were already developed in these
early air-breathing species. With evolution, the major
changes which have taken place have been in the neural circuits that shape the final motor output for respiration.
These changes have been related to the changes in the mechanical act of breathing.

Such arguments indicate that we may be able to take advantage of such species to elucidate mechanisms of respiratory rhythmogenesis. We have developed an *in vitro*
brainstem preparation of larval bullfrogs, *Rana catesbeiana*. The isolated brainstem of this species shows rhythmic
activity related to gill and lung ventilation. Gill ventilation
is blocked by removal of chloride ion while pulmonary ventilation continues. Thus, it seems likely that there are pacemaker cells for pulmonary ventilation. This *in vitro*
preparation may have important advantages since the thick-

ness of the tissue is about 800 μm and all neurons are close
to the dorsal surface.

ACKNOWLEDGMENTS

We are grateful to Mr. Daniel C. Barrett for help in preparing this manuscript. The studies reported here were supported in part by NIH grant HL-39975.

REFERENCES

1. Ballintijn, C.M. *Neural control of respiration in fish and
mammals in exogenous and endogenous influences on metabolic
and neural control,* ed. A.D.F. Addick and N. Sprack, 127-140.
Oxford, UK: Pergamon, 1982.

2. Ballintijn, C.M., B.L. Roberts, and P.G.M. Luiten. Respiratory responses to stimulation of branchial vagus nerve ganglia
of a teleost fish. *Resp. Physiol.* 51:241-257, 1983.

3. Bishop, I.R., and G.E.H. Foxon. The mechanism of
breathing in the South American lungfish, *Lepidosiren paradoxa*:
A radiological study. *J. Zool.* (London) 154:263-271, 1968.

4. Bullock, T.H. Comparative neuroscience holds promise for
quiet revolutions. *Science* 225:473-478, 1984.

5. Byrne, J.H., and J. Koester. Respiratory pumping: Neuronal control of a centrally commanded behavior in *Aplysia. Brain
Res.* 143:87-105, 1978.

6. Clark, F.J., and C. von Euler. On the regulation of depth
and rate of breathing. *J. Physiol.* (London) 222:267-295, 1972.

7. DeJongh, J.H., and C. Gans. On the mechanism of respiration in the bullfrog, *Rana catesbeiana*: A reassessment. *J. Mor-
phol.* 127:259-290, 1969.

8. DeLaney, R.G., and A.P. Fishman. Analysis of lung ventilation in the aestivating lungfish *Protopterus aethiopicus. Am. J.
Physiol.* 233:R181-R187, 1977.

9. DeLaney, R.G., P. Laurent, R. Galante, A.I. Pack, and
A.P. Fishman. Pulmonary mechanoreceptors in the dipnoi lungfish *Protopterus* and *Lepidosiren. Am. J. Physiol.* 244:R418-R428,
1983.

10. Feldman, J., and J.C. Smith. Cellular mechanisms underlying modulation of breathing pattern in mammals. *Ann. NY
Acad. Sci.* 563:114-130, 1989.

11. Feldman, J.L., J.C. Smith, H.H. Ellenberger, C.C. Connelly, G. Liu, J.J. Greer, A.D. Lindsey, and M.R. Otto. Neurogenesis of respiratory rhythm and pattern: Emerging concepts.
Am. J. Physiol. 259:R879-R886, 1990.

12. Fishman, A.P., R.J. Galante, and A.I. Pack. Diving Phys-
iology: Lungfish. In *Comparative Pulmonary Physiology,* ed.
S.C. Wood, vol. 30, *Lung Biology in Health and Disease,* ed. C.
Lenfant, 645-676. New York: Marcel Dekker Inc., 1989.

13. Florey, P.L. Relationships of lungfishes. In *The biology
and evolution of lungfishes,* ed. W.E. Bemis, W.M. Burggren,
and N.E. Kemp, 75-81. New York: Alan R. Liss, 1987.

14. Grigg, G.C. Studies on the Queensland lungfish, *Neoceratodus fosteri* (Krefft). *Aust. J. Zool.* 13:243-253, 1965.

15. Grillner, S., P. Wallen, A.D. McClellan, K. Sigvardt, T.
Williams, and J. Feldman. The neural generation of locomotion in
the lamprey: An incomplete account. In *Neural origin of rhythmic
movements,* ed. A. Roberts and B.L. Roberts, 285-303. Cambridge: Cambridge University Press, 1983.

16. Grunstein, M., M. Younes, and J. Milic-Emili. Control of tidal volume and respiratory frequency in anesthetized cats. *J. Appl. Physiol.* 35:463-476, 1973.

17. Hughes, G.M., and E.R. Weibel. Morphometry of fish lungs. In *Respiration of amphibious vertebrates*, ed. G.M. Hughes, 213-232. London: Academic Press, 1976.

18. Jesse, M.J., C. Shub, and A.P. Fishman. Lung and gill ventilation of the African lungfish. *Resp. Physiol.* 3:267-287, 1967.

19. Johansen, K., and C. Lenfant. Respiratory function in the South American lungfish, *Lepidosiren paradoxa* (Fitz). *J. Exp. Biol.* 46:205-218, 1967.

20. Johansen, K., and C. Lenfant. Respiration in the African lungfish, *Protopterus aethiopicus*. II. Control of breathing. *J. Exp. Biol.* 49:453-468, 1968.

21. Kawasaki, R. Breathing rhythm-generation in the adult lamprey, *Entosphenus japonicus*. *Jpn. J. Physiol.* 29:327-338, 1979.

22. Kawasaki, R. Artificial pacemaking of breathing movements by medullary stimulation of adult lampreys. *Jpn. J. Physiol.* 31:571-583, 1981.

23. Knox, C.K.L. Characteristics of inflation and deflation reflexes during expiration in the cat. *J. Neurophysiol.* 36:284-295, 1973.

24. Krnjevik, K., E. Puil, and R. Werman. GABA and glycine actions on spinal motoneurons. *Can. J. Physiol. Pharmacol.* 55:658-669, 1977.

25. Liem, K.L. The biology of lungfishes: An epilogue. In *The biology and evolution of lungfishes*, ed. W.E. Bemis, W.M. Burggren, and N.E. Kemp, 299-303. New York: Alan R. Liss, 1987.

26. McMahon, B.R. A functional analysis of the aquatic and aerial respiratory movements of an African lungfish, *Protopterus aethiopicus*, with reference to the evolution of the lung-ventilation mechanism in vertebrates. *J. Exp. Biol.* 51:407-430, 1969.

27. Pack, A.I., and R.G. DeLaney. Response of pulmonary rapidly adapting receptors during lung inflation. *J. Appl. Physiol.* 55:955-963, 1983.

28. Pack, A.I., M.D. Ogilvie, R.O. Davies, and R.J. Galante. Responses of pulmonary stretch receptors during ramp inflations of the lung. *J. Appl. Physiol.* 61:344-352, 1986.

29. Pack, A.I., R.J. Galante, and A.P. Fishman. Control of interbreath interval in the African lungfish. *Am. J. Physiol.* 259:R139-R146, 1990.

30. Parker, W.N. On the anatomy and physiology of *Protopterus annectens*. *Trans. R. Irish. Acad.* 30:109-230, 1892.

31. Randall, D.J., W.W. Burggren, A.P. Farrell, and M.S. Haswell. *The evolution of air breathing in vertebrates*, Cambridge, U.K.: Cambridge University Press, 1981.

32. Richardson, C.A. Power spectra of inspiratory nerve activity with lung inflations in cats. *J. Appl. Physiol.* 64:1709-1720, 1988.

33. Romer, A.S. *The vertebrate body*, 4th ed. 644. Philadelphia: W.B. Saunders Co., 1970.

34. Rosen, D.E., P.L. Florey, B.G. Gardiner, and C. Patterson. Lungfishes, tetrapods, paleontology, and plesiomorphy. *Bull. Am. Mus. Nat. Hist.* 167:159-276, 1981.

35. Rovainen, C.M. Neural control of ventilation in the lamprey. *Fed. Proc.* 36:2386-2389, 1977.

36. Rovainen, C.M. Generation of respiratory activity by the lamprey brain exposed to picrotoxin and strychnine, and weak synaptic inhibition in motoneurons. *Neuroscience* 10:875-882, 1983.

37. Sant'Ambrogio, G., G. Miserocchi, and J. Mortola. Transient responses of pulmonary stretch receptors in the dog to inhalation of carbon dioxide. *Resp. Physiol.* 22:191-197, 1974.

38. Schultz H.-P. Dipnoans as sarcopterygioans. In *The biology and evolution of lungfishes*, ed. W.E. Bemis, W.M. Burggren, and N.E. Kemp, 39-74. New York: Alan R. Liss, 1987.

39. Smith, J.C., J.J. Greer, G. Liu, and J.L. Feldman. Neural mechanisms generating respiratory pattern in mammalian brainstem–spinal cord *in vitro*. I. Spatiotemporal patterns of motor and medullary neuron activity. *J. Neurophysiol.* 64:1149-1169, 1990.

40. Suzue, T. Respiratory rhythm generation in the *in vitro* brainstem–spinal cord preparation of the neonatal rat. *J. Physiol.* (London) 354:173-183, 1984.

41. Syed, N.I., A.G.M. Bulloch, K. Lukowiak. *In vitro* reconstruction of the respiratory central pattern generator of the mollusk *Lymnaea*. *Science* 250:282-285, 1990.

42. Thompson, K.J. Organization of inputs to motoneurons during fictive respiration in the isolated lamprey brain. *J. Comp. Physiol.* A 157:291-302, 1985.

43. West, N.H., and D.R. Jones. Breathing movements in the frog, *Rana pipiens*. I. The mechanical events associated with lung and buccal ventilation. *Can. J. Zool.* 53:332-344, 1975.

44. West, N.H., and W.W. Burggren. Reflex interactions between aerial and aquatic gas exchange in larval bullfrogs. *Am. J. Physiol.* 244:R770-R777, 1983.

45. Younes, M., P. Vaillancourt, and J. Milic-Emili. Interaction between chemical factors and duration of apnea following lung inflation. *J. Appl. Physiol.* 36:190-201, 1974.

III

Chemical Neuroanatomy

12

An Overview

Albert J. Berger

Chemical neuroanatomy deals with the localization of neurotransmitter substances within neural structures or pathways. The purpose of chemical neuroanatomical studies is to learn more about the associations of neurotransmitters, their synthetic machinery, and receptors with certain functionally defined structures. This is particularly important for chemical neuroanatomical studies that are designed to advance our understanding of the neural control of respiration. Although much is known about neural structures that have a role in respiration, many of these structures lie within portions of the nervous system that have diverse functions, such as control of circulation. It is imperative, therefore, that chemical neuroanatomical studies be designed so that the associations between structure and function may be unambiguously defined. Two of the papers in this section are particularly relevant to this point. In their paper, Ellenberger and Feldman (this volume) show how the use of tract tracing methods can reveal the rich interconnections of ponto-medullary structures having respiratory function. The paper by Lipski et al. (this volume) goes a step further by describing a variety of single cell approaches, including examination of ultrastructure following intracellular labeling to determine the kinds of transmitters in presynaptic processes that impinge upon functionally identified central respiratory neurons.

Chemical neuroanatomical studies lead ultimately to consideration of mechanisms by which neurotransmitters do their work. We can distinguish two general modes of action for neurotransmitter substances (1). In one mode, neurotransmitter-gated ion channels or ligand-gated channels are activated (fig. 12.1A). An example of this is the effect of GABA upon $GABA_A$ receptors in the activation of chloride channels (2). Further, activation of ligand-gated ionic channels is characterized by its brief duration, which is typically milliseconds. In the other mode, a neurotransmitter can activate ion channels by means of second-messenger systems (fig. 12.1B). Here the unifying concept is the effect of the transmitter-receptor complex on various G-protein systems, which in turn can alter second messengers in cells and ultimately, through (for example) protein kinases, can act on cellular effector proteins. In contrast to the ligand-gated channels, effects through second-messenger systems occur over long periods, usually seconds to minutes. This latter mode of action can affect ionic channels or even affect a cell's response to other neurotransmitters. An example of the longer term effects on ion channels is the long-lasting excitatory action of 5-HT on sensory neurons of *Aplysia*. The mechanism for this involves a decrease in an outward 5-HT-sensitive potassium conductance that comes about by activation of the second messenger, cAMP (3). In addition to their action on ion channels, these G-protein-coupled systems can intracellularly target biochemical enzymes, the cytoskeleton, membrane pumps, and genomic regulatory mechanisms.

Several criteria exist for classifying neurotransmitters (4); these include: 1) the presence of the substance, m-RNA, or synthetic enzymes within a neuron under study; 2) selective activation of a neuron produces release of the substance at the target site; 3) presence of the specific neurotransmitter receptor at the target site; 4) the response to the exogenously applied substance should mimic a response that follows activation of the synaptic pathway under investigation; and 5) pharmacological agents (agonist and antagonists) should produce expected effects as determined by exogenously applied agents and synaptic pathway-induced release of the substance. Ideally, for any substance to be classified as a neurotransmitter, all of the above criteria should be met. In reality, however, this usually is not the case.

Studies reported in this section largely focus on satisfying the first criterion, that is, showing that a substance, its m-RNA, or its synthetic enzymes actually exist in a specified respiratory-related neuron or pathway. Czyzyk-Krzeska et al. (this volume) for example, show that m-RNA for the rate-limiting enzyme tyrosine hydroxylase (TH) in the synthesis of catecholamines is present in carotid body Type I cells and that its expression is increased in carotid bodies that are exposed to hypoxia. Katz (this volume) also reports on the expression and regulation of TH by using immunocytochemical methods to reveal this synthetic enzyme. He shows that TH is present in petrosal ganglion sensory neurons and that TH expression is regulated by carotid sinus nerve innervation of the carotid body during development.

The main objective of chemical neuroanatomical studies is to localize both neurotransmitters and their target receptors along physiologically relevant pathways. Therefore, being able to unambiguously detect the neurotransmitter, m-RNA, or its synthetic enzymes, as well as its target receptors, is critical to the identification process. An ability to understand the role of neurochemicals in the organization of the nervous system as it relates to respira-

A. Ligand-Gated Ion Channel

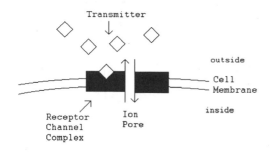

B. Second-Messenger Systems

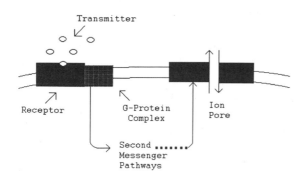

FIG. 12.1 Mechanisms by which transmitters cause changes in transmembrane ion fluxes. (Adapted from 1.)

tion has been dependent on the availability of appropriate methodologies. Recently some new methods have improved this ability.

The following several strategies are now available for identifying neurochemicals:

1. Radiolabeling: Typically this might be used with radiolabeling of an exogenously applied neurotransmitter, which then is detected on postsynaptic receptor sites.
2. Immunostaining: Here an antibody raised against a neurotransmitter, synthetic enzymes, or against the target receptor proteins is used to reveal the presence of a substance in a neuron or pathway.
3. m-RNA labeling: Because receptor proteins, neuropeptides, and synthetic enzymes are produced by transcription of the DNA template to mRNA and translation of the mRNA to protein, recently developed molecular biological methods involving *in situ* hybridization to specific mRNAs can reveal the presence of a substance in a neuron or pathway. Also the exciting question of genomic regulation of protein synthesis can be studied.

4. Some other methods are microdialysis, biochemical analysis of tissue samples, formaldehyde-induced fluorescence, and voltammetry.

A number of major issues need to be addressed using these techniques, the most important of which are the sensitivity and the specificity of the method. Further, with any of these methods, the anatomical and functional identification of the neuron where the transmitter is located, or upon which the transmitter is acting, must be determined. Without this knowledge and satisfaction of the criteria stated above for classifying a neurotransmitter, we cannot hope to understand completely the role of a neurotransmitter in a specific function. Consequently, such a substance is doomed to be relegated to the ignominious title of putative neurotransmitter.

The four papers presented in this section illustrate the use of several modern methods for neurotransmitter identification and regulation. They also utilize light and electron microscopic analysis of neurons, employing retrograde, anterograde, and intracellular labeling of cells. With these kinds of approaches, highly nonspecific, descriptive studies have given way to chemical neuroanatomic studies of such sophistication that data obtained from them can be used to formulate specific hypotheses, including those that enable us to understand basic mechanisms important in the neural control of respiration.

ACKNOWLEDGMENTS

This work was supported by a National Institutes of Health Javits Neuroscience Investigator Award NS 14857. Special thanks go to Hanna Atkins for editing the manuscript and to D.S. Berger for help with the illustrations.

REFERENCES

1. Hille, B. *Ionic Channels of Excitable Membranes.* Sunderland, Mass.: Sinauer Associates, 1984.
2. Jackson, M.B., H. Lecar, D.A. Mathers, and J.L. Barker. Single channel currents activated by gamma-aminobutyric acid, muscimol, and (−)-Pentobarbital in cultured mouse spinal neurons. *J. Neurosci* 2:889-894, 1982.
3. Klein, M., J. Camardo, and E.R. Kandel. Serotonin modulates a specific potassium current in the sensory neurons that show presynaptic facilitation in *Aplysia. Proc. Natl. Acad. Sci. USA* 79:5713-5717, 1982.
4. Siggins, G.R., and D.I. Gruol. Mechanisms of transmitter action in the vertebrate central nervous system. In *Handbook of Physiology.* ed. F.E. Bloom, Section 1, vol. 4, 1-114. Bethesda, Md.: American Physiological Society, 1986.

13

Neurotransmitter Content of Respiratory Neurons and Their Inputs: Double-Labeling Studies Using Intracellular Tracers and Immunohistochemistry

J. Lipski, C. Barton, D. de Castro, C. Jiang, I. Llewellyn-Smith,
G.S. Mitchell, P.M. Pilowsky, M.D. Voss, and H.J. Waldvogel

Studies of respiratory neurons using a combination of intracellular recording and labeling with horseradish peroxidase (HRP) have greatly extended our knowledge of the relationship between the function and structure of brainstem and spinal cord neurons involved in the control of respiratory motor output (e.g., 1, 2, 15, 23). Other studies utilizing the techniques of simultaneous extra- and intracellular recording from pairs of respiratory neurons and spike-triggered averaging have demonstrated monosynaptic connections between various subpopulations of respiratory neurons (e.g., 4, 6, 11, 14, 19). Although the latter studies show the direction of the synaptic influence (excitation or inhibition), they provide no information on the neurotransmitters involved. Other approaches are necessary to relate the structure and connectivity of respiratory neurons with their chemistry.

Until recently, information about neurotransmitters or neuromodulators of respiratory neurons largely originated from separate pharmacological, neurochemical, or immunohistochemical studies (3). Our recent investigations are aimed at identifying the chemical content of functionally and anatomically identified neurons and their inputs by combining three levels of analysis: (1) electrophysiological characterization with intracellular recording; (2) morphological examination following intracellular labeling with HRP or other tracers; and (3) immunohistochemistry using antibodies against putative neurotransmitters or their synthesizing enzymes. The examples outlined below illustrate the potential of this new approach in assessing the neurotransmitter content of respiratory neurons or their afferent inputs. Experiments were conducted on anaesthetized cats or rats. The general experimental procedures are summarized in figure 13.1.

The aim of the study, described in detail elsewhere (12, 21, 26), was to examine contacts between serotonergic fibers and three groups of respiratory neurons: phrenic, hypoglossal, and inspiratory neurons of the ventrolateral subnucleus of the nucleus of the solitary tract (dorsal respiratory group). The procedure is summarized in figure 13.1A. Following intracellular impalement, neurons were identified by antidromic activation and recording depolarizing membrane potential shifts in phase with inspiratory activity recorded from the phrenic nerve. After injection of neurons with HRP and 1–8-hour survival times, the ani-

mals were perfused transcardially with fixative and 50 μm sections from appropriate parts of the brain were cut with a vibratome. The neurons were visualized using standard HRP histochemistry (8). Serotonin-immunoreactive boutons were detected by incubating sections in (1) polyclonal rabbit anti-serotonin antibody, (2) biotinylated sheep anti-rabbit antibody, and (3) avidin-HRP conjugate. The reaction product of this immunoperoxidase procedure was usually produced using diaminobenzidine (DAB) intensified with nickel. This resulted in a dark blue or black reaction product, clearly distinct (by light microscopy) from the brown reaction product observed in intracellularly labeled neurons.

Immunoreactive boutons were found in close apposition to labeled neurons, with a greater density on distal dendrites than on proximal dendrites or cell bodies. In addition, the density of contacts was found to be substantially higher on phrenic motoneurons than on respiratory neurons of the dorsal respiratory group (21, 26). Electron microscopy confirmed that serotonin-immunoreactive boutons formed synapses with the identified phrenic motoneurons (21).

Three advantages of this approach, compared with retrograde labeling combined with immunohistochemistry (9, 25) are the following: (1) Contacts can be examined between immunoreactive boutons and central neurons which have been electrophysiologically characterized. In contrast, when retrograde labeling is used, definite functional identification is possible only in motoneurons, (2) Examined neurons can be reconstructed, (3) The distribution of contacts can be studied over the entire dendritic tree, including distal dendrites which cannot usually be visualized with retrograde labeling. There are two potential limitations to this technique. First, one may confuse immunoreactive boutons and terminals of filled neurons. A search must therefore be made for recurrent axon collaterals. Second, the reaction product in strongly HRP-labeled neurons may obscure details of postsynaptic densities during ultrastructural analysis.

Identification of immunoreactivity in terminals (or in cell bodies) provides no more than an *indication* that a substance may be involved in synaptic processes. Other approaches are needed to confirm its activity as a neurotransmitter, such as studies of release and inactivation, as-

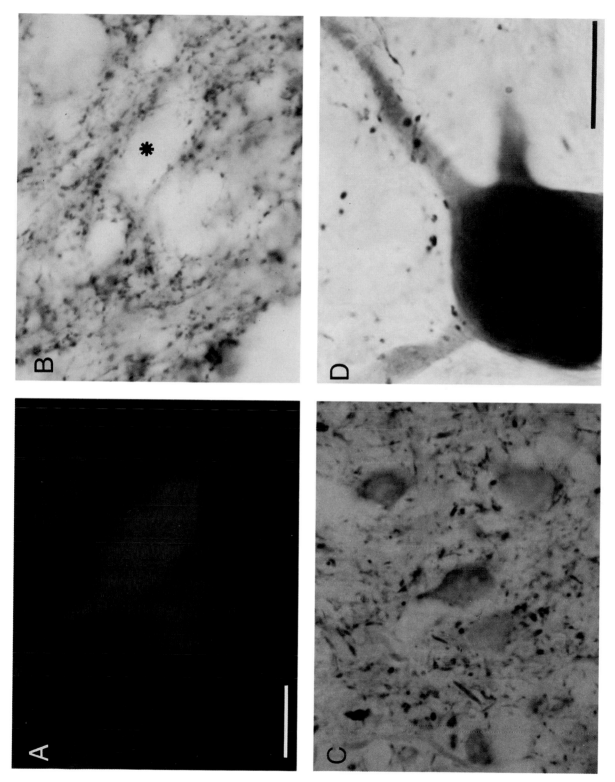

FIG. 13.3 GABAergic input to respiratory neurons in the ventrolateral medulla of the cat. (A) Texas Red fluorescence of an expiratory neuron in the Böt-zinger Complex, labeled with biocytin. (B) Bright-field photomicrograph of the same area (injected neuron marked with asterisk) showing lack of GABA immunoreactivity in the labeled cell body, but presence in surrounding boutons. (C) Examples of GABA-immunoreactive cell bodies in the dorsomedial part of the medulla oblongata. (D) Apposition of immunoreactive boutons and a HRP-filled inspiratory laryngeal motoneuron. Calibration bar: 25μm. (From Barton, Jiang, Lipski, and Pilowsky, unpublished.)

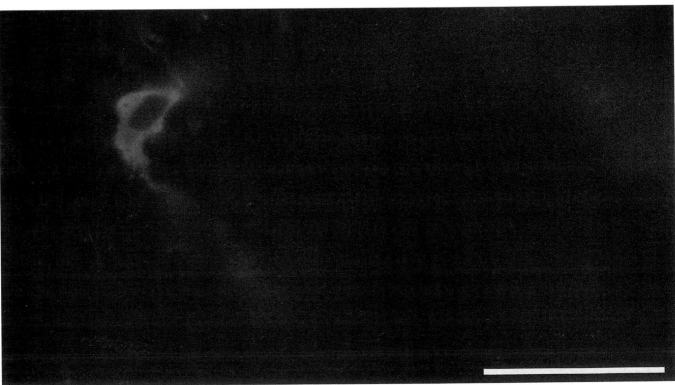

FIG. 13.4 Photomicrographs illustrating lack of TH-immunoreactivity in an LY-filled respiratory neuron in the rostral ventrolateral medulla in the rat. *Top*: LY-filled neuron. *Bottom*: Same site showing tyrosine hydroxilase- (TH-) immunoreactive neuron (rhodamine fluorescence). Calibration bar: 50μm. (Adapted from 21, with permission.)

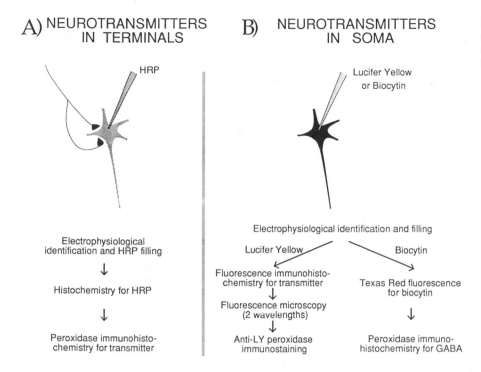

A) NEUTRANSMITTERS IN TERMINALS

HRP

Electrophysiological identification and HRP filling
↓
Histochemistry for HRP
↓
Peroxidase immunohisto- chemistry for transmitter

B) NEUROTRANSMITTERS IN SOMA

Lucifer Yellow or Biocytin

Electrophysiological identification and filling

Lucifer Yellow ⟋ ⟍ Biocytin

Fluorescence immunohisto- chemistry for transmitter
↓
Fluorescence microscopy (2 wavelengths)
↓
Anti-LY peroxidase immunostaining

Texas Red fluorescence for biocytin
↓
Peroxidase immuno- histochemistry for GABA

FIG. 13.1 General procedures used to examine neurotransmitter content in ter- minals (A) and cell bodies (B). (For fur- ther explanations see text.)

sessment of pharmacological effects, identification of pre- and postsynaptic receptors, and demonstration of mRNA for receptors, the transmitter, or its synthesizing enzyme(s).

A combination of two approaches, summarized in figure 13.1A and B, was used to examine the hypothesis that gamma-aminobutyric acid (GABA) is involved in the inhi- bition of medullary inspiratory neurons by augmenting ex- piratory neurons of the Bötzinger Complex (Böt-Aug). This hypothesis was based on two previous findings: (1) Spike- triggered averaging experiments revealed monosynaptic inhibitory actions of Böt-Aug neurons on several subpopu- lations of respiratory neurons (7, 11, 19), and (2) some GABA-immunoreactive neurons in the region of the Böt- zinger Complex could be retrogradely labeled after injecting of HRP into the region of the dorsal respiratory group (17).

In the initial stage of the study (16) we used intracellular HRP labeling of inspiratory neurons in the dorsal respira- tory group and immunohistochemistry for GABA. Follow- ing the procedure in figure 13.1A, contacts between immunoreactive boutons and the dendrites and cell bodies of these neurons could be demonstrated at the light micro- scopic level (fig. 13.2A–C). Electron microscopic analysis confirmed the presence of synapses (16 and fig. 13.2D). Similar contacts were found between GABA-immunoreac- tive boutons and inspiratory neurons of the ventral respira- tory group (fig. 13.3D, and Barton, Jiang, Lipski, and Pilowsky, unpublished).

Subsequently, we attempted to demonstrate GABA im- munoreactivity in Böt-Aug neurons (Fig. 13.1B, and Bar- ton, Jiang, Lipski, and Pilowsky, unpublished). Following intracellular injection of biocytin and transcardiac fixation

with a mixture of 2% glutaraldehyde and 1% formaldehyde, 40 μm parasagittal sections of the medulla were incubated in monoclonal mouse anti-GABA antibody (18) diluted 1:1000 for 2 days and in StreptAvidin Texas Red (Sigma, 1:200) for 4 hours. Sections with fluorescent cell bodies were incubated with a goat anti-mouse antibody (1:100, overnight) and mouse peroxidase-antiperoxidase (1:200, 4 hours), followed by DAB-Ni staining. Following dehydra- tion, clearing in xylene, and covering with depex, injected Böt-Aug neurons retained the fluorescence. Switching be- tween fluorescence and standard microscopy allowed exam- ination of biocytin-labeled cell bodies for immunoreactivity.

Eleven labeled Böt-Aug neurons were examined (fig. 13.3 A, B). None showed GABA immunoreactivity (fig. 13.3B,*). Although themselves not immunoreactive, the cell bodies of these neurons were surrounded by immunor- eactive boutons, some of which appeared to form close ap- positions with labeled cell bodies and their proximal dendrites.

This finding is not compatible with the hypothesis that Böt-Aug neurons are GABAergic but nevertheless could be a false-negative result and should be interpreted with cau- tion. First, this protocol may not be sensitive enough to detect the usually small amounts of GABA in the cell bod- ies of GABAergic neurons without colchicine pretreat- ment, even though GABA-immunoreactive cell bodies were observed in other parts of the medulla (fig. 13.3C). Second, it is known that some intracellularly injected labels inter- fere with subsequent immunohistochemical protocols (24), although such interference has not been reported for biocy- tin (10, 13, see also 20).

The Lucifer Yellow (LY) protocol in figure 13.1B was

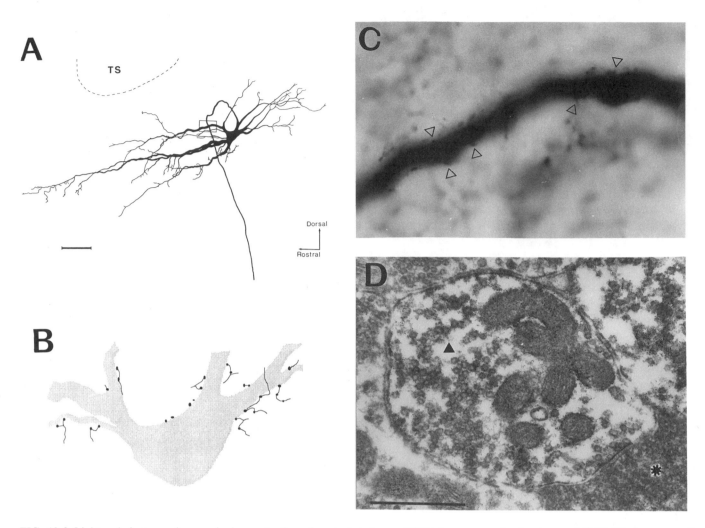

FIG. 13.2 Light and electron microscopic demonstration of contacts between GABA-immunoreactive boutons and HRP-filled neurons of the dorsal respiratory group in the cat. (A) Reconstruction of the labeled neuron. (B) Camera-lucida drawing showing appositions of immunoreactive boutons with the cell body. (C) Photomicrograph of the region shown in A by the box. Contacts between immunoreactive boutons and the labeled dendrite are indicated by open triangles. (D) Electron micrograph showing GABA-immunoreactive bouton (filled triangle) synapsing with HRP-filled dendrite (*). Calibration bar in A, 100 μm (corresponding to 10 μm in C); in D, 0.5 μm. (Adapted from 15, with permission.)

used in rats to examine the morphology of respiratory neurons in the rostral ventrolateral medulla and to study their relationship to catecholamine-containing neurons of the C1 group (22). The advantage of using LY as a label is that it can be visualized directly in injected neurons using fluorescence microscopy. This allows selection of sections containing labeled cell bodies for immunohistochemical processing. These sections were used for an immunofluorescence procedure with rhodamine (TRITC)-labeled secondary antibodies to reveal tyrosine hydroxylase (TH)-immunoreactivity. Sections were reexamined by changing between appropriate filter blocks to assess TH-immunoreactivity of LY-filled neurons. After photography (fig. 13.4), sections containing labeled cell bodies and adjacent sections were incubated with LY antiserum, and LY-immunoreactivity was revealed with standard immunoperoxidase staining. This final stage allowed camera-lucida reconstruction of labeled neurons and detailed examination of their morphology.

Using this procedure we could demonstrate (22) that none of the 16 LY-labeled neurons was immunoreactive for TH, although these neurons were often intermingled with catecholamine-containing neurons. Three-dimensional reconstructions of the axonal and dendritic morphology of labeled neurons showed axonal arborizations within the ventrolateral medulla in the vicinity of the C1 group, among other respiratory neurons and near neurons reported to have a cardiovascular function (5). The dendrites of some neurons radiated widely through the ventrolateral medulla and frequently approached the ventral surface.

CONCLUSIONS

A combination of intracellular recording and labeling of respiratory neurons with immunohistochemistry for putative neurotransmitters can be used to relate their function, structure, and chemistry. Although this type of analysis is technically demanding and not free from limitations (e.g., some intracellular tracers may interfere with immunohistochemical staining), this approach should help to fill the gap in our knowledge between what is known about the chemical anatomy of various regions of the central nervous system involved in respiratory control, and the properties of individual neurons.

ACKNOWLEDGMENTS

This work was supported by the New Zealand Medical Research Council; the Wellcome Trust Foundation, U.K.; the National Heart Foundations of New Zealand and Australia; the Auckland Medical Research Foundation; the New Zealand Lottery Grants Board; and the National Health and Medical Research Council of Australia.

REFERENCES

1. Berger, A.J., D.B. Averill, and W.E. Cameron. Morphology of inspiratory neurons located in the ventrolateral nucleus of the tractus solitarius of the cat. *J. Comp. Neurol.* 224:60-70, 1984.

2. Cameron, W.E., D.B. Averill, and A.J. Berger. Morphology of cat phrenic motoneurons as revealed by intracellular injection of horseradish peroxidase. *J. Comp. Neurol.* 219:70-80, 1983.

3. Dempsey, J.A., E.B. Olson, Jr., and S.B. Skatrud. Hormones and neurochemicals in the regulation of breathing. In *Handbook of Physiology.* Section 3, vol. 2, ed. N.S. Cherniack and J.G. Widdicombe, 181-222. Bethesda, Md.: American Physiological Society, 1986.

4. Duffin, J., and J. Lipski. Monosynaptic excitation of thoracic motoneurones by inspiratory neurones of the nucleus tractus solitarius in the cat. *J. Physiol.* 390:415-431, 1987.

5. Ellenberger, H.H., J.L. Feldman, and W.-Z. Zhan. Subnuclear organization of the lateral tegmental field of the rat. II: Catecholamine neurons and ventral respiratory group. *J. Comp. Neurol.* 294:212-222, 1990.

6. Ezure, K., and M. Manabe. Monosynaptic excitation of medullary inspiratory neurons by bulbospinal inspiratory neurons of the ventral respiratory group in the cat. *Exp. Brain Res.* 74:501-511, 1989.

7. Fedorko, L., J. Duffin, and S. England. Inhibition of inspiratory neurons of the nucleus retroambigualis by expiratory neurons of the Bötzinger Complex in the cat. *Exp. Neurol.* 106:74-77, 1989.

8. Hanker, J.S., P.E. Yates, C.B. Metz, and A. Rustioni. A new specific sensitive and non-carcinogenic reagent for the demonstration of horseradish peroxidase. *J. Histochem.* 9:789-792, 1977.

9. Holtman, J.R., Jr., W.P. Norman, L. Skirboll, K.L. Dretchen, C. Cuello, T.J. Visser, T. Hökfelt, and R.A. Gillis. Evidence for 5-hydroxytryptamine, substance P, and thyrotropin-releasing hormone in neurons innervating the phrenic motor nucleus. *J. Neurosci.* 4:1064-1071, 1984.

10. Horikawa, K., and W.E. Armstrong. A versatile means of intracellular labeling: Injection of biocytin and its detection with avidin conjugates. *J. Neurosci. Methods* 25:1-11, 1988.

11. Jiang, C., and J. Lipski. Extensive monosynaptic inhibition of ventral respiratory group neurons by augmenting neurons in the Bötzinger complex in the cat. *Exp. Brain Res.* 81:639-649, 1990.

12. Jiang, C., G.S. Mitchell, and J. Lipski. Prolonged augmentation of respiratory discharge in hypoglossal motoneurons following superior laryngeal nerve stimulation. *Brain Res.* 538:215-225, 1991.

13. Kitai, S.T., G.R. Penny, and H.T. Chang. Intracellular labeling and immunocytochemistry. In *Neuroanatomical tract-tracing methods.* vol. 2, *Recent Progress,* ed. L. Heimer and L. Záborszky, 173-199. New York: Plenum Press, 1989.

14. Lipski, J., L. Kubin, and J. Jodkowski. Synaptic action of R_β neurons on phrenic motoneurons studied with spike-triggered averaging. *Brain Res.* 228:105-118, 1983.

15. Lipski, J., and R.L. Martin-Body. Morphological properties of respiratory intercostal motoneurons in cats as revealed by intracellular injection of horseradish peroxidase. *J. Comp. Neurol.* 260:423-434, 1987.

16. Lipski, J., H.J. Waldvogel, P.M. Pilowsky, and C. Jiang. GABA-immunoreactive boutons make synapses with inspiratory neurons of the dorsal respiratory group in the cat. *Brain Res.* 529:309-314, 1990.

17. Livingston, C.A., and A.J. Berger. Immunocytochemical localization of GABA in neurons projecting to the ventrolateral nucleus of the solitary tract. *Brain Res.* 494:143-150, 1989.

18. Matute, C., and P. Streit. Monoclonal antibodies demonstrating GABA-like immunoreactivity. *Histochem.* 86:147-157, 1986.

19. Merrill, E.G., J. Lipski, L. Kubin, and L. Fedorko. Origin of the expiratory inhibition of nucleus tractus solitarius inspiratory neurones. *Brain Res.* 263:43-50, 1983.

20. Mulloney, B., and W.M. Hall. Only two of the four accessory neurons of the crayfish MRO are GABAergic: Phenotyping neurons by combining biocytin backfills with immunocytochemistry. *Soc. Neurosci. Abstr.,* 16:633, 1990.

21. Pilowsky, P.M., D. de Castro, I. Llewellyn-Smith, J. Lipski, and M.D. Voss. Serotonin immunoreactive boutons make synapses with feline phrenic motoneurons. *J. Neurosci.* 10:1091-1098, 1990.

22. Pilowsky, P.M., C. Jiang, and J. Lipski. An intracellular study of respiratory neurons in the rostral ventrolateral medulla of the rat and their relationship to catecholamine containing neurons. *J. Comp. Neurol.* 301:604-617, 1990.

23. Sasaki, H., K. Otake, H. Mannen, K. Ezure, and M. Manabe. Morphology of augmenting inspiratory neurons of the ventral respiratory group in the cat. *J. Comp. Neurol.* 282:157-168, 1989.

24. Scharfman, H.E., D.D. Kunkel, and P.A. Schwartzkroin. Intracellular dyes mask immunoreactivity of hippocampal interneurons. *Neurosci. Lett.* 96:23-28, 1989.

25. Skirboll, L.R., K. Thor, C. Helke, T. Hökfelt, R. Robertson, and R. Long. Use of retrograde fluorescent tracers in combination with immunohistochemical methods. In *Neuroanatomical tract-tracing methods.* Vol. 2, *Recent progress,* ed. L. Heimer and L. Záborsky, 5-18. New York: Plenum Press, 1989.

26. Voss, M.D., D. de Castro, J. Lipski, P.M. Pilowsky, and C. Jiang. Serotonin immunoreactive boutons form close appositions with respiratory neurons of the dorsal respiratory group in the cat. *J. Comp. Neurol.* 295:208-218, 1990.

14

Induction of Tyrosine Hydroxylase Gene in Carotid Body by Hypoxia

Maria F. Czyzyk-Krzeska, Douglas A. Bayliss, and David E. Millhorn

The carotid body (*glomus caroticum*) is a chemosensitive organ located at the bifurcation of the common carotid artery. The mammalian carotid body detects alterations in the partial pressures of oxygen (PO_2), carbon dioxide (PCO_2) and pH in arterial blood and transduces these signals into electrical impulses in primary sensory fibers of the carotid sinus nerve. Although the actual mechanism by which changes in blood gases are detected by the carotid body remains unknown, it is now generally believed that chemosensory signals are transmitted from Type I (glomus) cells to closely apposed sensory terminals (15) by release of a chemical transmitter (6).

A number of classical neurotransmitters (3, 7, 11) and neuropeptides (4, 13, 14) have been identified in cell bodies as well as in sensory and sympathetic fibers in the carotid body. Thus far, the best evidence that one of these compounds might actually mediate chemosensory signalling between Type I cells and primary sensory terminals supports involvement of the catecholamine neurotransmitter dopamine. Biochemical studies have revealed that dopamine is synthesized in Type I cells (2) and released in response to a reduction in arterial PO_2, that is, hypoxia (12). Moreover, the activity (V_{max}) of tyrosine hydroxylase (TH), the first and rate-limiting enzyme in the biosynthesis of catecholamines, is substantially increased in Type I cells by hypoxia (8, 10). The activity of dopamine-β-hydroxylase, the enzyme that converts dopamine to norepinephrine, is unaffected by hypoxia (10). The increase in V_{max} of TH activity could result from either recruitment of previously synthesized (but nonfunctional) enzyme or from *de novo* synthesis of new enzyme. The latter possibility would involve increased gene expression for tyrosine hydroxylase.

The present study was undertaken to test the hypothesis that the increase in TH activity during hypoxia results, at least in part, from an increase in TH gene expression. If this hypothesis is correct, exposure to hypoxia would cause an increase in the concentration of TH messenger RNA (mRNA) in carotid body Type I cells. The concentration of TH mRNA in the carotid body in control and test animals was determined by *in situ* hybridization. *In situ* hybridization is an extremely powerful molecular technique that provides a means for identification and quantification of specific mRNAs in individual cells. Although there are a number of other techniques for measuring mRNA in tissue (e.g. Northern analysis, RNA protection assay), these require relatively large amounts of tissue and do not provide cellular resolution. However, *in situ* hybridization is ideally suited for studying gene regulation in small organs such as the carotid body and in heterogeneous tissue such as the nervous system.

In this report we demonstrate that exposure to 10% O_2 for as little as 1 hour caused a substantial increase in the concentration of TH mRNA in the carotid body Type I cells. In addition, we found that hypercapnia, another natural stimulus of the carotid body, did not enhance TH gene expression in Type I cells. Thus, TH gene expression is regulated in both a tissue- and stimulus-specific manner in the carotid body by hypoxia.

METHODS

Individual adult male Sprague-Dawley rats (200–400 g) were placed in an environmental chamber and exposed to either 10% O_2 for 1–48 hr or to air (21% O_2) for the same durations. During exposures of long duration (12–48 hr), normal light-dark cycles were maintained and the animal received food and water *ad libitum*. Following the experiment, the animals were removed from the environmental chambers and anesthetized. The carotid body, superior cervical sympathetic ganglia, adrenal glands, and petrosal ganglia were removed surgically and frozen immediately over dry ice. The tissues were cut (10 μm) on a microtome in a cryostat, thaw-mounted onto gelatin-coated microscope slides, and either stored at $-70°C$ or processed immediately for *in situ* hybridization as described previously (1, 5). Briefly, sections were warmed to room temperature, fixed in 4% paraformaldehyde, rinsed extensively in 0.1 M phosphate buffered saline (PBS), and dehydrated and delipidated through graded ethanol and chloroform rinses. Sections were then hybridized to 0.5×10^6 cpm of probe (see below) in a buffer that contained 50% deionized formamide, $4 \times SSC$ ($1 \times SSC$ is 0.15 M NaCl/0.015 M sodium citrate, pH 7.2), 10% dextran sulfate, 0.02% each of Ficoll, polyvinylpyrrolidone, and bovine serum albumin, 500 μg/ml denatured salmon sperm DNA, 250 μg/ml yeast tRNA, and 100 mM dithiothreitol overnight at 37°C. The sections were washed in $1 \times SSC$ for an hour at 55°C (4 × 15 min

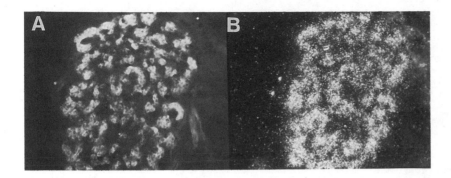

FIG. 14.1 Photomicrograph showing carotid body cells that are immunostained for tyrosine hydroxylase (TH) (*A*) and contain label for TH mRNA (*B*). A combination of immunohistochemistry for TH enzyme and *in situ* hybridization for TH mRNA was performed on the same tissue. Notice that the same cells that contain TH enzyme (*A*) also contain the mRNA that encodes TH (*B*).

rinses) and for 1 hour at room temperature. The sections were then dipped briefly in water and ethanol (95%), air dried, and apposed to X-ray film (Hyperfilm-βmax, Amersham) for 3–10 days. The slides were then dipped in nuclear track emulsion (Kodak NTB2). After exposure for 1–3 weeks, the emulsion was developed and fixed, and the sections were counterstained with toluidine blue before being analyzed with light- and dark-field microscopy. Quantification of silver grain density was performed with a counting device (Artek) interfaced with a microscope and custom software.

Two oligodeoxyribonucleotide (oligonucleotide) probes (TH$_1$, 49-mer; TH$_2$, 30-mer) directed against different regions (1441–1488 and 1230–1259, respectively) of rat TH cDNA (9) were synthesized (Milligen DNA synthesizer) and used to detect TH mRNA. The TH$_2$ probe was used in most experiments; however, in some cases a mixture of TH$_1$ and TH$_2$ were applied to tissue sections as a cocktail. This strategy is used to increase the sensitivity of the technique. The DNA for TH$_2$ and corresponding TH cDNA sequence are shown below. The probe sequences chosen showed no significant homology with other published cDNA sequences (GenBank).

TH cDNA (mRNA): 5′GAG CCT GAG GTC CGA GCC TTT GAC CCA GAC 3/
TH$_2$ probe: 3′CTC GGA CTC CAG GCT CGG AAA CTG GGT CTG 5′

Oligonucleotides were labelled at the 3/ end with α-thio[^{35}S]-dATP (New England Nuclear; >1000 Ci/mmol) and terminal deoxynucleotidyl transferase (Bethesda Research Laboratories) to specific activities of 2–6 × 10^6 cpm/pmol. The labelled probe was separated from unincorporated nucleotide by gel filtration (Sephadex G50; Pharmacia), dried in a vacuum concentrator, and resuspended in hybridization buffer (5 × 10^6 cpm/ml).

In some cases, a combination of TH immunohistochemistry and *in situ* hybridization was performed on the same tissue. In these cases, the animals were anesthetized and perfused transcardially with 2% paraformaldehyde. The carotid bodies were removed, frozen over dry ice, and *in situ* hybridization was performed as described above. However,

prior to dipping slides in nuclear emulsion, either rabbit polyclonal or mouse monoclonal antibodies against TH were applied to the tissue and detected by the indirect immunofluorescence technique. A more detailed description of this technique is provided in previously published papers from our laboratory (see 16). The combination of *in situ* hybridization and immunohistochemistry allowed direct visualization of both TH mRNA and TH protein in the same cells. This is an excellent control to show that the probes used for the *in situ* hybridization are specific for the mRNA of interest.

RESULTS

In the present study, TH mRNA was found in individual cells of the carotid body, medulla of the adrenal gland, superior cervical sympathetic ganglia, and petrosal ganglia. In unrelated studies in our laboratory in which the same probes were used, TH mRNA was also found in areas of the brain that contain catecholamine-synthesizing enzymes.

In a number of experiments, a combination of TH *in situ* hybridization and immunohistochemistry was performed on the same carotid bodies. Figure 14.1 shows a tissue section of carotid body from one of those experiments. TH-like immunoreactivity (IR) was observed in most Type I cells (fig. 14.1A). This was certainly not an unexpected finding since it had previously been shown that Type I cells are rich in dopamine (2, 7, 12). Of particular interest was the finding that the individual Type I cells that contain TH-IR also express TH mRNA (fig. 14.1B). The silver grains over the tissue denote hybridization of the probe with TH mRNA. Note the cellular resolution of the hybridization signal. It is important to recognize that cells that synthesize TH mRNA translate this message into TH protein. As mentioned above, localization of both the mRNA and its cognate protein in the same cells attests to the specificity of our probes.

Figure 14.2 shows sections of carotid bodies taken from animals that were exposed to either room air (Fig. 14.2A) or 10% O$_2$ for 6 hr (fig. 14.2B), 12 hr (fig. 14.2C), and 24 hr (fig. 14.2D). It is clear from this figure that TH mRNA is

FIG. 14.2 Photomicrographs showing tyrosine hydroxylase (TH) mRNA levels in carotid bodies taken from a control animal (*A*, exposed only to room air) and from animals exposed to 10% O_2 for 4 hr (*B*), 12 hr (*C*), and 24 hr (*D*). Notice that the density of silver grains (indicating presence of TH mRNA) is substantially enhanced in the animals exposed to hypoxia and that the level of TH gene expression in carotid body remains elevated during the relatively long exposure.

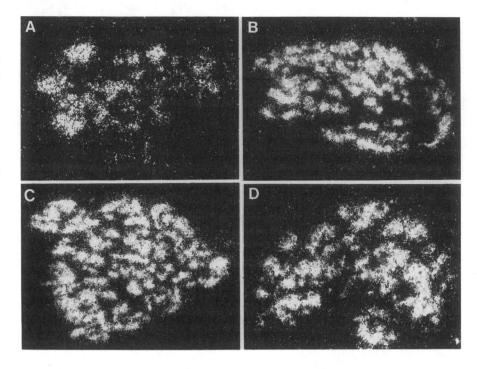

constitutively expressed in the carotid body. The level of TH mRNA was substantially increased (notice increased density of silver grains) in the carotid bodies (fig. 14.2*B*–*D*) that were taken from rats exposed to 10% O_2. In similar experiments, the induction of TH mRNA by hypoxia was quantitated. Briefly, we found that exposure to 10% O_2 lasting as little as 1 hr was sufficient to induce a near doubling of TH mRNA; peak expression of TH mRNA in the carotid body was measured (an increase of ca. 500%) in animals exposed to 10% O_2 for 6 hr. The concentration of TH mRNA in carotid body was enhanced by 200–300% in animals exposed to hypoxia for longer durations (24–48 hr).

In several experiments we examined the possibility that gene expression for dopamine-β-hydroxylase (DBH), the enzyme that converts dopamine to norepinephrine, might also be induced by hypoxia. We detected a very low level of constitutively expressed DBH mRNA in carotid body during control conditions; the concentration of DBH mRNA was not increased by exposure to hypoxia (not shown).

To determine if the increased TH gene expression in the carotid body is an inherent property of Type I cells, we performed experiments in which the sensory innervation, sympathetic innervation, or both were eliminated by cutting the carotid sinus nerve and removing the superior cervical ganglion at least 7 days before exposing the animal to hypoxia. Figure 14.3 shows findings from experiments in which the neural innervation of carotid body was intact (fig. 14.3*A*, *B*) and completely denervated (fig. 14.3*C*, *D*). There was a constitutive level of TH gene expression in the carotid bodies of control animals (Fig. 14.3*A*, *C*). Hypoxia stimulated TH gene expression to a similar degree in both the intact (fig. 14.3*B*) and denervated (Fig. 14.3*D*) carotid bodies.

Thus, neural innervation of the carotid body is not required for the induction of TH gene expression in Type I cells by hypoxia.

We also examined the effect of hypoxia on the TH gene expression in other catecholamine-synthesizing tissue (e.g., adrenal medulla, superior cervical ganglia, and petrosal ganglia). Hypoxia caused a slight increase in TH mRNA in the catecholamine-containing cells of the adrenal medulla when the adrenal nerve was intact but not in animals in which the adrenal gland had been previously denervated (not shown). Thus, the hypoxia-induced increase in TH gene expression in the adrenal medulla appears to require synaptic input. TH gene expression in the superior cervical ganglion and petrosal ganglion was not enhanced by hypoxia.

Finally, we examined the possibility that hypercapnia might induce TH gene expression in the carotid body. Rats were exposed to a mixture of 10% CO_2 and air for 6 hr. In no case did we detect an increase in TH mRNA (not shown) indicating that TH gene expression is not induced by hypercapnia.

DISCUSSION

In the present study *in situ* hybridization was used to measure TH mRNA concentration in the carotid body and other catecholamine-synthesizing tissues during hypoxia. This is the first experimental evidence that the increase in TH activity measured previously in the carotid body during hypoxia (10, 12) is indeed associated with an increase in TH mRNA. TH gene expression in other tissues (adrenal medulla, superior cervical ganglion, and petrosal ganglion)

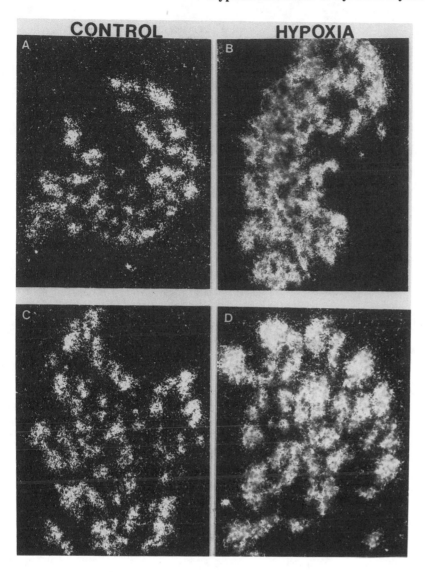

FIG. 14.3 Photomicrographs showing the effect of hypoxia on TH gene expression in innervated (*A,B*) and denervated (*C,D*) carotid body. Panels *A* and *C* show constitutive level of TH mRNA in carotid bodies that were taken from animals that were exposed only to room air. Panels *B* and *D* are carotid bodies taken from animals that were exposed to 10% O_2 for 6 hr. This figure clearly shows that denervation of the carotid bodies had no effect on hypoxia induction of TH gene expression.

was not induced directly by hypoxia. The cellular mechanisms that mediate induction of TH gene expression in Type I cells by hypoxia are currently under investigation in our laboratory.

We also found that the hypoxia-induced increase in TH mRNA in carotid body does not require innervation (and thus synaptic input) by either fibers of the carotid sinus nerve or sympathetic fibers of the ganglioglomerular nerve. Thus, intrinsic to Type I cells are mechanisms that are activated by hypoxia and mediate increases in TH gene expression. Moreover, the increase in TH gene expression in carotid body cells is stimulus-specific. Exposure to hypercapnia, another natural stimulus of carotid body activity, failed to induce an increase in TH gene expression in Type I cells.

The present experiments were not undertaken to address mechanisms by which carotid body cells detect alterations in the chemical composition of arterial blood. Nevertheless, findings from our study do suggest that dopamine plays an important role in O_2 chemoreception. Another im-

portant feature of this research is that it represents a rare example of an alteration in gene expression in response to an environmental or natural stimulus (i.e., hypoxia) for a molecule that is implicated in mediating the physiological response to the stimulus.

ACKNOWLEDGEMENTS

This work was supported by grants from the National Institutes of Health (HL33831), the American Heart Association (National; 88–1108), and the American Lung Association. DEM is a career investigator of the American Lung Association. DAB was supported by a fellowship from Glaxo Inc.

REFERENCES

1. Bayliss, D.A., Y.-M. Wang, C.A. Zahnow, D.R. Joseph, and D.E. Millhorn. Localization of histidine decarboxylase mRNA in rat brain. *Molecular and Cellular Neurosci.* 1:3-9, 1990.

2. Bolme, P., K. Fuxe, T. Hökfelt, and M. Goldstein. Studies on the role of dopamine in cardiovascular and respiratory control: Central versus peripheral mechanisms. *Adv. Biochem. Psychopharmacol.* 16:281-290, 1977.

3. Chiocchio, S.R., M.P. King, L. Carballo, and E.T. Angelakos. Monoamines in the carotid body cells of the cat. *J. Histochem. Cytochem.* 19:621-626, 1971.

4. Cuello, A.C., and D.S. McQueen. Substance P: A carotid body peptide. *Neurosci. Lett.* 17:215-219, 1980.

5. Czyzyk-Krzeska, M.F., D.A. Bayliss, K.B. Seroogy, and D.E. Millhorn. Gene expression for peptides in neurons of the petrosal and nodose ganglia in rat. *Exp. Brain Res.* 83:411-418, 1991.

6. Eyzaguirre, C., and P. Zapata. Perspectives in carotid body research. *J. Appl. Physiol.* 57:931-957, 1984.

7. Fidone, S.J., S. Weintraub, and W. Stavinoha. Acetylcholine content of normal and denervated cat carotid bodies measured by pyrolysis gas chromatography/mass fragmentography. *J. Neurochem.* 26:1047-1049, 1976.

8. Gonzalez, C., Y. Kwok, J. Gibb, and S. Fidone. Effects of hypoxia on tyrosine hydroxylase activity in rat carotid body. *J. Neurochem.* 33:713-719, 1979.

9. Grima, B., A. Lamouroux, F. Blanot, N.F. Biguet, and J. Mallet. Complete coding sequence of rat tyrosine hydroxylase mRNA. *Proc. Natl. Acad. Sci.* USA 82:617-621, 1985.

10. Hanbauer, I., W. Lovenberg, and E. Costa. Induction of tyrosine 3-monooxygenase in carotid body of rats exposed to hypoxic conditions. *Neuropharmacol.* 16:277-282, 1977.

11. Hellström, S. Putative neurotransmitters in the carotid body: Mass fragmentographic studies. *Adv. Biochem. Psychopharmacol.* 16:257-263, 1977.

12. Hellström, S., I. Hanbauer, and E. Costa. Selective decrease of dopamine content in rat carotid body during exposure to hypoxic conditions. *Brain Res.* 118:352-355, 1976.

13. Heym, C., and W. Kummer. Immunohistochemical distribution and colocalization of regulatory peptides in the carotid body. *J. Electron Microscopy Tech.* 12:331-342, 1989.

14. Lundberg, J.M., T. Hökfelt, J. Fahrenkrug, A. Nilsson, and L. Terenius. Peptides in the cat carotid body (glomus caroticum): VIP-, enkephalin- and Substance P-like immunoreactivity. *Acta Physiol. Scand.* 107:279-281, 1979.

15. McDonald, D.M., and R.A. Mitchell. The innervation of glomus cells, ganglion cells and blood vessels in the rat carotid body: A quantitative ultrastructural analysis. *J. Neurocytol.* 4:177-230, 1975.

16. Millhorn, D.E., T. Hökfelt, A.A.J. Verhofstad, and L. Terenius. Individual cells in the raphe nuclei of the medulla oblongata in rat that contain immunoreactivities for both serotonin and enkephalin project to the spinal cord. *Exp. Brain Res.* 75:536-542, 1989.

15

Expression and Development of Transmitter Properties in Carotid Body Afferent Neurons

David M. Katz

Physiologic studies have demonstrated that peripheral chemoreflexes change markedly during development, profoundly altering respiratory responses to hypoxia (5, 9, 14, 15, 18, 19, 35). In the fetus, for example, the carotid chemoreceptors are relatively ineffective in increasing respiration during hypoxia (5, 7, 19, 35) and hypoxic stimulation leads to depression of respiratory movements (5). In neonates, on the other hand, hypoxia produces a transient hyperventilation, followed by a prolonged hypoventilation (5, 7, 9, 14, 15, 32, 35). In adults, however, hypoxia evokes a relatively sustained increase in ventilation, primarily by acting on the carotid bodies (10). Mechanisms that underlie these developmental changes are unknown, though neural, metabolic and mechanical factors have all been postulated to play a role (5, 9, 14, 15, 18, 19, 35). One approach to this issue has been the identification of cellular elements in chemoreflex pathways that undergo significant developmental changes coincident with physiological maturation. Many cell groups may be involved in regulating the development of chemo-responsiveness, including the peripheral chemoreceptors themselves, primary afferent neurons, and brain and spinal cord respiratory neurons.

This chapter focuses on the biochemical maturation of primary sensory neurons, located in the petrosal and jugular cranial sensory ganglia, that innervate the carotid body. These cells project peripherally in the carotid sinus nerve (CSN) to innervate glomus cells within the carotid body. In addition, carotid body afferents project centrally to the brainstem nucleus tractus solitarius and ventrolateral medulla, as well as other sites (11), forming the afferent link between the carotid body chemoreceptors and central neural pathways. Therefore, transmission of carotid body stimulation to the central nervous system is critically dependent upon the maturity of neurochemical properties expressed by carotid body afferent neurons.

NEUROCHEMICAL CHANGES EXTRAUTERINE BREATHING

Recent studies have begun to identify neurochemical changes in chemoreceptor pathways that may influence functional maturation. Hertzberg, et al., for example, found that dopamine turnover in the rat carotid body decreases markedly at birth, just prior to the emergence of peripheral chemoreflexes (17). These authors hypothesize that the decrease in turnover reflects decreased dopamine release from carotid body glomus cells, and that this process contributes to the resetting of chemoreceptor sensitivity in accord with the demands of the *ex utero* environment. Peptidergic properties expressed by glomus cells also exhibit significant perinatal changes. In the cat carotid body, for example, substance P (SP) immunoreactivity is not detectable until after birth and increases significantly in the postnatal period (33). Perinatal alterations in transmitter properties have also recently been described in the nucleus tractus solitarius (NTS), the primary brainstem locus of second-order neurons in the carotid body afferent pathway. Srinivasan, et al., found that levels of preprotachykinin messenger RNA, which encodes the tachykinin peptides substance P and neurokinin A, increase markedly in the rabbit NTS at birth (34). This increase is only seen if animals are allowed to breath room air for at least 2 hours after birth, suggesting an association with the onset of respiration. Although the physiologic significance of these neurochemical changes in the carotid body and NTS remains to be established, these observations underscore the high degree of biochemical plasticity in respiration-related neural structures at birth.

TRANSMITTER PROPERTIES OF CAROTID BODY AFFERENT NEURONS

Visceral sensory neurons in general express a wide spectrum of classical sensory transmitter candidates, including the neuropeptides substance P (SP; 4, 16, 22, 29), calcitonin gene–related peptide (CGRP; 6, 13, 29), vasoactive intestinal peptide (16, 29), somatostatin (16, 29), and cholecystokinin (16, 29). In addition, some nodose and petrosal ganglion cells express monoaminergic transmitter properties not previously associated with sensory neurons. In the nodose and petrosal ganglia of adult rats, for example, a subpopulation of sensory neurons express catecholaminergic (CA) transmitter traits, including catalytically active tyrosine hydroxylase (TH), the rate-limiting enzyme in catecholamine biosynthesis, formaldehyde-induced catecholamine fluorescence, and a monoamine oxidase–like pathway for CA metabolism (24). These cells exhibit morphologic features typical of primary sensory neurons, such as an initial axon glomerulus and a single primary neurite that branches into a central and peripheral axonal process (24). TH-containing petrosal neurons are readily distinguished from sympathetic and small intensely fluorescent cells by cytochemical, morphometric, and pharmacologic criteria (24). For example, CA sensory neurons are insensitive to neonatal treatment with the neurotoxin 6-hydroxydopamine, thereby distinguishing them from sympathetic neurons (24). The CA neurons in the rat nodose and petrosal ganglia appear to synthesize dopamine, as they contain tyrosine hydroxylase and dopa decarboxylase (24) but do not express immunoreactivity for dopamine-β-hydroxylase, the enzyme that converts dopamine to norepinephrine (24). TH-containing neurons are found in a wide variety of species including rat, guinea pig (27), cat (23), and dog (36).

Of the many transmitter properties expressed by visceral sensory neurons, only the CA phenotype has been shown to be selectively associated with carotid body afferent neurons. By combining immunocytochemical staining with retrograde tracing methods, Katz and Black (21) found that expression of CA properties by petrosal ganglion (PG) afferents is highly correlated with innervation of the carotid body. In these experiments, carotid body afferent neurons in the PG were labeled by retrograde transport of fluorescent tracers applied either to the carotid sinus nerve or selectively infused into the carotid body (22). Cryostat sections of the PG were then stained with antiserum against TH (30) and examined for colocalization of the retrograde marker and antibody labeling. These studies demonstrated that 93% of the TH-containing cells in the PG project peripherally in the carotid sinus nerve (CSN) and 84% innervate the carotid body (21). TH is therefore a highly selective marker for carotid body afferents in the rat PG. Similar findings have recently been reported in the guinea pig (27).

The fact that some carotid body afferents exhibit dopaminergic properties suggests that dopamine plays a previously unrecognized role in peripheral chemoreceptor pathways, not only as a transmitter or modulator released from glomus cells but also as a transmitter or modulator of the afferent neurons. Possible sites of action of dopamine in this system include both the central synapses of PG afferents in NTS as well as peripheral terminals in the carotid body. Evidence for a central site of action includes the recent demonstration that carotid body stimulation by hypoxia or NaCN and electrical stimulation of the CSN evoke dopamine release in NTS (12); it remains to be determined, however, whether the source of the amine is peripheral or central. The possibility that afferents release transmitter peripherally is supported by ultrastructural studies showing reciprocal synapses between vesicle-containing afferent terminals and glomus cells (31). Moreover, Almaraz and Fidone (2) have shown that electrical stimulation of the cut peripheral end of the cat sinus nerve evokes dopamine release from the carotid body *in vitro*. Here too, however, it is unknown whether the dopamine was released directly

from sinus nerve terminals in the carotid body or from glomus cells activated transsynaptically following CSN stimulation. The possibility that dopamine may be released by peripheral sensory terminals is supported by more recent studies showing dopamine synthesis by carotid sinus nerve afferents *in vitro* (23).

In addition to dopaminergic afferents, the carotid body also receives innervation from peptidergic sensory neurons. A small number of substance P- (SP-) containing cells in the jugular ganglion of the rat, for example, can be retrogradely labeled by tracer injections into the vascularly isolated carotid body (Finley and Katz, unpublished observations). Similarly, the guinea pig carotid body contains calcitonin gene–related peptide- (CGRP-) and SP–immunoreactive fibers that appear to arise from cells in the petrosal and jugular ganglia (25, 26). Unlike the catecholaminergic markers, however, CGRP and SP are not specifically localized to carotid body afferents and are expressed by cells innervating diverse visceral targets (25). Moreover, these peptides do not colocalize with TH in either rat (Finley and Katz, unpublished observations) or guinea pig (27) PG neurons, indicating that the carotid body receives sensory innervation from at least two neurochemically distinct populations of afferents; catecholaminergic and tachykinin peptidergic. We speculate that these two afferent populations may subserve different functions; one possibility is that peptidergic and catecholaminergic fibers innervate different cell types within the carotid body or may project to different sites within the brainstem.

DEVELOPMENT OF TRANSMITTER PROPERTIES IN CAROTID BODY AFFERENT NEURONS

The highly selective localization of CA traits to carotid body afferents within the rat PG provided us with sensitive markers for monitoring the biochemical development of these cells. To begin investigating transmitter ontogeny, immunocytochemical and biochemical methods were used to define the appearance and maturation of tyrosine hydroxylase in PG cells in the rat (20). Immunocytochemical studies demonstrated that the TH cells found in the adult PG first become detectable around embryonic day (E) 16.5 (birth = E22.5). Interestingly, this is the same age at which SP-containing cells become detectable (4), suggesting that neurochemical development of diverse ganglion cell subpopulations may be coordinately regulated at this age. The number of detectable TH cells subsequently rises to 70% of adult levels by E21.5, the day before birth, and then an additional 50% to reach adult values by postnatal day one (P1). As neuronal cell division ends in the PG by E14.5 (3), these increases in TH cell number most likely reflect an increase in TH levels per cell above the threshold for immunostaining.

The perinatal increase in TH staining suggested that a rapid induction of TH protein per cell occurs around birth. To quantify the magnitude of this induction, the relative amount of TH protein in E21.5 and P1 ganglion homogenates was compared by immunoblot analysis (20). Samples containing equal numbers of ganglia per volume were probed with a mouse monoclonal TH antibody and compared by densitometric scanning of nitrocellulose filters. These studies revealed that on average, TH levels per cell rose approximately 3.5-fold between E21.5 and P1. Thus, the development of this specific CA trait in carotid body afferents appears to be highly regulated around birth.

Although adult numbers of TH neurons are present by P1, the amount of TH protein per cell continues to increase during the first few postnatal weeks. Western blot analysis demonstrated an approximate fourfold rise in TH levels per ganglion between P1 and 3–4 weeks of age. Preliminary observations indicate that the postnatal increase in TH protein is accompanied by increased catecholamine levels. On the basis of these findings we conclude that carotid body afferent neurons in the PG are biochemically immature at birth and may therefore be functionally immature as well. Afferent transmitter development during the postnatal period may contribute to the progressive increase in peripheral drives to ventilation that occurs after birth (17). One potential problem with this hypothesis is that dopamine is generally thought to be inhibitory to respiration (8) although this remains a controversial issue (8). On the other hand, there is growing evidence that during development monoamines may function not only as neurotransmitters but also as trophic regulators of neuronal maturation (28). It is possible, therefore, that during the early postnatal period, dopamine released from carotid body afferents is important as a developmental regulatory signal, in addition to its potential role as a transmitter.

MOLECULAR MECHANISMS OF CATECHOLAMINERGIC DEVELOPMENT IN CAROTID BODY AFFERENTS

The striking correlation between CA expression in adult PG neurons and innervation of the carotid body raised the possibility that target innervation plays a role in regulating development of the CA phenotype. To address this issue, immunohistochemical studies examined the temporal relationship between the appearance of TH in carotid body afferents on E16.5 and innervation of the carotid body. Immunostaining of cryostat sections of rat embryos with neurofilament protein antibodies was used to monitor development of the carotid sinus nerve pathway between the petrosal ganglion and the carotid body. These studies revealed that nerve fibers arrive in the carotid body anlage around embryonic day 13.5. By E16.5, both the carotid sinus nerve and carotid body are well differentiated, indicating that target development and innervation precede the appearance of TH in PG cell bodies. These findings are consistent, therefore, with the hypothesis that neuron-target interactions may play a role in regulating ganglion cell development at this stage.

To examine this possibility in more detail, explant cultures of the E16.5 PG were grown in the presence and absence of the carotid body and monitored for total neuronal survival and expression of TH. These studies revealed that cultures of the isolated PG contained relatively few neurons, and virtually no TH cells, after 3 days to 2 weeks *in vitro*. In contrast, co-culture with the carotid body resulted in approximately a 3-fold greater survival of TH cells as compared with the increase in survival of all neuronal cells. Although further studies are required to characterize the nature and specificity of this effect, these preliminary observations suggest that, in addition to its role as a sensory receptor, the carotid body plays a trophic role in regulating maturation of PG afferent neurons during embryogenesis.

ACKNOWLEDGMENTS

Supported by NIH HL-42131 and the Dysautonomia Foundation.

REFERENCES

1. Acker, H., D.W. Lubbers, M.J. Purves, and E.D. Tan. Measurement of partial pressure of oxygen in the carotid body of fetal sheep and newborn lambs. *J. Dev. Physiol.* 2:323-338, 1980.

2. Almaraz, L., and S. Fidone. Carotid sinus nerve C-fibers release catecholamines from the cat carotid body. *Neurosci. Lett.* 67:153-158, 1986.

3. Altman, J., and S. Bayer. Development of the cranial nerve ganglia and related nuclei in the rat. *Adv. Anat. Embryol. Cell Biol.* 74:1-90, 1982.

4. Ayer-LeLievre, C.S., and A. Sieger. Development of substance P-immunoreactive neurons in cranial sensory ganglia of the rat. *Int. J. Dev. Neurosci.* 2:451-463, 1984.

5. Bryan, A.C., G. Bowes, and J.E. Maloney. Control of breathing in the fetus and the newborn. In *Handbook of Physiology.* Section 3, vol.2, ed. N.S. Cherniack and J.G. Widdicombe, 621-647. Bethesda, Md.: Americal Physiological Society, 1986.

6. Cadieux, A., D.R. Springall, P.K. Mulderry, J. Rodrigo, M.A. Ghatei, G. Terenghi, S.R. Bloom, and J.M. Polak. Occurrence, distribution and ontogeny of CGRP immunoreactivity in the rat lower respiratory tract: Effect of capsaicin treatment and surgical denervations. *Neuroscience* 19:605-627, 1986.

7. Dawes, G.S. The central control of fetal breathing and skeletal muscle movements. *J. Physiol.* 346:1-18, 1984.

8. Dempsey, J., E.B. Olson Jr., and J.B. Skatrud. Hormones and neurochemicals in the regulation of breathing. In *Handbook of Physiology.* Section 3, vol. 2, ed. N.S. Cherniack and J.G. Widdicombe, 181-221. Bethesda, Md.: American Physiological Society, 1986.

9. Eden, G.J., and M.A. Hanson. The effect of hypoxia from birth on the biphasic respiratory response of the newborn rat to acute hypoxia. *J. Physiol.* 366:59P, 1985.

10. Fidone, S.J., and C. Gonzales. Initiation and control of chemoreceptor activity in the carotid body. In *Handbook of Phys-

iology, Section 3, vol. 2, ed. N.S. Cherniack and J.G. Widdicombe, 247-312. Bethesda, Md.: American Physiological Society, 1986.

11. Finley, J.C.W., and D.M. Katz. The central projections of carotid body afferent neurons to the brainstem of the rat. Submitted for publication.

12. Goiny, M., H. Lagercrantz, M. Srinivasan, U. Ungerstedt, and Y. Yamamoto. Hypoxia-mediated *in vivo* release of dopamine in the nucleus tractus solitarii of the rabbit. *J. Appl. Physiol.* 70:2395-2400, 1991.

13. Green, T., and G.J. Dockray. Calcitonin gene-related peptide and substance P in afferents to the upper gastrointestinal tract in the rat. *Neurosci. Lett.* 76:151-156, 1987.

14. Haddad, G.G., and R.B. Mellins. Hypoxia and respiratory control in early life. *Ann. Rev. Physiol.* 46:629-643, 1984.

15. Hanson, M.A. Maturation of the peripheral chemoreceptor and CNS components of respiratory control in perinatal life. In *Neurobiology of the Control of Breathing,* ed C. von Euler and H. Lagercrantz, 59-65. New York: Raven Press, 1986.

16. Helke, C.J., and K.M. Hill. Immunohistochemical study of neuropeptides in vagal and glossopharyngeal afferent neurons in the rat. *Neuroscience* 26:539-51, 1988.

17. Hertzberg, T., S. Hellstrom, H. Lagercrantz, and J.-M. Pequignot. Development of the arterial chemoreflex and turnover of carotid body catecholamines in the newborn rat. *J. Physiol.* (London) 425:211-225, 1990.

18. Hertzberg, T., and H. Lagercrantz. Postnatal sensitivity of the peripheral chemoreceptors in newborn infants. *Arch. Dis. Child.* 62:1238-1241, 1987.

19. Jansen, A.M., and V. Cherniack. Development of respiratory control. *Physiol. Rev.* 63:437-483, 1983.

20. Katz, D.M., and M.J. Erb. Developmental regulation of tyrosine hydroxylase expression in primary sensory neurons of the rat. *Dev. Biol.* 137:233-242, 1990.

21. Katz, D.M., and I.B. Black. Expression and regulation of catecholaminergic traits in primary sensory neurons: Relationship to target innervation *in vivo. J. Neurosci.* 6:983-989, 1986.

22. Katz, D.M., and H.J. Karten. Substance P in the vagal sensory ganglia: Localization in cell bodies and pericellular arborizations. *J. Comp. Neurol.* 193:549-564, 1980.

23. Katz, D.M., J.C.W. Finley, L. Stensaas, and S. Fidone. Dopaminergic primary sensory neurons: Neurochemical and ultrastructural studies of peripheral target innervation. In Preparation.

24. Katz, D.M., K.A. Markey, M. Goldstein, and I.B. Black.

Expression of catecholaminergic characteristics by primary sensory neurons in the normal adult rat *in vivo. Proc. Natl. Acad. Sci.* USA, 80:3526-3530, 1983.

25. Kummer, W. Calcitonin gene-related peptide-immunoreactive nerve fibers in carotid body and in carotid sinus. *Exp. Brain Res.* Series 16:84-88, 1987.

26. Kummer, W. Retrograde neuronal labelling and double-staining immunohistochemistry of tachykinin- and calcitonin gene-related peptide-immunoreactive pathways in the carotid sinus nerve of the guinea pig. *J. Autonom. Nerv. Sys.* 23:131-141, 1988.

27. Kummer, W., I.L. Gibbins, P. Stefan, and V. Kapoor. Catecholamines and catecholamine-synthesizing enzymes in guinea-pig sensory ganglia. *Cell Tiss. Res.* 261:595-606, 1990.

28. Lipton, S.A., and S.B. Kater. Neurotransmitter regulation of neuronal outgrowth, plasticity and survival. *Trends Neurosci.* 12:265-270, 1989.

29. Lundberg, J.M., T. Hökfelt, G. Nilsson, L. Terenius, J. Rehfeld, R. Elde, and S. Said. Peptide neurons in the vagus, splanchnic and sciatic nerves. *Acta Physiol. Scand.* 104:499-501, 1978.

30. Markey, K.A., S. Kondo, and M. Goldstein. Purification and characterization of tyrosine hydroxylase from a clonal pheochromocytoma cell line. *Mol. Pharmacol.* 17:79-85, 1980.

31. McDonald, D. M., and R.A. Mitchell. The innervation of glomus cells, ganglion cells and blood vessels in the rat carotid body: A quantitative ultrastructural analysis. *J. Neurocytol.* 4:177-230, 1975.

32. Saetta, M., and J.P. Mortola. Interaction of hypoxic and hypercapnic stimuli on breathing pattern in the newborn rat. *J. Appl. Physiol.* 62:506-512, 1987.

33. Scheibner, T., D.J. Read, and C.E. Sullivan. Distribution of Substance P -immunoreactive structures in the developing cat carotid body. *Brain Res.* 453:72-78, 1988.

34. Srinivasan, M., Y. Yamamoto, H. Persson, and H. Lagercrantz. Birth-related activation of preprotachykinin-A mRNA in the respiratory neural structures of the rabbit. *Pediatric Res.* 29:369-371, 1991.

35. Walker, D. Peripheral and central chemoreceptors in the fetus and newborn. *Ann. Rev. Physiol.* 46:687-703, 1984.

36. Yoshida, M., Y. Kondo, N. Karasawa, K. Yamada, I. Takagi, and Nagatsu. Immunohistocytochemical localization of catecholamine-synthesizing enzymes in suprarenal, superior cervical and nodose ganglia of dogs. *Acta Histochem. Cytochem.* 14:588-595, 1981.

16

Intrinsic Organization and Pontomedullary Connections of Rat Ventral Respiratory Group

Howard H. Ellenberger and Jack L. Feldman

The medullary lateral tegmental field (LTF) is critically important for neural control of respiration. Our knowledge of the remarkably complex intrinsic organization of this region and its network connections with other respiratory neuron populations has been increasingly elaborated over the past decade. Recognition of these complexities is essential in order to understand the functional role of this region and for designing and appropriately interpreting experiments. A major focus of our recent research has been to determine the organization of cell columns within the medullary lateral tegmental field that are involved in the control of breathing. We briefly summarize the most important results based on anatomical studies in rats and then offer our view as to their relevance to the functional organization of the LTF in respiratory regulation.

The ventral respiratory group (VRG), a cell column of the lateral tegmental field, is the most extensive respiratory neuron population in the rat brainstem. It plays a central role in integration of cardiopulmonary afferent inputs, generation of respiratory pattern (and perhaps rhythm), and transmission of respiratory drive to spinal motoneurons. These diverse VRG functions require equally diverse classes of constituent neurons with the appropriate functional properties, morphology and synaptic contacts to carry out these tasks. Although the subdivisions of VRG are often considered to be homogeneous, recent physiological evidence suggests a microorganization that has functional consequences (10). We provide anatomical evidence in this report for a heterogeneous organization of bulbospinal and propriobulbar neurons that might underlie the functional diversity within the VRG.

Many VRG functions are likely to involve interactions with other pontomedullary cell groups in addition to local interactions within the VRG cell column. The connectivity pattern of VRG neurons is therefore an important determinant of their function and must be characterized to understand the network underlying the formation of the complex spatiotemporal pattern of respiratory motoneuron activity.

We characterized the intrinsic organization of the VRG cell column, its anatomical relationship to adjacent cell columns (i.e., nucleus ambiguus, A1/C1 catecholamine cell columns) and its connections with other pontomedullary respiratory groups in a series of neuronal tracing/immunohistochemistry experiments. Spectrally distinct fluorescent retrograde tracers were used to label bulbospinal pre-motor and propriobulbar interneurons of the VRG and vagal motoneurons of nucleus ambiguus. In subsequent studies, bulbospinal and propriobulbar neurons of the VRG and catecholamine neurons of the A1 and C1 cell groups were simultaneously labeled in the rat medulla by a combination of retrograde tracing and immunohistochemical detection. Combined retrograde and anterograde neuronal tracing experiments were performed to label the brainstem connections of the VRG.

METHODS

The pontomedullary neuronal labelling patterns described below are based on neuronal tracer injections into physiologically identified sites within inspiratory spinal (phrenic nucleus) or medullary (rostral VRG) neuron populations. The methods for injections of neuronal tracers, catecholamine immunohistochemistry, and data analysis have been previously described (3, 4, 5).

RESULTS

Intrinsic VRG organization. Injections of fluorescent retrograde tracer into the phrenic nucleus and rostral (r) VRG labeled cell somata in a cell column extending the entire length of the medullary LTF, from the rostral C1 segment up to the caudal edge of the facial nucleus. Vagal motoneurons, labeled after fast blue application to the cervical vagus nerve, formed a parallel cell column in the medullary LTF. At the most caudal medullary level, distinctly labeled propriobulbar and bulbospinal neurons were coextensive in the region of nucleus retroambigualis at the level of the pyramidal decussation. This level corresponds to the physiologically identified caudal (c) VRG as described in the cat (7). Both classes of VRG neurons increased in number, and labeled vagal motoneurons also began to appear between the levels of the pyramidal decussation and the obex. The peak density of all three classes of neurons spanned the level of the area postrema. All three classes of neurons decreased in number rostral to obex except for a ventrolateral subdivision of VRG propriobulbar neurons (see below), but then increased again at the level of the compact division of rostral nucleus ambiguus. The facial nucleus formed the rostral boundary of each type of labeled neuron; only a few labeled neurons of each class were found dorsal to the caudal portion of the facial nucleus. Labeled vagal motoneurons of the cervical vagus nerve formed a bimodal rostrocaudal distribution. These two divisions of the vagal motoneuron population correspond to the external and loose division of caudal nucleus ambiguus, and the external and compact divisions of rostral nucleus ambiguus. Neurons within the semicompact division of nucleus ambiguus at an intermediate rostrocaudal level were not labeled since this division contains mainly pharyngeal motoneurons whose axons travel in the glossopharyngeal nerve and the pharyngeal ramus of the vagus nerve (1). Labeled bulbospinal and propriobulbar VRG neurons also formed two rostrocaudal divisions that paralleled the caudal and rostral divisions of nucleus ambiguus. Based on comparison with the cat, these two divisions of VRG neurons represent the rVRG and Bötzinger Complex (BötC), respectively (7).

Subnuclear organization of the VRG. Labeled neurons at the level of nucleus retroambigualis (caudal to nucleus ambiguus) were clustered to form a single ventrolateral to dorsomedial band. At the caudal border of area postrema, labeled bulbospinal and propriobulbar neurons both were clustered into distinct ventrolateral and dorsomedial subdivisions within the VRG that were distinguished by the morphology and orientation of their constituent neurons. Labeled neurons of all three types were found in both subdivisions; bulbospinal neurons were the most numerous type, followed by propriobulbar neurons, and lastly by vagal motoneurons. Propriobulbar neurons usually formed a continuous band throughout the two subdivisions, but more rostrally (around the level of obex) they were often clustered separately within these groups as the ventrolateral division became more fully developed. Vagal motoneurons were clustered within a more confined region of these groups than bulbospinal or propriobulbar neurons and were sometimes concentrated between the ventrolateral and dorsomedial divisions (corresponding to the loose formation of caudal nucleus ambiguus). Vagal motoneurons that were more broadly scattered through the two VRG subdivisions formed the external division of caudal nucleus ambiguus (1). At the level just caudal to rostral nucleus ambiguus, labeled bulbospinal neurons and vagal motoneurons fell to minimum numbers, whereas propriobulbar neurons rose to peak numbers. This VRG region (immediately caudal to BötC) may form a functionally distinct division of VRG, containing a large pool of interneurons that project to the more caudal level of rVRG that contains peak numbers of bulbospinal neurons. We apply the term pre-Bötzinger Complex (pre-BötC) to this VRG level to emphasize the differential distribution of propriobulbar and bulbospinal neurons in the rostral versus caudal portions of rVRG.

At the level of rostral nucleus ambiguus, labeled neurons formed three distinct groups. One group, the compact division of rostral nucleus ambiguus, was composed entirely of densely packed labeled vagal motoneurons. Medial to this group was a dorsomedial subdivision of BötC composed mainly of small to medium sized labeled propriobulbar neurons, and very few labeled bulbospinal neurons. The third group of neurons formed a larger cluster corresponding to the main division of BötC and was characterized by a diffuse scattering of labeled vagal motoneurons ventral to the compact division of rostral nucleus ambiguus (corresponding to the external division of rostral nucleus ambiguus) intermingled with labeled bulbospinal and propriobulbar neurons.

VRG and catecholamine neurons. Retrogradely labeled propriobulbar and bulbospinal VRG neurons and the catecholamine immunoreactive neurons of the A1/C1 groups formed adjacent, parallel cell columns extending from the level of the pyramidal decussation to the facial nucleus. At the level of the pyramidal decussation, A1 neurons (dopamine-β-hydroxylase-[DBH-] immunoreactive) were ventral to cVRG neurons. From the level of the pyramidal decussation to the caudal border of area postrema, the A1 group and cVRG formed separate dense clusters, the A1 group being ventral and lateral to cVRG. At the level of area postrema, neurons of the rVRG and A1 group increased in number and covered a larger area of the ventrolateral medulla, with rVRG neurons nested immediately dorsal to A1/C1 neurons. In the rostral medulla, neurons of the BötC were dorsal and lateral to most C1 neurons (phenylethanolamine N-methyltransferase-[PNMT-] immunoreactive). The C1 neurons were distributed over a larger area within the lateral paragigantocellular nucleus (PGCL), so individual C1 neurons could be found medial, ventral, and lateral to BötC neurons. The facial nucleus formed the rostral border of both the BötC and C1 group, although a few BötC neurons were labeled dorsal and a few C1 cells were labeled ventral to the caudal facial nucleus.

Most VRG neurons were clustered dorsal to the A1/C1 groups, but at the level of rVRG and BötC, A1 and C1 neurons intermingled with rVRG and BötC neurons. Some A1/C1 neurons were displaced from the main group and were located within the rVRG or BötC. These displaced A1/C1 neurons could not be distinguished from neighboring rVRG or BötC neurons on the basis of cell size or morphology. Despite the intermingling of DBH- and PNMT-immunoreactive neurons with retrogradely labeled VRG neurons, there were no neurons double-labeled with the retrograde tracer and the immunohistochemical reaction product.

Neuronal projections to rVRG injection sites. The Kölliker-Fuse nucleus (K-F) contained the highest density of retrogradely labeled cell bodies in the pons after rhodamine bead injections centered in the region of rVRG. Labeled neurons densely filled the K-F region, forming a narrow, continuous dorsoventral band of cells extending from the ventrolateral tip of the brachium conjunctivum downward to the A6 catecholamine cell group. At the dorsal border of K-F, labeled cells merged with those in the medial and lateral parabrachial nuclei (PB) where a much lower density of labeled cells was located. A small number of labeled cells were located medial to K-F and ventral to the medial PB within the subceruleus region.

In the caudal pons, labeled neurons formed a single, diffusely organized and sparsely populated column in the ventrolateral portion of the pontine lateral tegmental field dorsal to the superior olive or between the superior olive and the fibers of the facial nerve in the region of the A5 catecholamine cell group. A few somata were also labeled in the raphe magnus in the caudal pons.

Cell somata were labeled in the rostral ventrolateral medulla forming a small cluster between the facial nucleus and the fibers of the rubrospinal tract running along the ventrolateral medullary surface. Some cells were located superficial to the fiber tract immediately adjacent to the ventrolateral surface of the medulla. A homologous cell group termed the retrotrapezoid nucleus (RTN) was originally described by anatomical means in the cat (13). The RTN has been subsequently studied by electrophysiological methods in the cat (2) and rat (11) so we apply that term to labeled cells in this region in the rat. Cell somata were also labeled in the rostral division of the PGCL medial to the facial nucleus.

Cell somata were also labeled in the retrofacial division of PGCL. One group had a diffuse distribution throughout the PGCL, while the other was confined to the regions ventral and medial to the compact division of the rostral nucleus ambiguus. Neurons in the latter location have previously been designated as the BötC in the cat (7, 13) and rat (3, 4). Labeled cell somata extended caudally from BötC the entire length of the medulla to the level of the pyramidal decussation, forming the continuous bilateral longitudinal VRG cell columns in the lateral tegmental field.

Labeled cell somata were also located in the dorsomedial medulla, within the area postrema and several subnuclei of the nucleus of the solitary tract (NTS). Labeled cells were located in the ventrolateral and intermediate NTS subnuclei and in a continuous band extending from the dorsomedial tip of the tractus solitarius to the border of area postrema in dorsomedial NTS. Cell soma labelling in these subnuclei extended from the medullary level just rostral to the area postrema caudally to merge with labeled cell somata in the commissural NTS subnucleus. Labeled cells were only occasionally observed in the medial NTS subnucleus.

Labeled cell somata were also located within the raphe magnus, pallidus and obscurus, in the magnocellular tegmental field and occasionally in the spinal trigeminal nucleus. Highly localized depositions of *phaseolus vulgaris* leucoagglutinin into the rVRG labeled axons, terminal arborizations and presumptive synaptic varicosities in several pontomedullary regions. Labeled axons emerged both rostrally and caudally from injection sites and formed dense arborizations with *en passant* varicosities throughout the rostrocaudal length of the ipsilateral medullary LTF. Fibers that exited the lateral tegmental field primarily followed one of four principal trajectories. One route coursed caudally down the ipsilateral spinal cord. A second group separated from the first and coursed dorsally, entering NTS and leaving a few *en passant* varicosities before decussating to the contralateral medulla. Individual axons could not be traced continuously beyond this decussation, but the general pattern of the route appeared to include terminal arborizations in the contralateral lateral tegmental field in a region homologous to the ipsilateral terminations, and a component coursed caudally to the contralateral spinal cord. The bilateral terminal arborizations in the LTF appeared to overlap with the regions containing rhodamine-labeled cell somata, corresponding to all levels of VRG. In the rostral medulla, the terminal arborizations broadened beyond this region, especially ipsilaterally, to leave varicosities in the region of PGCL. A third trajectory left the ipsilateral LTF and decussated in the rostral medulla to arborize within the homologous contralateral LTF and to a small extent in the facial nucleus. The fourth trajectory coursed rostrally in the ventrolateral medulla and left *en passant* varicosities in the lateral portions of the facial nucleus before continuing an ascent to the rostral pons, where the K-F region was filled with extremely dense arborizations with terminal varicosities. Minor terminations extended from K-F into medial and lateral PB and the subceruleus region. Some labeled fibers crossed the midline at this level and made terminations to a much lesser extent in the K-F/PB region.

DISCUSSION

Neuronal tracing techniques have revealed an anatomical subnuclear organization of the VRG cell column that includes three principal rostrocaudal subdivisions (four including the pre-BötC), as well as distinct ventrolateral and dorsomedial subdivisions of the rVRG and BötC (3). Physiological studies demonstrate a functional heterogeneity of neurons within different regions of the VRG column. This heterogeneity is revealed by the variety of discharge patterns of respiratory-related VRG neurons, including (1) excitatory (expiratory) bulbospinal neurons of the cVRG, (2) excitatory (inspiratory) bulbospinal neurons of the rVRG, and (3) inhibitory (expiratory) neurons of the BötC. Propriobulbar neurons with a variety of discharge patterns are distributed throughout the VRG cell column. The pre-BötC portion of VRG contains early (decrementing), plateau and late inspiratory neurons (6, 12). The pre-BötC may have an especially important interneuronal function via propriobulbar neurons antecedent to more caudally located VRG propriobulbar or bulbospinal neurons (3, 6, 12). Likely roles for these pre-BötC neurons include sensorimotor processing, pattern generation (7, 9), and perhaps rhythm generation (8; Smith et al., this volume). Functional heterogeneity of VRG neurons has also been revealed by focal stimulation of cell bodies within the rVRG by pressure injection of small quantities of excitatory amino acids (10). Injections of glutamate produce site-specific effects on phrenic nerve activity when applied at different points within rVRG. Thus, the widely held view that the VRG is a functionally or anatomically homogeneous cell column can no longer be accepted.

Our combined retrograde tracing/immunohistochemistry studies demonstrate that the VRG, vagal motoneurons of nucleus ambiguus, and A1/C1 catecholamine groups are parallel and incompletely segregated cell columns in the medullary LTF. The proximal anatomical relationship between each of the identified classes of neurons with the possibility of overlapping of their dendritic fields suggests that neurons in these groups may receive common afferent inputs, and that local processing between neurons within these groups may couple the activity of these neurons. The proximity and co-mingling of VRG neurons, vagal motoneurons, and catecholamine neurons within the ventrolateral medulla is important to consider when investigating the neural function(s) of this region. Electrical or chemical stimulation and anatomical tracing studies with target sites in the ventrolateral medulla cannot, without stringent and difficult controls, provide clearly interpretable results because of the close proximity and incidental inclusion of functionally diverse neurons. Effector responses to stimulation observed for one system may be secondary to altered activity of the other system. Classification of neurons in this region based on activity pattern is not sufficient to distinguish respiratory from cardiovascular neurons, since the preganglionic efferent activity of sympathetic and parasympathetic neurons can have respiratory-modulated activity patterns; in fact, neurons in this region may have some role in generating the respiratory modulation of autonomic activity.

Based on results of both retrograde and anterograde experiments, the following relationship between the rVRG and other pontomedullary cell groups were established.

1. The rVRG has marked reciprocal connections with all levels of the VRG complex on both sides of the medulla and with the K-F/PB region in the pons.
2. The rVRG has modest reciprocal connections with NTS and PGCL and rare reciprocal connections with raphe, medial tegmental field, and the spinal trigeminal nucleus.
3. The rVRG has only efferent projections to the facial nucleus.
4. The rVRG receives only afferent projections from RTN, area postrema, and pontine lateral tegmental field.

The presence of either reciprocal or unidirectional connections between rVRG neurons and neurons of other nuclear groups suggest possible mechanisms for each type of connection in generating the pattern of breathing.

Reciprocal connections are a prerequisite for such mechanisms as reciprocal and recurrent excitation or inhibition between neuron populations. These mechanisms could play a role in generating the augmenting ramp of neuronal activity during inspiration, participate in phase transitions, or generate expiratory neuron activity (7). Reciprocal connections may also coordinate the timing of neuronal activity of the left and right brainstem respiratory circuitry, and the bilateral motor outputs to muscles of the upper airway, diaphragm, intercostal, and abdominal muscles.

Regions that receive only efferent rVRG projections may receive respiratory-modulated inputs but do not provide any direct (i.e., monosynaptic) feedback to rVRG neurons (e.g., facial motoneurons). Neurons that provide only afferent inputs to rVRG (e.g., area postrema, RTN, and pontine lateral tegmental field) may convey sensory information or descending drive to rVRG neurons that cannot be modulated by direct feedback from rVRG neurons.

Future experimental designs must take into consideration the heterogeneous organization of the VRG. A further understanding of the respiratory function of neurons in this region will ultimately require precise knowledge of the local organization, the connectivity patterns, and neurotransmitters or neuromodulators contained in each class of neurons in this region.

ACKNOWLEDGMENTS

Supported by NIH grants NS24742 and HL37941. We thank our colleagues in The Systems Neurobiology Laboratory, especially C.A. Connelly, J.C. Smith, and M.R. Otto.

References

1. Bieger, D., and D.A. Hopkins. Viscerotopic representation of the upper alimentary tract in the medulla oblongata in the rat: The nucleus ambiguus. *J. Comp. Neurol.* 262:546-582, 1987.

2. Connelly, C.A., H.H. Ellenberger, and J.L. Feldman. Respiratory activity in the retrotrapezoid nucleus of cat. *Am. J. Physiol.: Lung Cell. Mol. Physiol.* 258:L33-L44, 1990.

3. Ellenberger, H.H., and J.L. Feldman. Subnuclear organization of the lateral tegmental field of the rat. I. Nucleus ambiguus and ventral respiratory group. *J. Comp. Neurol.* 294:202-211, 1990.

4. Ellenberger, H.H., and J.L. Feldman. Brainstem connections of the ventral respiratory group of the rat. *Brain Res.* 513:35-42, 1990.

5. Ellenberger, H.H., J.L. Feldman, and W.-Z. Zhan. Subnuclear organization of the lateral tegmental field of the rat. II. Catecholamine neurons and ventral respiratory group. *J. Comp. Neurol.* 294:212-220, 1990.

6. Ezure, K., M. Manabe, and K. Otake. Excitation and inhibition of medullary inspiratory neurons by two types of burst inspiratory neurons in the cat. *Neurosci. Lett.* 104:303-308, 1989.

7. Feldman, J.L. Neurophysiology of breathing in mammals. In *Handbook of physiology,* Section 1, vol. 4, ed. F.E. Bloom, 463-524. Bethesda, Md.: American Physiological Society, 1986.

8. Feldman, J.L. Emergent properties of neural mechanisms controlling breathing in mammals. In *Respiratory Muscles and Their Neuromotor Control,* ed. G.C. Sieck, S.G. Gandevia and W.E. Cameron, p. 3-8. New York: Alan R. Liss, 1987.

9. Feldman, J.L., J.C. Smith, H.H. Ellenberger, M. Fournier, and C.A. Connelly. Respiration in mammals: Rhythm and pattern. In *Cellular and Neuronal Oscillators,* ed. J.W. Jacklet, 435-456. New York: Marcel Dekker, Inc., 1988.

10. McCrimmon, D.R., J.L. Feldman, and D.F. Speck. Respiratory motoneuronal activity is altered by picomole injections of glutamate in the cat brainstem. *J. Neurosci.* 6:2384-2392, 1986.

11. Pearce, R.A., R.L. Stornetta, and P.G. Guyenet. Retrotrapezoid nucleus in the rat. *Neurosci. Lett.* 101:138-142, 1989.

12. Segers, L.S., R. Shannon, S. Saporta, and B. Lindsey. Functional associations among simultaneously monitored lateral medullary respiratory neurons in the cat. I. Evidence for excitatory and inhibitory actions of inspiratory neurons. *J. Neurophysiol.* 57:1078-1100, 1987.

13. Smith, J.C., D.E. Morrison, H.H. Ellenberger, M.R. Otto, and J.L. Feldman. Brainstem projections to the major respiratory neuron populations in cat medulla. *J. Comp. Neurol.* 281:69-96, 1989.

PART IV

Central Integration of Respiratory Afferents

17

An Overview

K.M. Spyer

A large body of information is available on the range of afferent inputs that modify moment by moment the pattern of respiratory activity. Several chapters of this volume have been devoted to this issue and there are a number of excellent reviews on this topic (32, and others). It is, however, important to recognize that these same afferents influence other systems and that their major physiological role is the maintenance of cardio-respiratory homeostasis (9, 28). Given the importance of their role it is perhaps surprising that much less is known of the central processing of these inputs in achieving their objectives. The last decade has seen a dramatic increase in our understanding of the physiological actions of the central respiratory network in mediating these reflex responses (14) but it is premature to claim that a detailed picture of the synaptic processes has been obtained, or that the pharmacology of these interactions is understood. The purpose of this report is to highlight some of the achievements in this area of investigation and to identify those areas where one can expect progress in the next few years.

In compiling this review an attempt will be made to divide this broad canvas into distinct and relevant topics. These issues include afferent processing in the brainstem, supramedullary integration of pulmonary reflexes, and the central pharmacology of reflex respiratory control.

AFFERENT INPUTS TO THE MEDULLA

A wide range of afferents with endings in the airways and lungs relay to the medulla via the vagus. Considerable anatomical information exists in the literature concerning the diverse patterns of projection of these vagal afferents within the nucleus tractus solitarius (NTS) (19, 30). There are also physiological data indicating the interactions that occur between these afferents. To a degree the functional implications of their actions in the patterning of respiratory activity is becoming known. In addition the arterial baroreceptors and chemoreceptors both—those relaying via the vagus from the aortic arch and those relaying via the IXth cranial nerve from the carotid bifurcation—also send their fibers to defined regions of the NTS (24, 30). The gross anatomical picture that has been obtained with tracing techniques is often confusing, and indeed conflicting information has often been obtained by different groups for no easily explained reason (see 19 for discussion). However, with regard to slowly adapting vagal pulmonary stretch afferents (SARs), an extremely precise picture has emerged from the combined work of numerous laboratories.

The general vagal innervation of the NTS suggested that pulmonary stretch afferents projected into both the medial and the ventrolateral subnuclei of the NTS, as well as to other defined NTS subnuclei. Using antidromic mapping techniques, the pattern of projection of individual SARs was shown to conform to this pattern, although there appeared a predominance of input to the medial NTS (11). This observation was confirmed using a spike-triggered averaging technique (3). The more limited input to the ventrolateral and intermediate subnuclei have since been substantiated in the revealing studies of Richter and his colleagues (21, 22 as examples). Here the afferents were impaled intracellularly within the NTS and their patterns of termination mapped after horseradish peroxidase- (HRP-) labeling. Terminal branches of SARs were seen to arborize over considerable areas of the ventrolateral, ventral, and intermediate subnuclei and were shown ultrastructurally to contact neurons in these areas. This provides an anatomical substrate for the electrophysiological demonstrations of monosynaptic excitatory connections between SARs and a portion of the inspiratory neurons of the ventrolateral NTS (1, 2, 3) and onto pump or "P" cells (1) of the NTS (i.e., neurons with no central respiratory rhythm but receiving a lung inflation input). These neurons are more widely dispersed through the nucleus (see 10, McCrimmon et al. this volume). This approach of intracellular labeling of functionally defined afferents has been applied successfully to laryngeal mechanoreceptor and chemoreceptor afferents (see 29). Here the primary projection zone and site of termination was again the ventrolateral subnucleus, but a marked input of mechanoreceptor afferents to the dorsolateral NTS was observed. Laryngeal chemoreceptor afferents had more restricted projections close to the obex extending to the same general subnuclei of the NTS.

The distinctive patterns of projections of other afferents have been summarized at length elsewhere (see 30). It is, however, worthwhile detailing the case of the arterial chemoreceptors since they exert a potent influence on respiratory activity. Evidence has accrued to suggest that while they project exclusively to the NTS, they do not affect respiration by means of a monosynaptic connection with the dorsal respiratory neurons (see 23). Indeed studies have suggested that the most direct action of the chemoreceptor input is an inhibitory one, whilst overall reflexly they exert a powerful excitation to inspiration. Recent antidromic mapping studies have indicated that individual carotid body chemoreceptor afferents send a marked projection into the medial and commissural NTS at levels close to the obex with only limited input into the ventrolateral subnucleus, which contains the dorsal group of inspiratory neurons (12). Other electrophysiological studies show that numerous nonrespiratory neurons of the NTS, and particularly those in areas corresponding to this afferent projection zone, receive excitatory input from the arterial chemoreceptors (18, 25). Some potential second-order neurons have been labeled intracellularly with HRP; these were restricted to the commissural NTS overlying the tractus solitarius (31).

The major feature of these investigations is the demonstration that many nonrespiratory neurons of the NTS, particularly those localized in more dorsal regions of the nucleus, receive powerful inputs from a range of afferents that affect the respiratory system. The specific connections made by these interneurons and their integrative role remain to be elucidated, but evidence has been presented in this volume to suggest that the integrity of many of these neurons is essential for the functioning of the Hering-Breuer reflex (see McCrimmon et al., this volume). These regions of the NTS have profound, and often reciprocal, connections with areas of the brainstem concerned with both respiratory and autonomic function (see 15, 17).

BRAINSTEM CONNECTIONS IN AFFERENT INTEGRATION

There has been a long-held belief that the Hering-Breuer reflex involves a pontine relay. Such a relay was implicit in the von Euler model of respiratory rhythmogenesis that the inspiratory off-switch involved the pons and depended to an extent on the ascending lung stretch afferent input (13). The negation of this requirement in the three phase model developed by Richter for respiratory rhythm generation (27) does not dismiss the potential importance of pontine structures either in respiratory control in general or in the mediation of the pulmonary stretch reflex in particular. The abundant reciprocal connections between the NTS and the pontine Kölliker-Fuse nucleus and the parabrachial complex, and the equivalent connections into the ventral respiratory complex of the medulla attest to this possibility. Cohen and his colleagues, however, provide compelling evidence that inspiratory modulated pontine neurons do not contribute to the inspiratory off-switch and exert their influences on the medullary inspiratory population only via diffuse connections (Cohen et al., this volume). The pontine neurons themselves do not appear to receive a particularly direct synaptic input from either vagal or laryngeal afferents.

These observations and other data regarding the role of the pons in respiratory control may, however, have some considerable relevance given the fact that these pontine structures receive descending inputs from the cortex and diencephalon. Further the recent demonstration that the cerebellum has a respiratory representation and receives proprioceptive inputs from the thorax (Baker et al., this volume) merely adds more credence to this hypothesis.

In this context additional information has been obtained regarding the role of the cerebellum in eliciting cardiovascular and respiratory responses. The uvula of the posterior vermis (Lobule IXb) in both the cat and rabbit can modify both respiration and cardiovascular variables (4, 5) although it does not receive an afferent input from either vagal afferents or sinus and aortic baroreceptors (7). The pattern of evoked response is dependent on the presence of anaesthetic agents. In the anaesthetized preparation apnea, bradycardia, and a depressor response are elicited; but in the unanesthetized, decerebrate animal an apneusis, tachycardia, and pressor responses are seen. The appropriate regional blood flow changes were also observed in the two preparations. Interestingly, in the conscious rabbit, electrical stimulation of the uvula produced the responses seen in the decerebrate animal together with behavioural arousal (8). Anterograde tracing techniques have shown that the Purkinje cells of the uvula cortex project to the caudal region of the cerebellar fastigial nucleus, the pontine lateral parabrachial nucleus and the dorsal medulla (6). Activation of those regions of parabrachial nucleus that receive an innervation from the uvula evokes a pattern of response equivalent to that seen in the decerebrate unanesthetized animal when activating the uvula cortex (26). Bicuculline (a $GABA_A$ receptor antagonist) injected at this site abolishes the depressor response evoked from the uvula in the anaesthetized animal, consistent with the established inhibitory action of Purkinje axons. The physiological role of the uvula and the relationship of the pons in integrating inputs from the forebrain and cerebellum remains to be resolved. The potential is, however, significant since the parabrachial complex has important connections to the lower brainstem respiratory and cardiovascular cell groups and to the NTS.

PHARMACOLOGY OF CENTRAL RESPIRATORY CONTROL

There is an obvious scientific and clinical interest in establishing the chemistry of the synaptic connections that mediate central respiratory control. As yet we have only a rudimentary appreciation of the nature and diversity of the various neurotransmitters involved. Certain global indications of the role of excitatory and inhibitory amino acids in the reflex control of respiration have been obtained through the systemic administration of their various antagonists (see Speck et al., this volume) but the widespread action of these materials means that relatively little can be extracted from these data. In regard to pulmonary reflexes it is notable that afferent transmission in the NTS is considered to be largely glutaminergic, involving non-N-methyl-D-aspartate (non-NMDA) receptors (see 16). A selective antagonist at these receptors, 6-cyano-7-nitroquinoxaline-2, 3-dione (CNQX), antagonized the lung stretch reflex when injected into a restricted region of the NTS that contains ''P'' cells (McCrimmon et al., this volume), and the same was true of the non-specific amino acid antagonist kynurate. There is also compelling evidence that $GABA_A$ receptors in the NTS play a role in the regulation of cardiovascular reflexes (20). Other evidence has been cited regarding similar receptors influencing respiratory and cardiovascular mechanisms in the pons (see above). Details are also emerging on the chemical content of synaptic boutons on identified respiratory neurons, although the source of the afferent input has not yet been determined (see Lipski et al., this volume). There is clearly a requirement for a combination of electrophysiological and neuropharmacological approaches to establish the precise role of putative neurotransmitters in reflex function.

CONCLUSIONS

The understanding of the central organization of respiratory control is dependent on the use of a wide range of contemporary neuroscientific disciplines. The issues raised in this overview can only be addressed in this way, but it is essential to retain an awareness of the physiological consequences of the changes in respiratory activity that are induced from central structures. To determine the central basis of regulation, reflexes such as the pulmonary stretch reflex offer an ideal tool with which to test hypotheses. Experiments such as the ones discussed in this overview and described in the following chapters can be expected to reveal much information of fundamental and clinical importance.

ACKNOWLEDGMENTS

Original studies reported in this paper were supported by grants from the Medical Research Council and British Heart Foundation. Prof. K.M. Spyer is in receipt of a Nolfson University Award.

REFERENCES

1. Averill, D.B., W.E. Cameron, and A.J. Berger. Monosynaptic excitation of dorsal medullary respiratory neurons by slowly adapting pulmonary stretch receptors afferents. *J. Neurophysiol.* 52:771-785, 1984.

2. Backman, S.B., C. Anders, D. Ballantyne, N. Rohrig, H. Camerer, S. Mifflin, D. Jordan, H. Dickhaus, and K.M. Spyer. Evidence for a monosynaptic connection between slowly adapting pulmonary stretch receptor afferents and inspiratory beta neurones. *Pflügers Arch.* 401:129-136, 1984.

3. Berger, A.J., and D.B. Averill. Projection of single pulmonary stretch receptors to solitary tract region. *J. Neurophysiol.* 49:819-830, 1983.

4. Bradley, D.J., J.F.R. Paton, and K.M. Spyer. Cardiovascular responses evoked from the fastigial region of the cerebellum in anaesthetized and decerebrate rabbits. *J. Physiol.* 392:475-491, 1987.

5. Bradley, D.J., J.P. Pascoe, J.F.R. Paton, and K.M. Spyer. Cardiovascular and respiratory responses evoked from the posterior cerebellar cortex and fastigial nucleus in the cat. *J. Physiol.* 393:107-121, 1987.

6. Bradley, D.J., B. Ghelarducci, A. La Noce, J.F.R. Paton, L. Sebastiani, K.M. Spyer, and R.M. Sykes. Cardiovascular actions are exerted by the uvula cortex through two distinct efferent pathways in the anaesthetized or decerebrate rabbit. *J. Physiol.* 415:83P, 1989.

7. Bradley, D.J., B. Ghelarducci, A. La Noce, J.F.R. Paton, K.M. Spyer, and D.J. Withington-Wray. An electrophysiological and anatomical study of afferents reaching the cerebellar uvula in the rabbit. *Exp. Physiol.* 75:163-177, 1990.

8. Bradley, D.J., B. Ghelarducci, A. La Noce, and K.M. Spyer. Autonomic and somatic responses evoked by stimulation of the cerebellar uvula in the conscious rabbit. *Exp. Physiol.* 75:179-186, 1990.

9. Daly, M. de B. Interactions between respiration and circulation. In *Handbook of Physiology,* Section 3, vol. 2, ed. N.S. Cherniack and J.G. Widdicombe, 529-594. Bethesda, Md.: American Physiological Society, 1986.

10. Davies, R.O., L. Kubin, and A.I. Pack. Pulmonary stretch receptor relay neurones of the cat: Location and contralateral projections. *J. Physiol.* 383:571-586, 1987.

11. Donoghue, S., M. Garcia, D. Jordan, and K.M. Spyer. The brainstem projections of pulmonary stretch afferent neurones in cats and rabbits. *J. Physiol.* 322:353-363, 1982.

12. Donoghue, S., R.B. Felder, D.G. Jordan, and K.M. Spyer. The central projections of carotid baroreceptors and chemoreceptors in the cat: A neurophysiological study. *J. Physiol.* 347:397-409, 1984.

13. Euler, C. von. The functional organization of the respiratory phase-switching. *Fed. Proc.* 36:2375-2380, 1977.

14. Feldman, J.L. Neurophysiology of breathing in mammals. In *Handbook of Physiology,* Section 1, vol. 4., ed. F.E. Bloom, 463-524. Bethesda, Md.: American Physiological Society, 1987.

15. Fulwiler, C.E., and C.B. Saper. Subnuclear organization of the efferent connections of the parabrachial nucleus in the rat. *Brain Res. Rev.* 7:229-259, 1984.

16. Glaum, S.R., P.A. Brooks, S.M. Murphy, and R.J. Miller. Activation of 5-HT receptors causes pre- and postsynaptic effects in the nucleus tractus solitarius (NTS) of the rat *in vitro. Proc. of Physiological Society,* C121:146P, 1991.

17. Herbert, H., M.M. Moga, and C.B. Saper. Connections of the parabrachial nucleus with the nucleus of the solitary tract and the medullary reticular formation of the rat. *J. Comp. Neurol.* 293:540-580, 1990.

18. Izzo, P.N., R.J. Lin, D.W. Richter, and K.M. Spyer. Physiological and morphological identification of neurones receiving arterial chemoreceptive afferent input in the nucleus tractus solitarius of the cat. *J. Physiol.* 399:31P, 1988.

19. Jordan, D., and K.M. Spyer. Brainstem integration of cardiovascular and pulmonary afferent activity. In *Progress in Brain Research,* Vol. 67, ed. F. Cervero and J.F.B. Morrison, 295-314. New York: Elsevier Science Publishers, 1986.

20. Jordan, D.J., S.W. Mifflin, and K.M. Spyer. Hypothalamic inhibition of neurones in the nucleus tractus solitarius of the cat is GABA mediated. *J. Physiol.* 399:389-404, 1988.

21. Kalia, M., and D.W. Richter. Morphology of physiologically identified slowly adapting lung stretch receptor afferents stained with intra-axonal horseradish peroxidase in the nucleus of the tractus solitarius of the cat. I. A light microscopic analysis. *J. Comp. Neurol.* 241:503-520, 1985.

22. Kalia, M., and D.W. Richter. Morphology of physiologically identified slowly adapting lung stretch receptor afferents stained with intra-axonal horseradish peroxidase in the nucleus of the tractus solitarius of the cat. II. An ultrastructural analysis. *J. Comp. Neurol.* 241:521-535, 1985.

23. Lipski, J., R.M. McAllen, and K.M. Spyer. The carotid chemoreceptor input to the respiratory neurones of the nucleus of tractus solitarius. *J. Physiol.* 269:797-810, 1977.

24. Loewy, A.D. Central autonomic pathways. In *Central regulation of autonomic functions*, ed. A.D. Loewy and K.M. Spyer, 88-103. New York: Oxford University Press, 1990.

25. Mifflin, S. The arterial chemoreceptor input to nonrespiratory cells in the nucleus of the tractus solitarius (NTS). *Proceedings of the International Conference on the Modulation of Respiratory Pattern: Peripheral and Central Mechanisms,* 65, 1991.

26. Paton, J.F.R., and K.M. Spyer. Brain stem regions mediating the cardiovascular responses elicited from the posterior cerebellar cortex in the rabbit. *J. Physiol.* 427:533-552, 1990.

27. Richter, D.W. Generation and maintenance of the respiratory rhythm. *J. Exp. Biol.* 100:93-108, 1982.

28. Richter, D.W., and K.M. Spyer. Cardiorespiratory control. In *Central regulation of autonomic functions,* eds. A.D. Loewy and K.M. Spyer, 189-207. New York: Oxford University Press, 1990.

29. Schwarzacher, S.W., K. Anders, and D.W. Richter. Central projection of laryngeal afferents in the cat. *Proceedings of the International Conference on the Modulation of Respiratory Pattern: Peripheral and Central Mechanisms,* 59, 1991.

30. Spyer, K.M. The central nervous organization of reflex circulatory control. In *Central regulation of autonomic functions,* ed. A. D. Loewy and K.M. Spyer, 168-188. New York: Oxford University Press, 1990.

31. Spyer, K.M., P.N. Izzo, R.J. Lin, J.F.R. Paton, L.F. Silva-Carvalho, and D.W. Richter. The central nervous organization of the carotid body chemoreceptor reflex. In *Chemoreceptors and chemoreceptor reflexes,* ed. H. Akher, A. Trzebski, and R.G. O'Regan, 317-321. New York: Plenum Press, 1990.

32. Widdicombe, J.G. Pulmonary and respiratory tract receptors. *J. Exp. Biol.* 100:41-58, 1982.

18

The Breuer-Hering Reflex Requires Excitatory Amino Acid Neurotransmission in a Discrete Region of the Nucleus Tractus Solitarius

Donald R. McCrimmon, Ann C. Bonham, and Sharon K. Coles

In most mammalian species lung inflation during eupneic breathing activates slowly adapting pulmonary stretch receptors (SAR) thereby shortening inspiration and prolonging expiration. Although these reflex effects are often collectively referred to as the Breuer-Hering reflex, it is not clear that the central nervous system pathways giving rise to inspiratory termination are necessarily the same as those lengthening expiration (cf. 12). The focus of this discussion will be on the identity and synaptic pharmacology of interneurons mediating the expiratory lengthening response, which, for simplicity, we will refer to as the Breuer-Hering reflex.

Large myelinated afferent fibers arising from SAR course in the vagus nerve and terminate within the nucleus of the tractus solitarius (NTS). Within the NTS, SAR monosynaptically activate two classes of neurons, pump or P cells (4) and I(+) (9) or R_β neurons (3). Pump cells are strongly activated by lung inflation but do not receive a centrally generated inspiratory drive (6). In contrast, I(+) neurons receive a central inspiratory drive which is augmented by input from SAR. Since these are the only groups of neurons found to receive monosynaptic input from SAR, it is probable that activity in one or both groups is required for production of the Breuer-Hering reflex.

Attempts to identify the axonal trajectories of both groups of neurons have been partly successful, but no compelling evidence has been provided for a role of either group in the Breuer-Hering reflex. Many I(+) neurons monosynaptically activate phrenic motoneurons (2, 17). While this does not preclude a role for I(+) neurons in expiratory termination, it seems unlikely that the same neurons would participate in both the afferent and efferent sides of the control of respiratory pattern (17). In addition, activity induced in I(+) neurons by lung inflation during the expiratory period adapts too rapidly to account in a simple, direct manner for the increase in expiratory duration (4, 8). Additional evidence against the participation of I(+) bulbospinal neurons in the Breuer-Hering reflex derives from the lack of a change in respiratory pattern during antidromic activation of their axons (15, 23; but see 16). Thus, it seems unlikely that I(+) neurons are an obligatory component in the central pathway generating the Breuer-Hering reflex.

Most of our knowledge concerning the axonal projections of pump cells derives from the detailed work of Davies and co-workers (11). These authors identified two major populations of pump cells in the cat. One was located dorsolateral to the tractus solitarius while the second was centered ventromedial to the tractus solitarius. Axons of the dorsolateral but not the ventromedial group were found to project to the contralateral NTS. However, lesions of the contralateral NTS did not prevent the Breuer-Hering reflex, indicating that this projection was not required for production of the reflex (11). Axonal projections of pump cells in the ventromedial group have yet to be determined. Taken together, the evidence suggests that pump cells, with as yet unidentified projections, are required for the Breuer-Hering reflex.

We have recently undertaken experiments to identify neurons within the NTS which are required for the Breuer-Hering reflex, and to characterize the pharmacology of synaptic input to these cells. We began with the premise that second-order neurons were located within a relatively localized region of the NTS. If true, then within this region we should be able to (1) activate neurons and mimic the physiologically activated reflex, (2) block synaptic transmission and prevent the physiologically activated reflex, and (3) record neurons which are excited during SAR activation.

PROLONGATION OF EXPIRATION

The first step was to identify regions of the NTS containing neurons which when activated would lengthen the expiratory period and mimic the Breuer-Hering reflex. Studies were carried out in adult male Sprague-Dawley rats. Groups of neurons were activated by injecting small volumes (0.5 to 6 nl) of an excitatory amino acid (usually 1 to 20 mM DL-homocysteate [DLH] in 150 mM NaCl) in an attempt to activate somatodendritic membranes while minimizing the effect on axons of passage (7, 19). Ejection sites were subsequently reconstructed from marks made either by passing DC current (10 µA for up to 30 min) or by pressure ejection of a 2% solution of Chicago Sky Blue. Excitatory amino acid (EAA) injections were made at intervals of 50 to 200 µm in a region within the NTS and

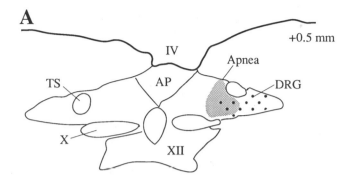

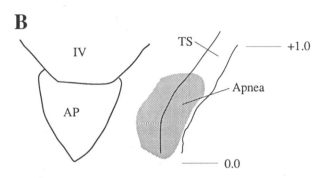

FIG. 18.1 Schematic frontal (*A*) and horizontal (*B*) views of the brainstem of a rat showing the region from which apnea was elicited by excitatory amino acid (EAA) injection. Apnea, region in which EAA injection produced apnea; DRG, region where respiratory activity was recorded; AP, area postrema; TS, tractus solitarius; X, dorsal motor nucleus of the vagus; IV, fourth ventricle; XII, hypoglossal nucleus.

proximal reticular formation which extends from 0.8 mm rostral, to 0.2 mm caudal to the calamus scriptorius. In this manner, a map was developed of NTS regions from which cardiorespiratory responses were elicited.

Expiratory lengthening was elicited by EAA injections into a discrete region of the NTS lying immediately medial to the tractus solitarius at the same rostrocaudal level as the area postrema (between about 0.1 and 0.6 mm caudal to the obex; fig. 18.1; 7). For simplicity this region will be referred to as the BH region. In the rostral one-half of the BH region, apnea was elicited with little or no detectable change in arterial blood pressure or heart rate. However, in the caudal half of the BH region, EAA injections elicited apnea and marked decreases in arterial pressure. If injections were made medial to the BH region, depressor responses were produced with little change in respiratory pattern. Injections immediately lateral to the BH region, including the tractus solitarius and adjacent reticular formation, had little or no effect on either respiratory pattern or arterial pressure.

The identification of a region from which apnea could be elicited is consistent with the involvement of neurons within this region in the production of apnea. However,

other reflexes such as swallowing can prolong the interval between inspiratory bursts on the phrenic neurogram, and it was necessary to determine whether neurons within the BH area were required for the physiologically activated Breuer-Hering reflex. To address this issue the apnea in response to maintained lung inflation was examined before, during and after recovery from the reversible blockade of synaptic transmission within the BH area.

ATTENUATION OF THE BREUER-HERING REFLEX

Synaptic transmission was blocked in unilaterally vagotomized rats by the injection of cobalt acetate (Co^{++} 100 mM, 3 to 24 nl) into the BH region ipsilateral to the intact vagus nerve. A double-barrel pipette containing DLH in one barrel and Co^{++} in the other was positioned within the BH area. Proper positioning was assured by determining that a 3 nl injection of DLH elicited an apnea lasting at least 3 sec. Prior to the injection of Co^{++}, control responses to lung inflations to at least two different distending pressures between 7.5 and 12 cm H_2O were determined. Each inflation was repeated twice with at least 90 seconds between inflations and the responses averaged. Co^{++} was then injected and lung inflations and DLH injection repeated. In all eight rats tested, Co^{++} markedly depressed the response to lung inflation but not to DLH injection (7). Almost full recovery occurred within 60 to 90 min. The depression of the response to lung inflation strongly suggested that neurons within this region were required for the physiologically activated Breuer-Hering reflex. The lack of a decrease in the response to DLH injection indicated that the post-synaptic membranes within the injection region were still excitable and that the effect was most likely due to an interruption of synaptic transmission. In a few animals the response to DLH injection was potentiated by the Co^{++} injection (e.g., see fig. 7 in ref. 7). This potentiated response was not examined in detail and did not occur in all animals; one possible explanation is that it resulted from blockade of inhibitory synaptic inputs to neurons within the Breuer-Hering reflex pathway.

In addition to blocking reflex responses to lung inflations, blockade of synaptic input from SAR should also alter the basic pattern of phrenic nerve activity. As shown in figure 18.2, Co^{++} injection increased both T_i and T_e; both returned toward control values within 1 hour.

NEURONS ACTIVATED BY SAR

Neurons within the BH area must receive lung volume–related input to have a role as interneurons in the Breuer-Hering reflex. Extracellular recording of single unit activity within the BH area indicated the presence of pump cells. These neurons had little or no spontaneous activity if lung inflation was withheld by turning the ventilator off at end-expiration, but they maintained their discharge with

FIG. 18.2 Cobalt-induced changes in respiratory pattern in a spontaneously breathing, unilaterally vagotomized rat. Cobalt (15 nl; 100 mM) injected in the NTS site in which DLH produced apnea significantly and reversibly lengthened inspiratory (T_i) and expiratory (T_e) times (asterisk indicates $P<0.05$).

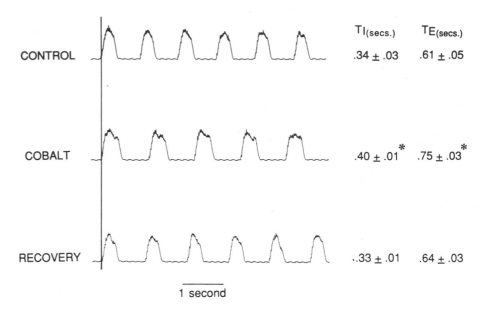

Within the BH region, pump cells were the most commonly encountered neuronal type. However, neurons with other discharge patterns were also recorded. Most other neurons with spontaneous activity had a tonic discharge pattern which was not modulated by lung inflation. A few neurons were found whose discharge was phase-locked to phrenic nerve discharge or the arterial pulse pressure, and one neuron appeared to receive chemoreceptor-related input (7). Of these neurons only those with a discharge pattern phase-locked to phrenic nerve discharge are likely to contribute to the Breuer-Hering reflex.

Several investigators have recently reported that there are few respiratory neurons other than pump cells in the nucleus tractus solitarius of rats (13, 22). However, we have recently identified a population of units with respiratory-related discharge patterns, independent of vagal afferent input, within the NTS of rats (unpublished observations). These units have small-amplitude action potentials, a predominantly inspiratory discharge pattern, and are concentrated ventral and ventrolateral to the tractus solitarius. Whether this respiratory activity arises from axons of passage or the somatodendritic membranes of small neurons located within this region is not yet clear. Even if this activity constitutes a DRG in the rat, there is a marked difference from the DRG in cats. In the cat the DRG consists of a column of relatively large neurons, most of which give rise to bulbospinal axons (5, 14). In contrast, neurons are

relatively small and only a few have bulbospinal axons in rats (25). Regardless of the role of neurons within the ventral and ventrolateral NTS in the rat, it is unlikely that neurons in this region are required for the Breuer-Hering reflex. Injecting EAAs into the ventral or ventrolateral NTS in either species has relatively little effect on expiratory duration (7, 20). Similarly, electrolytic lesions in the cat (21), or Co^{++}-induced block of synaptic transmission in the lateral NTS in the rat, have no detectable effect on the Breuer-Hering reflex (7). Thus, while the presence of a DRG in the rat is controversial, DRG neurons appear unnecessary for the Breuer-Hering reflex.

Taken together, these data strongly suggest that neurons, probably pump cells, within a region immediately medial to the tractus solitarius at the rostrocaudal level of the area postrema, are required for the production of the Breuer-Hering reflex. In addition, the ability of EAA injection to mimic the Breuer-Hering reflex and the likelihood that most fast excitatory synaptic responses in the NTS are mediated by the activation of EAA receptors (1, Champagnat et al., this volume) raise the possibility that SAR primary afferent fibers utilize an EAA neurotransmitter (possibly glutamate), as has been suggested for baroreceptor afferents (24). This possibility was pursued in a series of studies in which (1) agonists of subtypes of EAA receptors were compared for their ability to mimic the Breuer-Hering reflex and (2) antagonists of EAA transmission were injected into the BH area and examined for their ability to block the Breuer-Hering reflex and the synaptic input to single neurons in the BH area. These experiments are outlined below.

PHARMACOLOGY

There are at least three major categories of EAA receptors, generally referred to as the quisqualate (Quis) or D,L-

relatively little adaptation over several seconds with maintained lung inflation. Activity was considered to arise from somatodendritic membranes rather than axons of afferent fibers if (1) there was an inflection on the rising phase of the action potential, or (2) the unit did not follow 200 Hz stimulation (0.1 msec pulse duration) of the ipsilateral cervical vagus nerve, or 3) the unit increased its discharge rate in response to small DLH injections, which had no effect on phrenic nerve discharge.

α-amino-3-hydroxy-5-methylisoxazole-4-propionic acid (AMPA), kainate, and N-methyl-D-aspartate (NMDA) subtypes (10, 18). Agonists of each receptor type were found to alter respiratory pattern in a concentration-dependent manner. In these experiments, four-barrel electrodes were filled with a different concentration of a single agonist in each of the barrels and the respiratory response to equivolume ejections (usually 3 nl) of each concentration were compared.

Quisqualate, kainate, and NMDA injections all produced concentration-dependent prolongations of the expiratory duration. The threshold concentration for a 3 nl injection of Quis was about 10 μM (total injection amount was 30 femtomoles) and that of NMDA about 100 μM. Kainate (0.01 to 1 mM) injections always altered respiratory pattern but did not always produce apnea. In marked contrast, the equivolume injection of agonists of other neurotransmitter candidates, including acetylcholine, substance P, TRH, calcitonin gene-related peptide, serotonin, and norepinephrine, did not alter baseline respiratory pattern.

These findings confirm the presence of EAA receptors on neurons within the BH region. Excitatory amino acids are unique among the agents tested in their ability to produce an apnea. To determine whether EAAs were required for production of the Breuer-Hering reflex, the ability of selective antagonists to block the physiologically activated reflex as well as the response to exogenous agonists was tested.

The effectiveness with which EAA antagonists could block the Breuer-Hering reflex was tested using multibarrel electrodes. The electrode was considered to be correctly positioned when injection of ≤3 nl of an EAA elicited an apnea lasting at least 3 sec. The Breuer-Hering reflex was then tested at a series of tracheal pressures between 5 and 12.5 cm H₂O. An EAA antagonist was then pressure injected from a separate barrel of the same electrode. The effectiveness of receptor blockade was tested by injecting an EAA before repeating the lung inflations.

Kynurenic acid (KYN; 10 mM, 6 to 15 nl), a broad-spectrum EAA receptor antagonist, markedly attenuated both the Breuer-Hering reflex response to lung inflation and the apnea following Quis or NMDA injection. In contrast, 2-amino-5-phosphonovaleric acid, an antagonist with high selectivity for the NMDA receptor, effectively blocked the apnea in response to NMDA injection but had little or no detectable effect on either the reflex response to lung inflation or the apnea in response to Quis injection. The ability of a broad-spectrum EAA antagonist, but not an antagonist selective for the NMDA receptor, to block both the lung inflation and Quis responses strongly suggests that non-NMDA receptor activation is required for the production of the Breuer-Hering reflex.

Blocking non-NMDA EAA synaptic transmission within a restricted region of the NTS medial to the tractus solitarius interrupted the Breuer-Hering reflex. Because pump cells

were recorded within the BH area, and they are likely to be part of the pathway eliciting the Breuer-Hering reflex, the pharmacology of the synaptic input to these neurons was tested. Compound electrodes were used which consisted of a single-barrel recording pipette (filled with 3 M NaCl) glued to a double-barrel pipette with the tip of the recording barrel advanced 20 to 50 μm beyond the double-barrel pipette. An EAA agonist was placed in one barrel and its antagonist in the other. This electrode configuration permitted the use of electrodes with tip outside diameter < 1 μm, which aided in the isolation of small cells and also reduced pressure artifacts during drug ejection. Nevertheless, it was quite difficult to isolate the presumably small pump cells.

The pharmacology of the synaptic input to single neurons was similar in all neurons tested within the NTS. Three pump cells and four other neurons located in the same area increased their discharge rate in response to ejection of DLH (≤1 nl of 1–5 mM). KYN ejection completely blocked spontaneous discharge and greatly reduced or abolished the response to DLH. That all of these cells responded in a similar fashion to EAA agonists and antagonists is consistent with the findings of Champagnat et al. (this volume) in NTS slices from rat. These authors identified fast non-NMDA EAA synaptic inputs to all the NTS neurons they tested but found no evidence for fast excitatory potentials that were mediated via other transmitters.

The data presented here are consistent with the hypothesis that SAR primary afferent fibers release an EAA transmitter which activates non-NMDA receptors on pump cells mediating the Breuer-Hering reflex. However, alternative explanations include the possibility that the soma of neurons eliciting the apnea are located outside of the BH region and only have dendritic arbors extending into this region. This is unlikely, however, since EAA injections into surrounding regions, which would be likely to contain the soma, elicited little or no increase in expiratory duration (7 and Bonham, Joad, and Bric, unpublished observations). A second possibility is that pump cells receive EAA-mediated inputs from sources other than SAR, and blockade of these other inputs reduces the excitability of pump cells sufficiently to prevent the Breuer-Hering reflex. Pump cells, however, were strongly activated by lung inflation and had no spontaneous activity in the absence of lung inflation. Further, Berger and Dick (6) found no evidence of a modulation in the membrane potential of pump cells in cats in the absence of lung inflation. An additional possibility is that neurons, other than pump cells, within the BH region are required for the Breuer-Hering reflex. While the data linking pump cells to the Breuer-Hering reflex is only correlational, pump cells were the only neurons found within the BH region which increased their discharge rate during lung inflation and prolonged their period of discharge if lung inflation was maintained. Thus, pump cells remain the most likely candidates for mediating the Breuer-Hering reflex.

In summary, the apnea that occurs in response to maintained lung inflation was mimicked by injection of small volumes of dilute solutions of excitatory amino acid agonists into the NTS immediately medial to the tractus solitarius at the rostrocaudal level of the area postrema. This Breuer-Hering reflex-like response was not elicited by the agonists of several other non-EAA transmitter candidates. Injection of Co^{++} into this region greatly reduced the apnea in response to lung inflation but not the response to EAA injection, while injection of the EAA antagonist KYN blocked both the apnea in response to maintained lung inflation and the response to exogenous EAAs. Similarly, pump cells as well as other neurons within this region were excited by the injection of small volumes of EAAs, while their response both to lung inflation and exogenous EAAs was prevented by KYN. Taken together, these data suggest that an EAA is released by SAR afferents onto pump cells, which are an obligatory component in the Breuer-Hering reflex.

ACKNOWLEDGMENTS

We are grateful to Drs. Gordon Mitchell and Linda J. Larson-Prior for helpful comments on the manuscript. This work was supported by NIH grants HL40336 and NS 17489. ACB and SKC were supported by NIH/NRSA HL 07717 and HL 08298, respectively.

REFERENCES

1. Andresen, M.C., and M. Yang. Non-NMDA receptors mediate sensory afferent synaptic transmission in medial nucleus tractus solitarius. *Am. J. Physiol.* 259:H1307-H1311, 1990.

2. Averill, D.B., W.E. Cameron, and A.J. Berger. Neural elements subserving pulmonary stretch receptor-mediated facilitation of phrenic motoneurons. *Brain Res.* 346:378-382, 1985.

3. Baumgarten, R. von, and E. Kanzow. The interaction of two types of inspiratory neurons in the region of the tractus solitarius of the cat. *Arch. Ital. Biol.* 96:361-373, 1958.

4. Berger, A.J. Dorsal respiratory group neurons in the medulla oblongata of cat: Spinal projections, responses to lung inflation and superior laryngeal nerve stimulation. *Brain Res.* 135:231-254, 1977.

5. Berger, A.J., D.B. Averill, and W.E. Cameron. Morphology of inspiratory neurons located in the ventrolateral nucleus of the tractus solitarius of the cat. *J. Comp. Neurol.* 224:60-70, 1984.

6. Berger, A.J., and T.E. Dick. Connectivity of slowly adapting pulmonary stretch receptors with dorsal medullary respiratory neurons. *J. Neurophysiol.* 58:1259-1274, 1987.

7. Bonham, A.C., and D.R. McCrimmon. Neurones in a discrete region of the nucleus tractus solitarius are required for the Breuer-Hering reflex in rat. *J. Physiol.* (London) 427:261-280, 1990.

8. Camerer, H., D.W. Richter, N. Röhrig, and M. Meesmann. Lung stretch receptor inputs to Rβ-neurones: A model for "respiratory gating." In *Central nervous control mechanisms in breathing,* Wenner-Gren Ctr. Symp. Ser., ed. C. von Euler and H. Lagercrantz, vol. 32, 261-266. Oxford, U.K.: Pergamon, 1979.

9. Cohen, M.I., and J.L. Feldman. Discharge properties of dorsal medullary inspiratory neurons: Relation to pulmonary afferent and phrenic efferent discharge. *J. Neurophysiol.* 51:753-776, 1984.

10. Collingridge, G.L., and R.A.J. Lester. Excitatory amino acid receptors in the vertebrate central nervous system. *Pharmacol. Rev.* 41:143-210, 1989.

11. Davies, R.O., L. Kubin, and A.I. Pack. Pulmonary stretch receptor relay neurons of the cat: Location and contralateral medullary projections. *J. Physiol.* (London) 383:571-585, 1987.

12. Euler, C. von. Brain stem mechanisms for generation and control of breathing pattern. In *Handbook of Physiology,* Section 3, vol. 2, ed. N.S. Cherniack and J.G. Widdicombe, 1-67. Bethesda, Md.: American Physiological Society, 1986.

13. Ezure, K., M. Manabe, and H. Yamada. Distribution of medullary respiratory neurons in the rat. *Brain Res.* 455:262-270, 1988.

14. Feldman, J.L. Neurophysiology of breathing in mammals. In *Handbook of Physiology,* Section 1, vol. 4, ed. F.E. Bloom, 463-524. Bethesda, Md.: American Physiological Society, 1986.

15. Feldman, J.L., D.R. McCrimmon, and D.F. Speck. Effect of synchronous activation of medullary inspiratory bulbo-spinal neurones on phrenic discharge in the cat. *J. Physiol.* (London) 347:241-254, 1984.

16. Gauthier, P., and R. Monteau. Respiratory resetting induced by activation of inspiratory bulbo-spinal neurons. *Respir. Physiol.* 65:155-168, 1986.

17. Lipski, J., L. Kubin, and J. Jodkowski. Synaptic action of Rβ neurons on phrenic motoneurons studied with spike-triggered averaging. *Brain Res.* 288:105-118, 1983.

18. Mayer, M.L., and R.J. Miller. Excitatory amino acid receptors, second messengers and regulation of intracellular Ca^{++} in mammalian neurons. *Trends Pharmacol. Sci.* 11:254-260, 1990.

19. McCrimmon, D.R., J.L. Feldman, and D.F. Speck. Respiratory motoneuronal activity is altered by picomole injections of glutamate into cat brainstem. *J. Neurosci.* 6:2384-2392, 1986.

20. McCrimmon, D.R., J.L. Feldman, D.F. Speck, H.H. Ellenberger, and J.C. Smith. Functional heterogeneity of dorsal, ventral, and pontine respiratory groups revealed by micropharmacological techniques. In *Neurobiology of the control of breathing,* ed. C. von Euler and H. Lagercrantz, 133-138. New York: Raven Press, 1986.

21. McCrimmon, D.R., D.F. Speck, and J.L. Feldman. Role of the ventrolateral region of the nucleus of the tractus solitarius in processing respiratory afferent input from vagus and superior laryngeal nerves. *Exp. Brain Res.* 67:449-459, 1987.

22. Saether, K., G. Hilaire, and R. Monteau. Dorsal and ventral respiratory groups of neurons in the medulla of the rat. *Brain Res.* 419:87-96, 1987.

23. Speck, D.F. Respiratory resetting induced by spinal cord stimulation in the cat. *J. Appl. Physiol.* 65:1572-1578, 1988.

24. Talman, W.T., A.R. Granata, and D.J. Reis. Glutamatergic mechanisms in the nucleus tractus solitarius in blood pressure control. *Fed. Proc.* 43:39-44, 1984.

25. Yamada, H., K. Ezure, and M. Manabe. Efferent projections of inspiratory neurons of the ventral respiratory group: A dual labeling study in the rat. *Brain Res.* 455:283-294, 1988.

19

Connectivity of Rostral Pontine Inspiratory-Modulated Neurons as Revealed by Responses to Vagal and Superior Laryngeal Afferent Stimulation

Morton I. Cohen, Chen-Fu Shaw, and Russell Barnhardt

The classical experiments of Lumsden (15), in which transections at the level of the rostral pons produced apneusis (maintained inspiratory discharge), led to the concept that the region was the site of a "pneumotaxic center" that controls respiratory pattern. More modern hypotheses suggested that the pneumotaxic center facilitates the inspiratory off-switch (5). Subsequent lesion studies (20) resulted in a more precise localization of the pneumotaxic center to the region of the nucleus parabrachialis (NPBM) and the Kölliker-Fuse nucleus (KFN).

To further elucidate pneumotaxic center function, microelectrode explorations were done by several groups of investigators. The early study by Cohen and Wang (8) and subsequent studies by Hugelin and collaborators (1, 2) reported the presence of numerous respiratory-related neurons (RRNs) in the NPBM and KFN of paralyzed, vagotomized cats. The pontine RRN population was eventually designated as the pontine respiratory group (PRG) (12). It was found that the discharge patterns of pontine RRNs differ markedly from those of medullary RRNs. Whereas the great majority of medullary neurons discharge predominantly during one phase of the respiratory cycle, either inspiration (I) or expiration (E), the majority of the PRG neurons have tonic discharges with superimposed respiratory modulation.

Since a full fledged apneusis appears only with a combination of PRG lesions and vagotomy, the effect of lung afferent input on PRG RRNs was investigated by Feldman et al. (13) and more recently by St. John (19) and Shaw et al. (18). In decerebrate paralyzed cats having intact vagi and ventilated by a cycle-triggered pump, about 90% of PRG I-modulated neurons were strongly inhibited by lung inflation, as revealed by the "no-inflation test" (17).

In order to study the mechanisms and pathways of this inhibition, we used electrical stimulation of vagal afferents to mimic lung inflation. In addition, we studied the effects of afferent superior laryngeal stimulation, which produces inspiratory inhibition (14). Although both types of input produced marked changes of PRG RRN discharges, the effects had relatively long latencies (median of 170 msec for inspiratory inhibition). Locking of a neuron's discharge to individual stimuli was rare. These results indicate that connections of the PRG with caudal systems are multisynaptic and diffuse.

METHODS

Observations were made in midcollicular decerebrate cats (2.5–3.5 kg) after withdrawal of the halothane anesthesia used during surgical procedures. The cats were paralyzed by gallamine infusion and were ventilated with hyperoxic gas mixtures by a cycle-triggered pump system (6), which applied lung inflation during the central inspiratory (I) phase as monitored by phrenic (phr) discharge. Bilateral pneumothorax was produced to minimize motion artifacts and to avoid excitation of chest wall afferents. To prevent collapse of the lungs, an expiratory load of 1–2 cm H_2O was applied.

The brainstem was exposed with either a dorsal or ventral approach, and extracellular unit recordings were taken with tungsten microelectrodes (impedances 2–5 Mohm at 1000 Hz). Spikes of an isolated unit were used to derive standard pulses by means of a time-amplitude window discriminator.

In order to assess the influence of pulmonary afferents on neuron discharge, the no-inflation test (consisting of withholding inflation during one I phase, with resultant elimination of the phasic afferent discharge produced by lung inflation) was applied at intervals of 4–8 respiratory cycles.

Electrical stimulation (frequency 100/sec, pulse duration 0.05 msec, stimulus currents in the range 10–50 μA) was delivered through a bipolar electrode at the peripheral end of the whole superior laryngeal (SL) nerve or to a separated slip of the vagus (V) nerve (diameter one-third to one-half of the intact diameter). Stimulus trains were started 50–100 msec after onset of the I phase and were terminated at the end of I. The trains were applied during no-inflation I phases. With this protocol, the control I phases were those in which inflation was withheld but no stimulation was delivered.

Recordings were taken with an analog tape recorder or a video cassette recorder. After digitization (0.4 msec sampling interval), recordings were subjected to several types of analysis using a desktop computer.

The respiratory cycle-triggered histograms (CTH) were ensemble averages (15–30 cycles) of unit activity and half-wave rectified phrenic activity, with the onset of I or E as the synchronizing trigger. The change produced by a test was evaluated as the ratio of activity in corresponding time

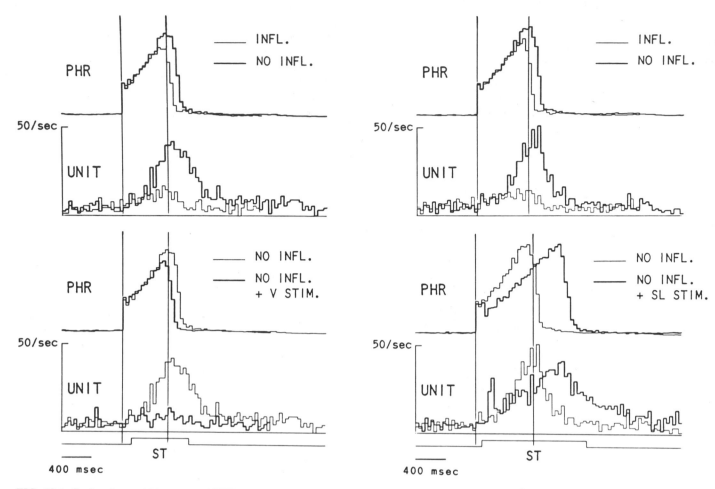

FIG. 19.1 Cycle-triggered histograms (CTHs) comparing responses of a tonic I-modulated neuron to afferent vagal (V) stimulation (*left*) and afferent superior laryngeal (SL) stimulation (*right*). PHR; phrenic activity. Stimulus trains (100/sec), delivered during no-inflation I phases, started 50 msec after I onset and were ended by I offset. Vertical pairs of lines indicate equivalent-time windows for comparison of inflation and no-inflation phases (*top*), and control and stimulation phases (*bottom*). *Top:* CTHs derived from inflation phases (thin lines) and no-inflation phases without stimulation (thick lines). Note that no-inflation converts unit pattern from very weak to strong I-modulation. *Bottom:* CTHs derived from no-inflation phases without stimulation (thin lines) and no-inflation phases with stimulation (thick lines). *Left:* V stimulation shortened the I phase, with little effect on PHR slope, and inhibited the unit's I-modulation. *Right:* SL stimulation lengthened the I phase, reduced PHR slope, and produced excitation followed by moderate inhibition of the unit. Number of trials: V, 22; SL, 26. 40-msec bins.

windows of test and control phases (1) for inflation tests during the no-inflation and inflation phases and (2) for stimulation tests during the no-inflation phases with stimulation and without stimulation.

Peristimulus histograms (PSHs) were computed as ensemble averages, with the first stimulus of each train as the synchronizing trigger. A control PSH was computed from activity in control phases, with the synchronizing trigger being a "dummy" pulse whose time in the phase corresponded to the time of the stimulus synchronizing trigger. Although the occurrence of a stimulus effect on unit activity was apparent on comparison of the control and test PSHs, it was difficult to ascertain the response latency. Therefore, latencies of unit responses were measured by use of a variant of cusum analysis (9). The cusum was calculated as the cumulative sum of test minus control activity, from which was subtracted the baseline difference activity

(calculated for a time of circa 100 msec preceding stimulation onset). The latency of a stimulus effect was taken as the point where the cusum went beyond 3 standard deviations of the baseline mean (cf. fig. 19.2).

Power spectral analysis was used to ascertain if there was short-term locking between neuron and phr activities (in control cycles) or between stimulus occurrence and phr or neuron activities (in stimulus cycles). Autospectra of signals and coherences between pairs of signals during appropriate time windows were computed with the fast Fourier transformer (FFT); details of computation methods have been given in earlier papers (4, 7).

RESULTS

In order to compare the effects of lung inflation with the effects of electrical stimulation of vagal (V) and superior

FIG. 19.2 Cumulative sum histograms showing response of the unit of figure 19.1 to V stimulation (*top*) and to SL stimulation (*bottom*). Horizontal lines: mean (thick line) and ± 3 S.D. of baseline counts. Cusums are derived from counts in peristimulus histograms (0.4 msec-bins), which were triggered from the first stimulus of each train (vertical line). Latencies, defined as time points where the histogram crosses the 3 S.D. line: V, inhibition at 190 msec; SL, excitation at 60 msec.

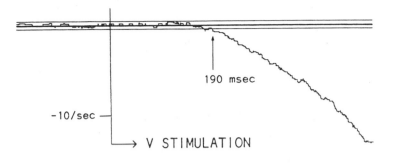

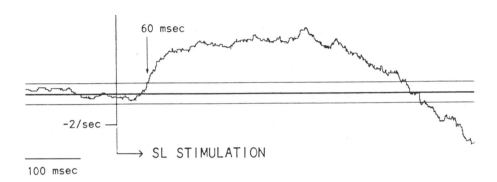

laryngeal (SL) afferents, stimulus trains were delivered during no-inflation I phases in a series of seven cats. The strength of V stimulation was adjusted to a level that produced shortening of I phase duration (T_I) with little or no excitation of phrenic discharge. The strength of SL stimulation was adjusted to a level that produced graded depression of phrenic discharge; this type of stimulation shortened T_I in five cats and lengthened T_I in two cats.

In figure 19.1, the effects of the two types of stimulation are compared for a tonic I-modulated PRG neuron. The CTHs comparing activity during inflation and no-inflation cycles (top) show that during inflation the unit's respiratory modulation was weak, though significant (verified statistically); during no-inflation cycles, respiratory modulation was greatly increased (62% increase of discharge during the comparison time window), so that the tonic I-modulated pattern became apparent. Afferent V stimulation applied during no-inflation I phases (bottom left) shortened T_I and inhibited unit activity to the extent that the unit's respiratory modulation was completely abolished.

SL stimulation (fig. 19.1, bottom right) produced more complex effects than did V stimulation. In this case, the usual reduction of phr activity (decreased slope of the CTH) was accompanied by lengthening of T_I. The effect on unit activity was biphasic: an initial excitation followed after a delay by a slowly increasing inhibition.

The time courses of the unit's responses to both types of stimulation are shown in the cusum difference histograms of figure 19.2: the latency of inhibition by V stimulation was 190 msec, and the latency for excitation by SL stimulation was 60 msec. The SL cusum histogram shows the mixed excitatory-inhibitory response: after the initial excitation there was no net activity change, as indicated by flatness of the histogram, until about 400 msec after the onset of stimulation, when a delayed inhibition of activity started.

The long latencies of the unit responses shown in figure 19.2 are typical of the responses of I-modulated (tonic or phasic) PRG neurons observed in this experimental series. Of twenty-three neurons tested with V stimulation, sixteen showed a pure inhibition, three showed pure excitation, and four showed an excitatory-inhibitory sequence. The latencies for inhibition ranged from 20 to 260 msec with a median of 170 msec. Inhibition started well before the premature inspiratory off-switch, whose latency ranged from 300 to 400 msec. Of thirty-six neurons tested with SL stimulation, twenty-one showed a pure excitation, nine showed a pure inhibition, and six showed an excitatory-inhibitory sequence. The latencies for excitation ranged from 3 to 374 msec, with a median of 70 msec; the latencies for inhibition ranged from 30 to 510 msec, with a median of 170 msec.

Thus, for both types of stimulation short-latency excitation and short-latency inhibition were rare. This contrasts with the high incidence of short-latency excitation and inhibition among medullary dorsal inspiratory neurons (10, 11). In peristimulus histograms, short-term locking of unit firing to individual stimuli was not apparent, although it was obvious in the PSHs of phr activity. In order to detect such locking, coherences between stimulus pulses and unit pulses were computed with the FFT; stimulus-phr coherences were similarly computed. Although significant (and often high) stimulus-phr coherences at the stimulus frequency were usually found, significant stimulus-unit coherences were rare: they were found in only 2 of 36 units with SL stimulation and in 1 of 23 units with V stimulation.

DISCUSSION

The analysis of timing relations between V or SL stimuli and I-modulated PRG neuron activity revealed that 1) the changes of unit activity (excitation or inhibition) usually had long latencies (median 170 msec for inhibition) and 2) locking of spike occurrence to stimulus occurrence was rare. These observations indicate that the afferent transmission pathways from medulla to pons are multisynaptic and diffuse.

This conclusion is congruent with additional observations indicating that pontine I-modulated neurons are "synaptically distant" from medullary I neurons. 1) In the larger study of PRG neurons (17), it was found that only a minority (about 25%) of phasic I neurons had high-frequency oscillations (HFO) in their discharges, as ascertained by coherence analysis; none of the PRG I-tonic neurons had HFO. This contrasts with the high incidence of HFO in medullary I neuron discharges (4, 6) and the ubiquity of HFO in I motor nerve discharges (7). 2) Short-latency cross-correlations between PRG and medullary RRNs are rare (16). 3) Only a small proportion of dorsal and ventral medullary I neurons have monosynaptic projections to the PRG region, as ascertained by antidromic stimulation (3).

ACKNOWLEDGMENT

This research was supported by N.I.H. Grant HL-27300.

REFERENCES

1. Bertrand, F., A. Hugelin, and J.F. Vibert. Quantitative study of anatomical distribution of respiration related neurons in the pons. *Exp. Brain Res.* 16:383-399, 1973.

2. Bertrand, F., A. Hugelin, and J.F. Vibert. A stereologic model of pneumotaxic oscillator based on spatial and temporal distributions of neuronal bursts. *J. Neurophysiol.* 37:91-107, 1974.

3. Bianchi, A.L., and W.M. St. John. Pontile axonal projections of medullary respiratory neurons. *Resp. Physiol.* 45:167-183, 1981.

4. Christakos, C.N., M.I. Cohen, W.R. See, and R. Barnhardt. Fast rhythms in the discharges of medullary inspiratory neurons. *Brain Res.* 463:362-367, 1988.

5. Cohen, M.I., and J.L. Feldman. Models of respiratory phase-switching. *Fed. Proc.* 36:2367-2374, 1977.

6. Cohen, M.I., and J.L. Feldman. Discharge properties of dorsal medullary inspiratory neurons: Relation to pulmonary afferent and phrenic efferent discharge. *J. Neurophysiol.* 51:753-776, 1984.

7. Cohen, M.I., W.R. See, C.N. Christakos, and A.L. Sica. High-frequency and medium-frequency components of different inspiratory nerve discharges and their modification by various inputs. *Brain Res.* 417:148-152, 1987.

8. Cohen, M.I., and S.C. Wang. Respiratory neuronal activity in pons of cat. *J. Neurophysiol.* 22:33-50, 1959.

9. Davey, N.J., P.H. Ellaway, and R.B. Stein. Statistical limits for detecting change in the cumulative sum derivative of the peristimulus time histogram. *J. Neurosci. Methods* 17:153-166, 1986.

10. Donnelly, D.F., A.L. Sica, M.I. Cohen, and H. Zhang. Dorsal medullary inspiratory neurons: Effects of superior laryngeal afferent stimulation. *Brain Res.* 491:243-252, 1989.

11. Donnelly, D.F., A.L. Sica, M.I. Cohen, and H. Zhang. Effects of contralateral superior laryngeal nerve stimulation on dorsal medullary inspiratory neurons. *Brain Res.* 505:149-152, 1989.

12. Feldman, J.L. Neurophysiology of breathing in mammals. In *Handbook of Physiology,* Section 1, vol. 4, 463-524. Bethesda, Md.: American Physiological Society, 1986.

13. Feldman, J.L., M.I. Cohen, and P. Wolotsky. Powerful inhibition of pontine respiratory neurons by pulmonary afferent activity. *Brain Res.* 104:341-346, 1976.

14. Iscoe, S., J.L. Feldman, and M.I. Cohen. Properties of inspiratory termination by superior laryngeal and vagal stimulation. *Resp. Physiol.* 36:353-366, 1979.

15. Lumsden, T. Observations on the respiratory centres in the cat. *J. Physiol.* (London) 57:153-160, 1923.

16. Segers, L.S., R. Shannon, and B.G. Lindsey. Interactions between rostral pontine and ventral medullary respiratory neurons. *J. Neurophysiol.* 54:318-334, 1985.

17. Shaw, C.-F. *Discharge patterns of rostral pontine respiratory-modulated neurons in relation to vagal and superior laryngeal afferent input.* Ph.D. diss., Albert Einstein College of Medicine, New York, 1990.

18. Shaw, C.-F., M.I. Cohen, and R. Barnhardt. Inspiratory-modulated neurons of the rostrolateral pons: Effects of pulmonary afferent input. *Brain Res.* 485:179-184, 1989.

19. St. John, W.M. Influence of pulmonary inflations on discharge of pontile respiratory neurons. *J. Appl. Physiol.* 63:2231-2239, 1987.

20. St. John, W.M., R.L. Glasser, and R.A. King. Apneustic breathing after vagotomy in cats with chronic pneumotaxic center lesions. *Resp. Physiol.* 12:239-250, 1971.

20
Respiratory Modulation of Afferent Transmission to the Cerebellum

S. Baker, C. Seers, and T.A. Sears

AUTOMATIC AND VOLUNTARY RESPIRATORY MOVEMENTS

The diaphragm, intercostal, and abdominal muscles form the boundary of the thorax and abdomen. Their coordinated activities power lung ventilation and contribute mechanical stability to the spine in posture and locomotion. In eupnea (effortless breathing) the respiratory movements satisfying metabolic demands normally occur automatically and without the need for conscious intervention even during changes in posture. Yet the slightest unexpected hindrance to breathing, such as an increase in elastic loading, is readily perceived (12). Breathing then shifts from the realm of "automatic" to "voluntary" and remains thus until the load is removed or, following habituation again becomes automatic and "eupneic".

In contrast, during their voluntary activation for speech, the respiratory muscles generate much higher subglottal pressures to overcome either the obstruction offered by the adducted vocal cords before phonation is initiated or the elevated flow-resistance during phonation itself, yet normal speech certainly occurs without a sense of dyspnea. The controlled exhalation of air during speech or song is, however, simply one component of a complete motor synergy also involving laryngeal and oropharyngeal movements, which constitutes a learned, highly skilled motor performance, acquired in infancy and practiced throughout life. Thus for each utterance the phonating larynx represents a highly predictable load on the respiratory muscles and gives rise to no obtrusive sensory phenomena, i.e., dyspnea.

Notwithstanding the fact that "automatic" breathing movements persist in sleep, under anaesthesia, and after decerebration, their nature in the awake state is different, as described above. Respiratory muscle activity is more similar to the voluntary activation of limb or other muscles than is generally recognized. For example, when one moves from the seated to the standing posture and walks, although this purposeful act is initiated by mental action, the maintenance of this intent is achieved through essentially automatic movements until further mental action determines otherwise. If an unexpected surface or load is encountered and perceived, full conscious attention is restored to the execution of the movement. The obverse, the rendering of movement automatic through habitual use, carries the implication that predictable afferent in-flows associated with it are prevented from obtruding into consciousness (34, 35).

The development of these ideas in relation to respiration arose from experiments utilizing changes in load on contracting intercostal muscles (30) and were aimed at evaluating the role of the "length" servo theory of muscular control (16, 27, 28) in respiratory muscle contraction in humans. In that theory, conceived originally as an "insentient" mechanism (29), changes in muscle spindle afferent discharge are used to detect the difference between intrafusal and extrafusal fiber contraction (or relaxation). This altered activity serves as a proportional error signal automatically calling forth more, or less, excitation of motoneurons to control the load.

A different concept was needed, however, to explain the early *inhibitory* effects of sudden loading of intercostal muscles in conscious humans, the delayed latency of the apparent stretch reflex, and the effects of prior instruction on the reflex (30). It was hypothesized that the occurrence of an unexpected load during a learnt movement caused automatic servo action at the segmental level to be withheld (or reduced) until, through neural events associated with the eventual perception of the load, segmental reflex compensation was allowed to proceed based on previous experience (30). It was suggested that during the control movement there is presynaptic inhibition of the Group Ib terminals onto inhibitory interneurons by corticospinal tract projections (3). Therefore, the autogenic inhibition by the Group Ib (tendon organ) afferent input signalling the time course of predicted changes in active tension (cf. 24) is suppressed. This allows the conjoint excitatory inputs (corticospinal and Ia) to the motoneurons carrying the executive (learnt) command for the control movement to be unopposed. With the unexpected load, however, autogenic inhibition would be exerted by the unmatched Ib input, thus suppressing excessive spindle feedback until control mechanisms with longer loop times, for example, via the cerebral or cerebellar cortices and attendant on "prior instruction" ("set"), have time to operate. This was important because the gain of the stretch reflex component was shown to be scaled to the current level of EMG activity (30). Thus overall, this mode of control has the merit of setting servo action within prescribed tension limits, has predictive properties, and allows reflex action to be the servant of volition (35).

Thus it is envisaged that voluntary motor commands not only specify the movements, but also the afferent signals

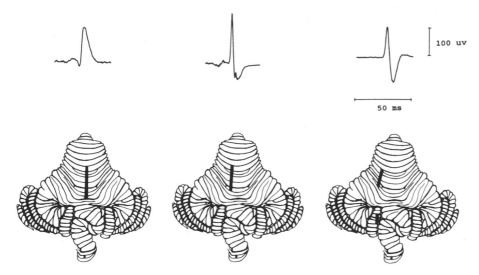

FIG. 20.1 Distribution of climbing fiber–evoked responses from the caudal
thoracic nerves (T9-T10). From left to
right, the vermal a zone, b zone, and C2
zone in the intermediate cortex
(contralateral response in C2 not shown).

used in their control. This is especially relevant for respiratory movements where presumably the changing but predictable mechanical loads offered by the lung and chest wall compliance, and the flow resistance of the airways would allow a high degree of automation. While certain categories of limb movement also employ gain control of afferent transmission (cf. 26), others are not immediately under afferent feedback control. Ballistic movements require a predictive control strategy and others are performed in an open loop mode, as exemplified by the vestibulooculomotor reflex (VOR).

As demonstrated by the wearing of dove prism goggles, prolonged mismatching of visual and vestibular information causes progressive changes in gain of the VOR to minimize retinal errors (19). In animal experiments, this adaptation is abolished by lesion of the flocculus (see 20 for references), suggesting the more general proposition that the cerebellum confers on a control system the capacity for "coordination, orthometria and compensation" (21), analogous to the multivariable, predictive and adaptive control mechanisms in engineering. Explicit models have been developed in which "motor learning" occurs in the cerebellar cortex as a result of an adaptive plasticity of the parallel fiber synapses on Purkinje cells (PCs) consequent on their conjunctive activation by climbing fiber (CF) afferents to that cell (1, 25). Direct experimental evidence is now available that long-term depression of parallel fiber transmission occurs following such conjunctive activation (14, 22, 23). Also, in animals performing a variety of tasks, the CF discharge of PCs at relevant sites of representation (microzones) is unaffected by the learnt movement, but responds specifically to perturbations by unexpected stimuli (5, 6, 17, 18). Under these circumstances the CF discharge is conceived as signalling an error in the motor performance and through the mechanism of adaptive plasticity described above plays a key role in motor learning (see 21). The error is not simply the proportional error signal from muscle spindle afferents automatically summoning forth reflex ac

tion but also carries the implication that the perceived, unexpected change in load may require an alternative strategy in the future.

In the light of these developments it was of interest to reexamine the representation of the thorax in the cerebellum. Previously Coffey et al. (13) had described discrete, intercostal-evoked CF responses in the intermediate cortex, but their investigation was directed primarily at the mossy fiber inputs and was made before the longitudinal organization of the spino-olivary CF inputs to the cerebellum was recognized (see 21 for references). Each longitudinal zone receives its CF afferents from a discrete olivary subnucleus and in turn projects to a discrete subcortical nucleus. Some zones have a detailed somatotopic organization and can be further subdivided into microzones. Thus a microzone receiving a CF input over spino-olivocerebellar pathways from the hindlimb in turn projects to that region of its target nucleus (e.g. lateral vestibular nucleus) that is connected to a hindlimb motor system (4). We have therefore investigated the spino-olivocerebellar projections from the thorax to determine first, the zonal representation of the thorax in the cortex and second, the relation between the execution of respiratory movements and afferent transmission to the zones.

CLIMBING FIBER RESPONSES

Climbing fiber responses (CFRs) were recorded from the surface following stimulation of a caudal intercostal nerve (or dorsal primary ramus) in anaesthetized or decerebrate cats, paralyzed and artificially ventilated with different gas mixtures as required. As illustrated in figure 20.1, typical, long-latency, initially positive-going CFRs (cf. 13) were present in two sagittal strips in the medial and lateral vermis, corresponding to the a and b zones, respectively, (4) and extending along the length of the exposed cortex of the anterior lobe (Lobule V) and to Lobule VI. In the a zone, thoracic CFRs overlapped with those from the

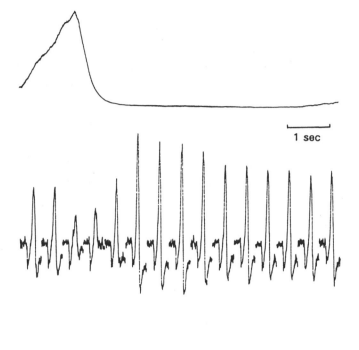

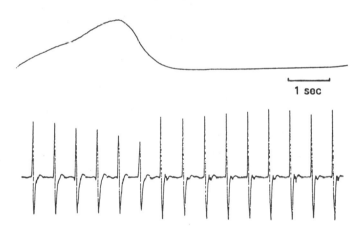

FIG. 20.2 *Upper traces:* Averaged inspiratory neurogram of the external intercostal nerve (T4). *Lower traces:* Climbing fiber responses from internal intercostal nerve T9, averaged from a total of 750 responses falling in sequential 500 μsec time bins of the respiratory cycle and plotted in respective bins of the cycle. Trace durations: 25 msec in the upper record and 50 msec in lower. Two examples from different experiments.

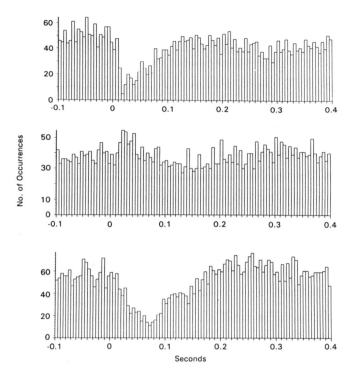

FIG. 20.3 Poststimulus time histograms of simple spike discharge of Purkinje cell in thoracic microzone of the b zone after stimulation of the superficial radial nerve (*top*), the intercostal nerve (*middle*), and the sciatic nerve (*bottom*).

hindlimb. However, consideration of the representation in the a zone of the neck (32) and splanchnic nerves (33), indicating that more rostral axial structures are represented in caudal folia of the anterior lobe and Lobule VI, means that the a zone can no longer be considered solely as a hindlimb zone but is also an axial zone (cf. 8). Within the b zone, the thoracic CFRs were found in the area between the fore and hindlimb-evoked responses as previously described (15).

In the intermediate cortex, bilateral thoracic CFRs were found in the anterior lobe and paramedian lobule corresponding to the C2 zone. The very localized projection from the vagus and superior laryngeal nerves was also contained within this area. Thus, although the limb inputs reveal no clear somatotopic organization within the C2 zone, the representation of axial structures there indicates an overlapping, rostrocaudal somatotopic gradient, with rostral structures represented in more caudal folia of the paramedian lobule. In the other zones of the intermediate cortex the thoracic representation is very restricted. In the C3 zone thoracic CFRs were only recorded in microelectrode penetrations and were found in a narrow region between face and hindlimb responses (15). Since CFRs from rostral thoracic nerves have also been recorded in the X zone (between the a and b zones of Lobules V and VI) the thorax is represented to some extent in each of the zones of the anterior lobe vermis and intermediate cortex.

RESPIRATORY MODULATION OF AFFERENT TRANSMISSION

From previous work by Aminoff and Sears (2) it was known that the intercostal-to-intercostal polysynaptic reflexes and the cortically evoked responses in the intercostal nerves are strongly modulated with the respiratory cycle. In the paralyzed decerebrate preparation we have found consistently that the intercostal-evoked CFRs in the vermal b zone are inhibited during the inspiratory phase (fig. 20.2). This in-

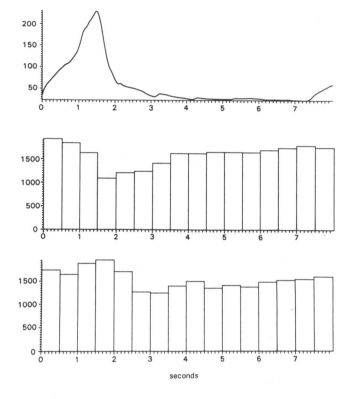

FIG. 20.4 Respiratory cycle histograms of spontaneous simple spike discharges of Purkinje cells in thoracic microzone within the b zone. Integrated inspiratory neurogram (*top, middle*), simple spike cycle histogram (*bottom*).

hibition occurs *pari passu* with that of the simultaneously evoked intercostal-to-intercostal reflex (not illustrated). Using near-threshold stimulation for the reflex, the CFRs also display significant latency modulation within the cycle, being of shortest latency during expiration (11).

During hypocapnic apnea, the CFRs (and the reflex) lose their phasic modulation and are then of relatively constant large amplitude and brief latency, as if facilitated during expiration. This probably reflects the fact that in hypocapnic apnea, expiratory motoneurons are in receipt of a brainstem-mediated, CO_2-dependent drive (9) causing them to discharge tonically. This drive, conveyed by expiratory bulbospinal neurons (10), appears also to have access to the interneurons mediating spino-olivary transmission. Such phasic modulation is consistent with the postulated role of this system as generating an "error signal." The phasic inhibition of transmission linked to the motor command would prevent olivary excitation by the "appropriate" afferent input generated by respiratory movement, whilst inputs relating to unexpected stimuli would evoke a CF discharge.

The coordination of the components of a complex movement requires the control system to receive appropriate information regarding the current status of sensory as well as motor components. This has been studied by extracellular

recording of simple spike (SS) activity of Purkinje cells in the vermis. As illustrated in figure 20.3, PCs recorded from the b zone of the lateral vermis respond to stimulation of thoracic and limb nerves with either biphasic excitation and inhibition or, in some cases, with a predominant inhibition of SS discharge.

In some PCs the spontaneous SS discharge is modulated during the respiratory cycle in the paralyzed decerebrate preparation, indicating a phasic modulation of the mossy fiber afferents. The precise phase relationship of the SS discharge to the respiratory cycle showed wide variation from cell to cell, but the pattern most commonly observed was the postinspiratory peak firing seen in the lower traces of figure 20.4. Since the central rhythm of breathing is unrelated to the pump rate (set high at 54/min) in these paralyzed preparations, the centrifugal motor command itself must have been responsible for a centripetal discharge in the spinocerebellar system(s) of mossy fiber afferents. Such an input clearly corresponds to the conceptual "efference copy" of a motor command. It would thus appear that centrifugal control is exerted in parallel on several afferent systems. Also, PC discharge in the lateral vermis is known to be phasically modulated during locomotion (7, 31).

The convergence in the cerebellum of mossy fiber and CF activity from the limbs and trunk provides a locus for an adaptive supraspinal control of their propriospinal connections and thus for the acquisition of skilled movements involving the trunk and limbs. Furthermore, this convergence, coupled with the respiratory-phased centrifugal modulation of afferent transmission, could provide an anatomical substrate for automation of the homeostatic adjustments of respiratory movements (and hence pulmonary ventilation) during changes in posture and during locomotion.

ACKNOWLEDGMENT

This work was supported by the Medical Research Council and the Brain Research Trust.

REFERENCES

1. Albus, J.S. A theory of cerebellar function. *Math. Biosci.* 1:25-61, 1971.

2. Aminoff, M.J., and T.A. Sears. Segmental integration of converging inputs to thoracic respiratory motoneurones. *J. Physiol.* 208:739-755, 1970.

3. Andersen, P., J.C. Eccles, and T.A. Sears. Cortically evoked depolarization of primary afferent fibres in the spinal cord. *J. Neurophysiol.* 27:63-77, 1964.

4. Andersson, G., and O. Oscarsson. Climbing fiber microzones in cerebellar vermis and their projection to different groups of cells in the lateral vestibular nucleus. *Exp. Brain Res.* 32:565-579, 1978.

5. Andersson, G., and D.M. Armstrong. Complex spikes in Purkinje cells in the lateral vermis (b zone) of the cat cerebellum during locomotion. *J. Physiol.* 385:107-134, 1987.

6. Apps, R., M. Lidierth, and D.M. Armstrong. Locomotion-related variations in the excitability of spino-olivocerebellar paths to the cat's cerebellar cortical C2 zone. *J. Physiol.* 424:487-512, 1990.

7. Armstrong, D.M., and S.A. Edgley. Discharge of Purkinje cells in the paravermal part of the cerebellar anterior lobe during locomotion in the cat. *J. Physiol.* 352:403-424, 1984.

8. Armstrong, D.M., R.J. Harvey, and R.F. Schild. Topographical localization in the olive-cerebellar projection: An electrophysiological study in the cat. *J. Comp. Neurol.* 154:287-302, 1974.

9. Bainton, C.R., P.A. Kirkwood, and T.A. Sears. On the transmission of the stimulating effects of carbon dioxide to the muscles of respiration. *J. Physiol.* 280:249-272, 1978.

10. Bainton, C.R., and P.A. Kirkwood. The effects of carbon dioxide on the tonic and the rhythmic discharges of expiratory bulbospinal neurones. *J. Physiol.* 296:291-314, 1979.

11. Baker, S.C., C.P. Seers, and T.A. Sears. The organization in the cerebellum of climbing fibre responses from the thorax and regulation of their afferent transmission. *Neurosci. Lett.* Suppl. 36:S86, 1989.

12. Campbell, E.J.M., S. Freedman, P.S. Smith, and M.E. Taylor. The ability of man to detect added elastic loads to breathing. *Clin. Sci.* 20:223-231, 1961.

13. Coffey, G.L., R.B. Godwin-Austin, B.B. MacGillivray, and T.A. Sears. The form and distribution of the surface evoked responses in cerebellar cortex from intercostal nerves in the cat. *J. Physiol.* 212:129-145, 1971.

14. Ekerot, C.F., and M. Kano. Long-term depression of parallel fibre synapses following stimulation of climbing fibres. *Brain Res.* 342:357-360, 1985.

15. Ekerot, C.F., and B. Larson. The dorsal spino-olivocerebellar system in the cat. II. Somatotopical organization. *Exp. Brain Res.* 36:219-232, 1979.

16. Eldred, E., R. Granit, and P.A. Merton. Supraspinal control of the muscle spindles and its significance. *J. Physiol.* 122:498-523, 1953.

17. Gellman, R., A.R. Gibson, and J.C. Houk. Inferior olive neurones in the awake cat: Detection of contact and passive body displacement. *J. Neurophysiol.* 54:40-60, 1985.

18. Gilbert, P.F.C., and W.T. Thach. Purkinje cell activity during motor learning. *Brain Res.* 128:309-328, 1977.

19. Gonshor, A., and G. Mellville Jones. Extreme vestibulo-ocular adaptation induced by prolonged optical reversal of vision. *J. Physiol.* 256:381-414, 1976.

20. Ito, M. Cerebellar control of the vestibulo-ocular reflex around the flocculus hypothesis. *Ann. Rev. Neurosci.* 5:275-296, 1982.

21. Ito, M. *The cerebellum and neural control.* New York: Raven Press, 1984.

22. Ito, M., and M. Kano. Long-lasting depression of parallel fibre Purkinje cell transmission induced by conjunctive stimulation of parallel fibres and climbing fibres in the cerebellar cortex. *Neurosci. Lett.* 33:253-258, 1982.

23. Ito, M., M. Sakurai, and P. Tongroach. Climbing fibre induced depression of both mossy fibre responsiveness and glutamate sensitivity of cerebellar Purkinje cells. *J. Physiol.* 324:113-134, 1982.

24. Jansen, J.K.S., and T. Rudjord. On the silent period and Golgi tendon organs of the soleus muscle of the cat. *Acta Physiol. Scand.* 62:364-379, 1964.

25. Marr, D. A theory of cerebellar cortex. *J. Physiol.* 202:437-470, 1969.

26. Marsden, C.D., P.A. Merton, and H.B. Morton. Servo action in the human thumb. *J. Physiol.* 257:1-44, 1976.

27. Merton, P.A. The silent period in a muscle of the human hand. *J. Physiol.* 114:183-198, 1951.

28. Merton, P.A. Speculation on the servo-control of movement. In *The Spinal Cord,* ed. G.E.W. Wolstenholme, 247-255, London: Churchill, 1953.

29. Merton, P.A. Human position sense and sense of effort. *Symp. Soc. Exp. Biol.* 18:387-400, 1964.

30. Newsom Davis, J., and T.A. Sears. The proprioceptive reflex control of the intercostal muscles during their voluntary activation. *J. Physiol.* 209:711-738, 1970.

31. Orlovsky, G.N. Work of the Purkinje cells during locomotion. *Biophysics* 17:935-941, 1972.

32. Robertson, L.T., K.D. Laxer, and D.S. Rushmer. Organization of climbing fiber input from mechanoreceptors to lobule V vermal cortex of the cat. *Exp. Brain Res.* 46:281-291, 1982.

33. Rubia, F.J., and W. Lange. The spatial distribution of climbing fibre suppression of Purkinje cell activity. In *The motor system: Neurophysiology and muscle mechanisms,* ed. M. Shahani, 247-259. Amsterdam: Elsevier, 1976.

34. Sears, T.A. Breathing: A sensori-motor act. *Sci. Basis Med. Ann. Revs.* 129-147, 1971.

35. Sears, T.A. Servo control of intercostal muscles. In *New developments in electromyography and clinical neurophysiology.* Vol. 3, ed. J.E. Desmedt, 404-417. Basel: Karger, 1973.

21

Respiratory Afferents and the Inhibition of Inspiration

Dexter F. Speck, Diane R. Karius and Liming Ling

Although many studies have examined the phenomena of inspiratory inhibitory reflexes, there is very little information available concerning the neural circuits and neurotransmitters utilized in mediating these inhibitions. There are at least two distinct types of inhibitory (or disfacilitatory) effects evident in the response of the respiratory motor output to perturbations elicited through respiratory-related afferents. The first type of inhibition involves a transient reduction of inspiratory motor output and may be observed after a single electrical shock delivered to either the superior laryngeal nerve (SLN; 2, 3, 15), the intercostal nerve (ICN; 8, 21) or the phrenic nerve (PN; 16, 22). A similar effect can be elicited by microstimulation within brainstem respiratory-related nuclei (24) or the ventrolateral cervical spinal cord (12).

A second type of inhibition is related to the termination of inspiration. This inspiratory-to-expiratory phase switching can be initiated by stimulus trains delivered to the vagus nerve (X), the SLN (15) and the ICN (21). A distinct mechanism for this inspiratory-terminating phenomenon has not yet been demonstrated. The stimulus-evoked transient reduction of inspiratory motor activity has generally been considered to be initiated by a mechanism(s) similar to that responsible for inspiratory termination, although the termination response typically requires both a higher intensity and a greater stimulation frequency. It is tempting to consider each type of inhibition as indicative of the activation of a single mechanism by the various afferents and central nuclei or tracts. It should be pointed out, however, that each afferent and each response may utilize its own separate circuitry.

Although recent *in vitro* mammalian studies suggest that Cl^--dependent inhibitory interactions are not required for rhythmogenesis (13), inhibitory mechanisms are important in mediating reflex motor responses. These reflexes are an integral part of the respiratory pattern generation in behaving animals. Chang (this volume) has shown in the conscious guinea pig that respiratory-related neurons undergo complex changes in discharge pattern in a discrete behavior-dependent fashion. Single units showed marked temporal variations in spike frequency and activity patterns. Steady-state rhythmic discharges typical of the anesthetized preparation were observed only when the animal assumed a motionless, resting posture. These results emphasize the physiologic importance of inhibitory (and excitatory) afferents in the genesis of respiratory patterns.

Various lesions and pharmacological manipulations have been conducted in our laboratory to attempt to localize and describe the underlying mechanisms of these different inhibitory reflexes.

STUDIES OF POSSIBLE NEUROTRANSMITTERS

Since glutamate has been implicated as a neurotransmitter in many afferent systems (14, 26, McCrimmon et al., this volume), the N-methyl-D-aspartate (NMDA) antagonist MK-801 was used to investigate the possibility that this neurotransmitter was involved in the production of these inhibitory reflexes (19). Systemic injection of MK-801 elicits an increase in the inspiratory duration and a reduced respiratory frequency. After injection of this drug, apneusis occurs if lung stretch receptor input is eliminated. Despite these marked central effects of MK-801, transient inspiratory inhibitory responses initiated by electrical stimulation of SLN, ICN, and PN persisted. In addition, microstimulation within the dorsal (DRG) and ventral respiratory groups (VRG) also continued to elicit transient inhibitory responses after drug administration. The inspiratory-terminating responses elicited by ICN, SLN, and vagal stimulation were also prominent after blockade of the NMDA receptor channels. These results suggest that the NMDA receptor is not essential for the production of these reflex inhibitions.

Since apneusis is induced by systemic injection of the NMDA receptor antagonist MK-801, it has been hypothesized that the pontine respiratory group (PRG) influence on inspiratory inhibitory mechanisms might be mediated through NMDA receptors. Therefore experiments were performed to determine if inhibitions elicited by pontine stimulation could be abolished after NMDA receptor antagonism with MK-801. The transient inhibition elicited by low-frequency PRG microstimulation was present with no significant change in thresholds or onset latencies at all doses. The duration of inhibition was increased after MK-801. Stimulus trains continued to elicit premature inspiratory termination even at doses of 1 mg/kg. We conclude that the inhibitory reflexes elicited by PRG stimulation do not depend on NMDA receptor-mediated neurotransmission. It is likely that the apneusis induced by systemic MK-801 involves NMDA receptors located at different sites, possibly proximal to the PRG neurons.

In those same studies, the short-latency excitation elicited by SLN and ICN stimulation was also examined. These excitations were unaltered following systemic administration of MK-801, suggesting that an NMDA receptor was not required in either the afferent or efferent pathway of these excitatory reflexes. Since the SLN excitation is believed to involve a monosynaptic projection onto DRG inspiratory neurons (1), it is unlikely that these afferents release glutamate to activate the NMDA receptors which are known to exist on the DRG pre-motor neurons.

Two major inhibitory transmitters are GABA and glycine. Both of these substances and their receptors have been localized within respiratory-related regions of the brainstem (20). In addition there is evidence for the release of glycine and GABA within the nucleus tractus solitarius of the rat (20). Both substances have a depressing effect on the spontaneous activity of brainstem respiratory-modulated neurons when applied locally (5, 9). Additional studies have indicated the involvement of glycine in the spinal inhibition of respiratory reflexes (10) and in the alteration of respiratory pattern (13). In a series of experiments (25), systemic injections of bicuculline (a $GABA_A$ antagonist) and strychnine (a glycine antagonist) have been utilized to determine if these neurotransmitters are involved in the circuitry mediating these afferent and central reflexes. With systemic application of drugs there is always concern whether the drug is reaching the necessary brainstem site to exert its desired effect. Therefore, the level of antagonist was incremented until obvious central nervous system effects were elicited in the form of convulsive discharges. Strychnine, which is a potent antagonist of glycine receptors (7,17), elicited the strongest convulsive-like discharges in our phrenic nerve recordings. Bicuculline, which is a competitive antagonist at the $GABA_A$ receptor (6,17), also elicited convulsive activity. Postdrug responses to stimulation were analyzed at the dosage immediately preceding the development of continuous convulsive activity and at convulsive doses in a few animals. This protocol ensured that antagonists were affecting central nervous system mechanisms. These experiments show no evidence for involvement of $GABA_A$ receptors in either the termination or the transient inhibitions evoked by SLN, ICN, DRG, or PN stimulation. Strychnine antagonism of glycine receptors did markedly delay the onset and prolong the duration of the evoked inhibitions. This finding is difficult to interpret since the increase in both parameters is not consistent with a simple decrease in the level of glycine-mediated inhibition. Despite relatively large doses of all antagonists, termination responses and transient inhibitions could still be elicited by all afferent inputs studied, thereby indicating that receptors for these specific neurotransmitters are not mandatory participants in the reflexes. The fact that all transient inhibitory reflexes were affected in a consistent fashion by the various neurotransmitter antagonists suggests that these inhibitory responses may share a final common pathway or mechanism.

ABLATION EXPERIMENTS

Selective electrolytic and/or chemical lesions have been performed to determine if specific brainstem regions are mandatory participants in any of these afferent-evoked inhibitions. Bonham and McCrimmon (4) have recently demonstrated that the medial nucleus of the tractus solitarius (mNTS) is involved in the Breuer-Hering reflex. Since this region also receives input from the SLN afferents, experiments were conducted to determine if the mNTS was involved in the production of SLN inhibitory reflexes. Procaine injections were made into the vicinity of the mNTS (23). This reversible blockade of cells and axons in the mNTS greatly increased the threshold of the SLN termination response with little or no effect on the SLN transient inhibitory response. This finding suggests that these two reflexes may involve separate circuitry with only the termination response relying upon structures within the region of the mNTS.

In other studies we examined the potential involvement of the PRG and the Bötzinger Complex (BötC) in these inhibitory reflexes. Although activation of pontine or Bötzinger Complex neurons can elicit similar transient inhibitions and inspiratory termination, lesion studies have suggested that these neurons are not essential for any of the reflexes studied to date. Both the transient inhibitions and the inspiratory-terminating reflexes persisted after bilateral lesions of the PRG (18). In the study of the BötC neurons (22), the transient inhibition of inspiratory activity elicited by phrenic afferent stimulation was abolished by electrolytic lesions of the BötC region. When the neurons in this nucleus were destroyed by the microinjection of kainic acid, however, the transient inhibition was not eliminated. These results suggest that axons important in this reflex pass through the BötC region, but that these axons do not require a synapse onto BötC neurons in order to elicit the reflex.

SUMMARY

Results from the experiments discussed above suggest that $GABA_A$ receptors and NMDA receptors for glutamate are unlikely to be involved in the circuitry responsible for the inhibitory reflexes studied. It does appear that glycine receptors may participate in the transient inhibitory responses, although there is likely to be at least one additional inhibitory neurotransmitter which can be involved. The ablation experiments have excluded several potential regions from the required circuitry. Obviously, further experiments are necessary to determine the underlying mechanisms of these important inhibitory reflexes.

Although the possibility exists that the transient inhibition and the inspiratory-terminating response discussed in this chapter may utilize similar mechanisms, several findings suggest the alternate hypothesis that these two types of inhibition may result from separate central mechanisms:

1. It is interesting to note that vagal stimulation results in only the inspiratory termination, while PN stimulation elicits only a transient inspiratory inhibition.
2. While stimulation of the SLN or ICN produces both transient responses and termination responses, the threshold intensities necessary for eliciting the inspiratory-terminating responses are consistently higher than those required for the transient responses.
3. Procaine injections into the mNTS diminished SLN-evoked inspiratory termination without affecting the SLN transient inhibition (23).
4. The potential involvement of glycine receptors in the transient inhibitions and not in the termination responses also suggest a possible difference in mechanisms.

Based on numerous findings, Feldman and colleagues (11) have proposed that the respiratory pattern generator involves two major components—a rhythm-generating system and an output amplitude–controlling system. This notion is consistent with speculation that the inhibitory reflexes also represent two systems. It is suggested that the transient reductions of inspiratory activity initiated by phrenic, intercostal, and SLN stimulation could represent reflexes associated with the control of the output amplitude. All three of these afferent systems are known to provide input into the region of the DRG, an important premotor respiratory population. Activation of these afferents (or a subset of the afferent population) could affect the amplitude of inspiratory discharges without necessarily influencing respiratory rhythms. Similarly, other afferents in these nerves could elicit changes in inspiratory and/or expiratory timing without influencing the pre-motor neurons directly. This potential separation of timing and amplitude would permit selective control of these mechanisms by the peripheral reflexes.

REFERENCES

1. Berger, A.J. Dorsal respiratory group neurons in the medulla of the cat: Spinal projections, responses to lung inflation and superior laryngeal nerve stimulation. *Brain Res.* 135:231-254, 1977.

2. Berger, A.J., and R.A. Mitchell. Lateralized phrenic nerve responses to stimulating respiratory afferents in the cat. *Am. J. Physiol.* 230:1314-1320, 1976.

3. Biscoe, T.J., and S.R. Sampson. An analysis of the inhibition of phrenic motoneurones which occurs on stimulation of some cranial nerve afferents. *J. Physiol.* (London) 209:375-393, 1970.

4. Bonham, A.C., and D.R. McCrimmon. Neurones in a discrete region of the nucleus tractus solitarius are required for the Breuer-Hering reflex in rat. *J. Physiol.* (London) 427:261-280, 1990.

5. Champagnat, J., M. Denavit-Saubié, S. Moyanova, and G. Rondouin. Involvement of amino acids in periodic inhibitions of bulbar respiratory neurones. *Brain Res.* 237:351-365, 1982.

6. Curtis, D.R., A.W. Duggan, D. Felix, and G.A.R. Johnston. Bicuculline, an antagonist of GABA and synaptic inhibition in the spinal cord of the cat. *Brain Res.* 32:69-96, 1971.

7. Curtis, D.R., A.W. Duggan, and G.A.R. Johnston. The specificity of strychnine as a glycine antagonist in the mammalian spinal cord. *Exp. Brain Res.* 12:547-565, 1971.

8. Decima, E.E., and C. von Euler. Intercostal and cerebellar influences on efferent phrenic activity in the decerebrate cat. *Acta Physiol. Scand.* 76:148-158, 1969.

9. Denavit-Saubié, M., and J. Champagnat. The effect of some depressing amino acids on bulbar respiratory and non-respiratory neurons. *Brain Res.* 97:356-361, 1975.

10. Eldridge, F.L., D.E. Millhorn, and T. Waldrop. Spinal inhibition of phrenic motoneurones by stimulation of afferents from leg muscle in the cat: Blockade by strychnine. *J. Physiol.* (London) 389:137-146, 1987.

11. Feldman, J.L. Neurophysiology of respiration in mammals. In *Handbook of Physiology,* Section 1, vol. 4, ed. F.E. Bloom, 463-524. Bethesda, Md.: American Physiological Society, 1986.

12. Feldman, J.L., D.R. McCrimmon, and D.F. Speck. Effect of synchronous activation of medullary inspiratory bulbo-spinal neurones on phrenic nerve discharge in cat. *J. Physiol.* (London) 347:241-254, 1984.

13. Feldman, J.L., and J.C. Smith. Cellular mechanisms underlying modulation of breathing pattern in mammals. *Ann. NY Acad. Sci.* 563:114-130, 1989.

14. Granata, A.R., A.F. Sved, and D.J. Reis. *In vivo* release by vagal stimulation of L-[3H]-glutamic acid in the nucleus tractus solitarius preloaded with L-[3H]-glutamine. *Brain Res. Bull.* 12:5-9, 1984.

15. Iscoe, S., J.L. Feldman, and M.I. Cohen. Properties of inspiratory termination by superior laryngeal and vagal stimulation. *Resp. Physiol.* 36:353-366, 1979.

16. Jammes, Y., B. Buchler, S. Delpierre, A. Rasidakis, C. Grimaud, and C. Roussos. Phrenic afferents and their role in inspiratory control. *J. Appl. Physiol.* 60:854-860, 1986.

17. Johnston, G.A.R. Neuropharmacology of amino acid inhibitory transmitters. *Ann. Rev. Pharmacol. Toxicol.* 18:269-289, 1978.

18. Karius, D.R., L. Ling, and D.F. Speck. Lesions of the rostral dorsolateral pons have no effect on afferent evoked inhibition of inspiration. *Brain Res.* 559:22-28, 1991.

19. Karius, D.R., L. Ling, and D.F. Speck. Blockade of N-methyl-D-aspartate receptors has no effect on certain inspiratory reflexes. *Am. J. Physiol.* 261:L443-L448, 1991.

20. Meeley, M.P., M.D. Underwood, W.T. Talman, and D.J. Reis. Content and *in vitro* release of endogenous amino acids in the area of the nucleus of the solitary tract of the rat. *J. Neurochem.* 53:1807-1817, 1989.

21. Remmers, J.E., and I. Marttila. Action of intercostal muscle afferents on the respiratory rhythm of anesthetized cats. *Resp. Physiol.* 24:31-41, 1975.

22. Speck, D.F. Bötzinger Complex region role in phrenic-to-phrenic inhibitory reflex of cat. *J. Appl. Physiol.* 67:1364-1370, 1989.

23. Speck, D.F. Attenuation of inspiratory inhibitory reflexes by small injections of procaine within the brainstem of cats. *FASEB J.* 3:A404, 1989.

24. Speck, D.F., and J.L. Feldman. The effects of microstimulation and microlesions in the ventral and dorsal respiratory groups in medulla of cat. *J. Neurosci.* 2:744-757, 1982.

25. Speck, D.F., D.R. Karius, and L. Ling. Effects of intravenous bicuculline and strychnine on transient inhibitory responses in the cat. *Soc. Neurosci. Abstr.* 15:100, 1989.

26. Talman, W.T. Kynurenic acid microinjected into the nucleus tractus solitarius of rat blocks the arterial baroreflex but not responses to glutamate. *Neurosci. Lett.* 102:247-252, 1989.

Part V

Modulation of Respiratory Pattern by Peripheral Afferents

22

An Overview

Hazel M. Coleridge

Respiratory patterns are modulated by peripheral neural feedback to the central respiratory networks. The inputs discussed in the following chapters include a description of input from the larynx, diaphragm, and exercising muscle, and an account of the special properties of chemosensitive C fibers in the bronchial branches of the vagus nerve. By way of introduction, I will discuss the functional significance of these peripheral inputs and give a brief description of input from the lower respiratory tract.

The papers in this session emphasize that the afferent fibers comprising anatomically defined peripheral inputs that modulate breathing are not homogeneous. Afferent fibers from all the regions considered here are of several modalities. These various modalities of afferents cause breathing pattern to change with great flexibility, and there is no doubt that a detailed investigation of the central connections of any one of them would tell us a good deal about the synaptic interconnections of the respiratory networks as a whole.

From what is known about the various inputs that modulate breathing pattern, and from what the contributors to this conference tell us, there is a major difference in the functional significance of afferent feedback from skeletal muscle and afferent feedback from the respiratory apparatus itself. Input from skeletal muscle has the primary effect of increasing alveolar ventilation. The studies of Dr. Kaufman and his colleagues (this volume) have increased our understanding of the properties of sensory endings in skeletal muscle and have contributed information about their spinal pathways. The endings that provide respiratory neurons with an excitatory input that relates to the intensity of exercise are supplied by small myelinated and nonmyelinated fibers, representative of somatic sensory Groups III and IV. Because this input increases the overall level of ventilation, it probably influences breathing through central mechanisms different from those recruited by input from the respiratory apparatus.

Afferent input from the respiratory apparatus itself, including the upper and lower respiratory tract, the chest wall, and the diaphragm, seems to act primarily to change the pattern of respiratory motor output rather than to control the level of alveolar ventilation. This modulation of pattern can be loosely classified as either regulatory or defensive. Nerve endings, including, for example, the slowly adapting stretch receptors that supply phasic, volume-related feedback from the lungs, and the muscle spindles

and tendon organs that supply proprioceptive feedback from the diaphragm, subserve regulatory reflexes concerned with normal breathing pattern. Their sensitivity is appropriate to the signalling of the normal, mechanical respiratory events, and they are connected to the central nervous system by myelinated fibers with relatively rapid conduction velocities. When conduction in these fibers is prevented from reaching the central respiratory networks, the emerging rhythm is that of the networks themselves. Other nerve endings that supply the respiratory apparatus have a tonic discharge of very low frequency and become active only in unusual situations. They are often chemosensitive and are supplied by small myelinated or nonmyelinated fibers, the latter being in the majority. Their reflex effects have an emergency or defensive character and may temporarily interrupt alveolar ventilation.

The rich innervation of the larynx by afferents of different modalities, described by Dr. Sant'Ambrogio (this volume), seems appropriate to a structure at the entrance to the airway proper, immediately below a region common to the functions of both respiration and alimentation. Although input from laryngeal proprioceptors seems to have at most a minor influence on the pattern of breathing, cough, adduction of the vocal cords, and defensive changes in breathing pattern are readily evoked from the larynx by inhaled irritants. An initial apnea and accompanying depression of cardiac activity is common and resembles that originating from the lower airways. The work of Dr. Jammes and others shows that defensive modulations of breathing are also evoked when small myelinated and nonmyelinated chemosensitive phrenic afferents are stimulated by intense diaphragmatic activity. These may reduce the diaphragmatic contribution to ventilation by reducing phrenic nerve discharge.

In investigations of the normal, on-going regulation of breathing pattern, it has been customary for at least a hundred years to demonstrate the influence of lung volume–related vagal input by cutting or cooling the vagus nerves. Alternatively, pulmonary stretch receptor input has been increased by electrical stimulation of the vagus at a threshold just sufficient to inhibit central inspiratory activity or by static lung inflation to a volume sufficient to produce a similar effect. The difference between the temporal characteristics of the input produced by the last two methods and the normal profile and timing of pulmonary stretch receptor input, and the likelihood that other types of vagal afferent will also be stimulated, has been generally regarded as relatively unimportant. It is now well accepted that the timing and frequency profile of input from the respiratory apparatus in general is a major factor in modifying the activity of the rhythmically firing central neurons. Hence use of the cycle-triggered ventilator has been an important aid in interpreting the regulatory influence of volume-related feedback from the lungs because it maintains the normal temporal relationship between the motor act of breathing and the input profile from lower airway stretch receptors.

The regulatory influence of phrenic nerve afferents on breathing pattern has been recognized only recently. This phrenic influence can be demonstrated in the absence of vagal and thoracic spinal input, when the phrenic nerves are cooled sufficiently to block conduction in myelinated fibers from the diaphragmatic proprioceptors (Jammes and Balzamo, this volume). There is evidence that these proprioceptors, in a manner somewhat analogous to the slowly adapting pulmonary stretch receptors, provide inhibitory input to inspiratory neurons and decrease inspiratory time. The tonic input in small myelinated and nonmyelinated phrenic afferents is thought to have no influence during quiet breathing. This fits in well with the general hypothesis that the large afferent fibers that innervate the respiratory apparatus subserve regulatory reflexes and that the small afferent fibers, including nonmyelinated fibers, have, in the main, a defensive function. There is some evidence, however, that even in the absence of abnormal events, the tonic, low-frequency discharge in vagal, nonmyelinated fibers from the lungs and lower airways affects expiratory time. Thus in experiments in anesthetized dogs, the vagus nerves were cooled to $-1\ °C$ at a rate sufficiently slow to allow the influence of nonmyelinated afferent fibers to be distinguished from that of myelinated afferents. The typical prolongation of expiratory time seen after vagotomy was not complete at vagal temperatures several degrees lower than those required to block conduction in myelinated fibers, but became complete when the nerves were cooled to $-1\ °C$, or the pulmonary branches were cut (8).

When full account is taken of the many modalities of afferent input from the respiratory apparatus as a whole, it could be argued that investigators have been unduly preoccupied with the modulations of breathing pattern produced by vagal input from the lower airways. This preoccupation is to some extent justified, however, on the basis of the evolutionary development of respiratory modulation. Vagal feedback from the lower respiratory tract seems to have acquired a major influence on breathing pattern at an early stage of vertebrate evolution. A regulatory Hering-Breuer inspiration-inhibitory reflex or its equivalent is present in all air breathing vertebrates and can be seen in forms that represent the earliest stage of lung development (see Pack et al., this volume). In lower vertebrates such as fish a defensive type of vagal chemoreflex originates in the gills and is virtually identical with that in mammals in causing a

brief cessation of ventilatory movements with inhibition of cardiac activity (10).

The possibility that a third modality of vagal input from the lower airways, supplied by rapidly adapting receptors, can modulate breathing pattern during eupnea remains an open question. The pulmonary and bronchial branches of the vagus carry not only inspiration-inhibitory input from slowly adapting mechanoreceptors, but also inspiration-excitatory input from rapidly adapting ones. Rapidly adapting receptors are supplied by myelinated vagal fibers. They have a relatively high threshold to lung inflation and have been thought to be virtually inactive during quiet breathing. They were first identified by their rapidly adapting response to inflation, and their input was associated with a burst of activity in phrenic motoneurons (3). The special characteristics of rapidly adapting receptors at the tracheal bifurcation identified them as cough receptors (11). Those elsewhere in the airways were found to become active in experimental models of lung disease and were thought to cause hyperpnea and bronchoconstriction rather than cough (5). They were given the alternative title "irritant receptor." For a time, rapidly adapting or irritant receptors were thought to be mainly of importance in airway disease, but a quantitative examination of their dynamic properties showed that these were consistent with the provision of an excitatory feedback to central inspiratory neurons as the volume and rate of lung inflation increases in exercise (6). Nevertheless, the prolonged stimulation of rapidly adapting receptors by bronchoconstrictor agents and its ready reversal by hyperinflation of the lung (9) suggested a specific sensitivity to changes in lung mechanics that might be of significance during normal, quiet breathing.

It was discovered that in the absence of any irritant stimulus the activity of rapidly adapting receptors at resting tidal volume increases progressively when lung compliance decreases, and that some receptors are sensitive to decreases of as little as 10–15% (7, 12). Lung compliance is known to decrease by 30% or more during normal periods of quiet breathing. Thus increases in lung stiffness in the physiological range cause rapidly adapting receptors to discharge regular, high-frequency bursts of impulses at the peak of each inflation. This discharge is abolished when compliance is restored by hyperinflating the lung (fig. 22.1). Hence as the lungs become stiffer during quiet breathing, an excitatory vagal input from rapidly adapting receptors may well increase the activity of inspiratory neurons, and when this input reaches a critical level, trigger the sighs or augmented breaths that serve to restore compliance to optimum.

The chemosensitive C fibers of the vagus nerve, mentioned already as a source of defensive reflex input to the central respiratory networks, supply all levels of the lower respiratory tract from the trachea to the most distal division of the bronchial tree. Stimulation of these fibers by bolus injection of micromolar amounts of capsaicin and other

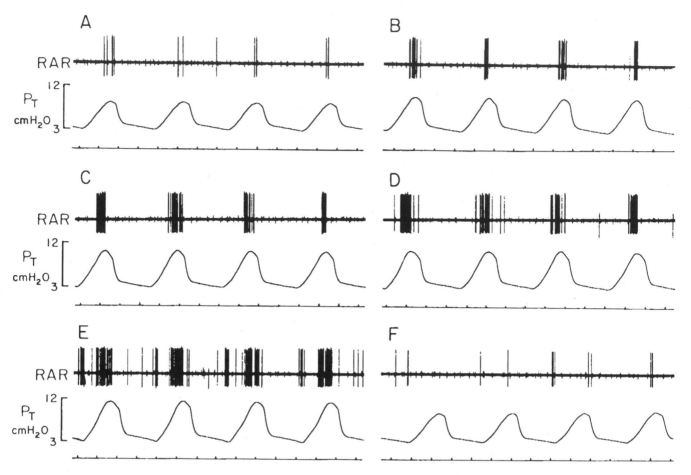

FIG. 22.1 Stimulation of a rapidly adapting receptor (RAR) in a rabbit by progressive reduction of lung compliance. The lungs were ventilated at constant tidal volume. P_T, tracheal pressure, time marks 1 sec. (A) Control, lung compliance maximal; (B-E) Lung compliance successively reduced to 68% of control (at E). Between E and F lung compliance was restored to maximal by hyperinflating the lungs. (F) activity when lung compliance was restored. (From 12.)

irritants into the pulmonary or bronchial arteries evokes an initial apnea, succeeded by an often prolonged period of rapid shallow breathing (1). The central component of this apnea was described by Koepchen et al. (4) as an inhibition of both medullary inspiratory and expiratory neurons. This differs from the apnea of the Hering-Breuer reflex, in which inhibition of inspiratory neurons is accompanied by a reciprocal excitation of expiratory ones. The rapid, shallow breathing that follows the apnea of the airway chemoreflex was described as having, as its basis, a rapid succession of inspiratory neuron bursts with long-lasting inhibition of expiratory activity (fig. 22.2). The initial total inhibition of central respiratory activity was thought to be related in some fashion to an accompanying overall depression of somatic motor activity (2, 4), but the subsequent prolonged and apparently specific depression of expiratory neurons argues for more complex and specific central respiratory effects. Results of investigation of the central sites involved in this response are presented in an abstract by Kubin and Davies presented at this symposium and by Bonham et al. (this volume) and are a promising begin-

ning to our understanding of the phenomenon. Kubin and Davies describe modality-specific regions of the nucleus of the solitary tract, and find a high density of substance P–containing neurons in the region to which bronchopulmonary C fibers project. Bonham et al. define discrete relay sites in the caudomedial solitary tract nucleus associated with the rapid shallow breathing described above.

Interest in the vagal chemosensitive C fibers that supply the conducting airways has acquired a new impetus, because it has been demonstrated that, like the chemosensitive C fibers that supply the skin, they exhibit a substance P–like immunoreactivity. Dr. Lundberg and his colleagues (this volume) have presented compelling evidence that stimulation of airway C fibers not only brings about central transmission along axons, with reflex changes in breathing pattern and autonomic effects on airway function, but also a peripheral, Ca^{++}-dependent, "axon-reflex" transmission, with release of neuropeptides into the airway mucosa. These neuropeptides have local effects on airway structures and induce secondary release of other mediators. To date axon-reflex effects on airways have been demonstrated

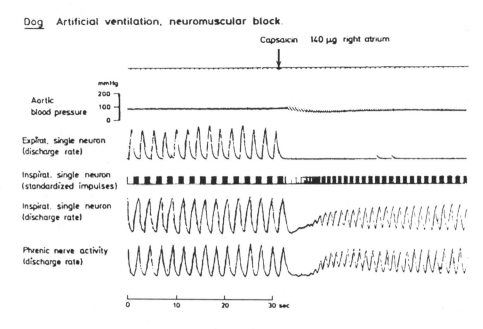

Dog Artificial ventilation, neuromuscular block.

Capsaicin 140 μg right atrium

Aortic blood pressure

mmHg
200
100
0

Exspirat. single neuron (discharge rate)

Inspirat. single neuron (standardized impulses)

Inspirat. single neuron (discharge rate)

Phrenic nerve activity (discharge rate)

0   10   20   30 sec

FIG. 22.2 Effect of right atrial injection of capsaicin on arterial blood pressure, the discharges of one expiratory and one inspiratory single unit, and integrated phrenic nerve activity, recorded in an anesthetized, artificially ventilated dog. The activity of the expiratory neuron resumed after the end of this recording. (From 4.)

mainly in guinea pigs and rats. There may be species differences in the peripheral response since bronchoconstrictor axon-reflex effects are best studied in the guinea pig, and rats are much less sensitive. Dr. Lundberg's group has been unable to demonstrate an axon-reflex increase in airway vascular permeability in cats and dogs. An increase in bronchial blood flow of axon-reflex origin could be readily demonstrated in pigs, however, and seemed to be a major determinant of changes in bronchial blood flow in that species. Hence, although to date few of the airway axon-reflex phenomena have been demonstrated in larger mammals, they may be of major significance in human airway disease.

REFERENCES

1. Coleridge, J.C.G., and H.M. Coleridge. Afferent vagal C fibre innervation of the lungs and airways and its functional significance. *Rev. Biochem. Pharmacol.* 99:1-110, 1984.

2. Ginzel, K.H., and E. Eldred. Reflex depression of somatic motor activity from heart, lungs and carotid sinus. In *Krogh centenary symposium on respiratory adaptations, capillary exchange and reflex mechanisms,* ed. A.S. Paintal and P. Gill-Kumar, 358-394. Delhi: Vallabhbhai Patel Chest Institute, 1977.

3. Knowlton, G.C., and M.G. Larrabee. A unitary analysis of pulmonary volume receptors. *Am. J. Physiol.* 147:100-114, 1946.

4. Koepchen, H.P., M. Kalia, D. Sommer, and D. Klussendorf. Action of type J afferents on the discharge pattern of med

ullary respiratory neurons. In *Krogh centenary symposium on respiratory adaptations, capillary exchange and reflex mechanisms,* ed. A.S. Paintal and P. Gill-Kumar, 407-425. Delhi: Vallabhbhai Patel Chest Institute, 1977.

5. Mills, S.E., H. Sellick, and J.G. Widdicombe. Activity of lung irritant receptors in pulmonary micro-embolism, anaphylaxis and drug-induced bronchoconstrictions. *J. Physiol.* (London) 203:337-357, 1969.

6. Pack, A.I., and R.G. DeLaney. Response of pulmonary rapidly adapting receptors during lung inflation. *J. Appl. Physiol.* 55:955-963, 1983.

7. Pisarri, T.E., A. Jonzon, J.C.G. Coleridge, and H.M. Coleridge. Rapidly adapting receptors monitor lung compliance in spontaneously breathing dogs. *J. Appl. Physiol.* 68:1997-2005, 1990.

8. Pisarri, T.E., J. Yu, H.M. Coleridge, and J.C.G. Coleridge. Background activity in pulmonary vagal C-fibers and its effects on breathing. *Resp. Physiol.* 64:29-43, 1986.

9. Sampson, S.R., and E.H. Vidruk. Properties of 'irritant' receptors in canine lung. *Resp. Physiol.* 25:9-22, 1975.

10. Satchell, G.H. The J reflex in fish. In *Krogh centenary symposium on respiratory adaptations, capillary exchange and reflex mechanisms,* ed. A.S. Paintal and P. Gill-Kumar, 432-437. Delhi: Vallabhbhai Patel Chest Institute, 1977.

11. Widdicombe, J.G. Receptors in the trachea and bronchi of the cat. *J. Physiol.* (London) 123:71-104, 1954.

12. Yu, J., J.C.G. Coleridge, and H.M. Coleridge. Influence of lung stiffness on rapidly adapting receptors in rabbits and cats. *Resp. Physiol.* 68:161-176, 1987.

23

Laryngeal Sensory Modalities and Their Functional Significance

Giuseppe Sant'Ambrogio, James W. Anderson, and Franca B. Sant'Ambrogio

The larynx has a very rich sensory supply (1, 4), which plays an important role in defensive reflexes as well as the regulation of breathing. On the basis of their activation during upper airway breathing, tracheostomy breathing, upper airway occlusion, and tracheal occlusion, respiratory modulated laryngeal endings have been classified as cold, pressure, and "drive" receptors (16).

Cold receptors are activated during upper airway breathing and remain silent during tracheal breathing, upper airway occlusion, and tracheal occlusion (fig. 23.1). These receptors are silent at body temperature and are activated during inspiration when temperature in the laryngeal lumen decreases (17). They have been localized to a discrete region of the vocal folds, at the level of the vocal process.

Laryngeal pressure receptors are stimulated strongly during upper airway occlusion at end inspiration or expiration, depending on whether the appropriate stimulus is distending or collapsing pressure (fig. 23.1). Usually these receptors are active during upper airway breathing and most of them are activated by collapsing pressure. Besides their primary response to transmural pressure, many of these endings show a residual modulation during tracheal breathing and tracheal occlusion, that is, in the absence of any pressure stimulation (16).

Laryngeal "drive" receptors are stimulated phasically during breathing, even in the absence of airflow and pressure (fig. 23.1). They generally show some degree of pressure detection, more often being inhibited by collapsing pressure and stimulated by distending pressure. Reversible laryngeal paralysis, by cold blocking either the recurrent nerve or the external branch of the superior laryngeal nerve, demonstrated that intrinsic laryngeal muscle contraction is the most frequent factor for their activation (18). Tracheal tug (motion due to the chest wall muscles transmitted through the trachea) was also found to be the stimulus for some of the endings (18). The term "drive" describes the dependence of the activation of these receptors on the outputs of the respiratory center that "drive" both laryngeal and chest wall respiratory muscles (16).

Recent studies have evaluated, in anesthetized dogs, the relative contribution of laryngeal cold, pressure, and "drive" receptors to the regulation of the pattern of breathing and the maintenance of upper airway patency (15). In these experiments no significant change in breathing pattern could be attributed to cold receptors; however, laryngeal cooling was found to induce bronchoconstriction in cats (5) and ventilatory depression in newborn dogs (12) as well as in adult guinea pigs (13). Cooling of the larynx, besides stimulating specific cold receptors, inhibits both pressure and "drive" receptors (19), which could therefore contribute to the observed responses. The importance of cold receptor stimulation, however, can be inferred from experiments in guinea pigs in which 1-menthol, a specific stimulant of cold receptors (14), was also capable of depressing ventilation in the absence of changes in laryngeal temperature (13).

The function of laryngeal pressure receptors in the regulation of breathing pattern and upper airway muscle activity has been estimated either by comparing the responses to upper airway and tracheal occlusion (fig. 23.2) or following the application of pressure changes to the isolated upper airway. In either case it was found that collapsing pressure in the upper airway prolongs inspiratory duration without markedly affecting peak inspiratory activity, and decreases inspiratory drive (11, 15). At the same time there was a marked activation of various upper airway dilating muscles (9, 15, 20). Since all the responses to upper airway pressure changes become substantially weaker or are abolished by anesthetization of the laryngeal mucosa or section of the superior laryngeal nerves, they are attributed to pressure sensitive laryngeal receptors (10, 15, 20).

The reflex function of "drive" receptors can be inferred by comparing the responses to tracheal occlusion before and after section of the superior laryngeal nerve (fig. 23.2), that is, in a condition in which the larynx is subjected to the activity of its own muscles and the tracheal tug in the absence of pressure and cold stimuli (15). No alteration in breathing pattern or in upper airway muscle activity was found between the two situations, and thus no reflex effects could be attributed to these receptors. However, since many "drive" receptors are affected by laryngeal intrinsic muscle activity they could have an important function for the fine coordination of these muscles, as required in vocalization. These findings suggest that the afferent activity from the larynx plays a role in overcoming oropharyngeal obstruction through a reflex recruitment of upper airway muscles in conditions such as obstructive sleep apnea.

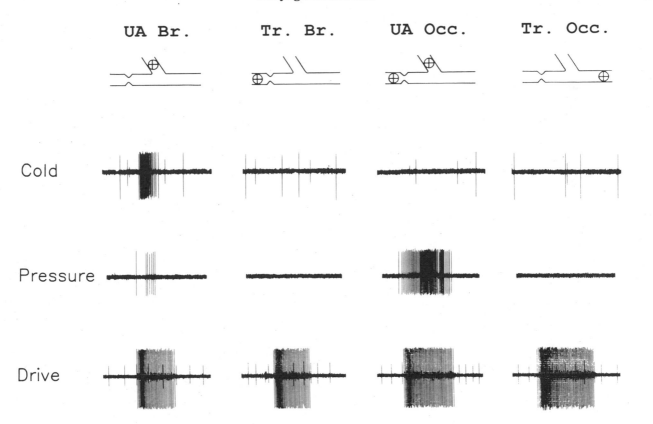

FIG. 23.1 Behavior of laryngeal cold, pressure, and "drive" receptors during the following experimental conditions: upper airway breathing (UA Br.), tracheostomy breathing (Tr. Br.), upper airway occlusion (UA Occ.), and tracheal occlusion (Tr. Occ.).

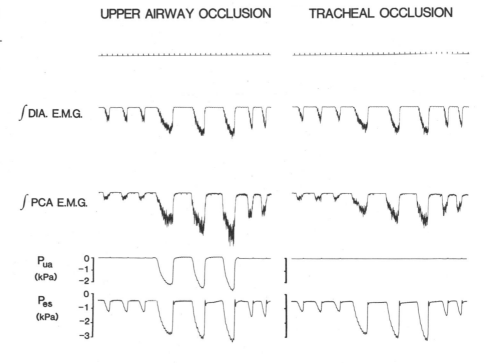

FIG. 23.2 Activity of the diaphragm and posterior cricoarytenoid muscle to upper airway occlusion (*left*) and tracheal occlusion (*right*). Traces from top to bottom are time in seconds, integrated diaphragmatic activity ($\int$DIA. E.M.G.), integrated activity of the posterior cricoarytenoid muscle ($\int$PCA E.M.G.), pressure in the upper airway (P_{ua}), and esophageal (P_{es}) pressures in kiloPascal (kPa). Note that upper airway occlusion elicits a stronger activation of the PCA than tracheal occlusion.

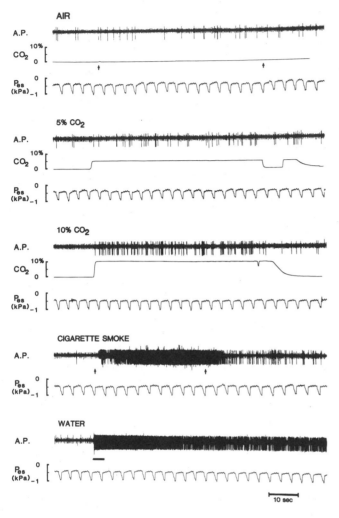

FIG. 23.3 Effect of warm air, carbon dioxide (5% and 10%), cigarette smoke, and water on a laryngeal "irritant" receptor. In each panel traces are, from top to bottom, action potentials recorded from the superior laryngeal nerve (A.P.), carbon dioxide concentration (first three panels), and esophageal pressure (P_{es}). Whereas air does not affect the receptor discharge, carbon dioxide causes a clear increase in its activity, especially at a 10% concentration. Cigarette smoke (between arrows) and water (time of delivery indicated by the thick line) are very potent stimulants for this receptor.

In addition to the afferent activity closely related to the breathing cycle, there are laryngeal endings that are either silent or randomly active in control conditions but are promptly recruited whenever the laryngeal mucosa is exposed to mechanical and/or chemical irritants. In fact, these "irritant" type receptors respond to several tussigenic stimuli (fig. 23.3) and therefore can be considered to provide an important triggering mechanism of the cough reflex from the larynx (6).

Recently it was found that a significant proportion of pressure and "drive" receptors are stimulated by solutions of low osmolality and inhibited by carbon dioxide (2, 3), which could presumably act by increasing the hydrogen ion

concentration. On the other hand, laryngeal "irritant" receptors are affected by the ionic composition of solutions introduced into the laryngeal lumen. In particular, they are stimulated by solutions lacking permeant anions, such as chloride (fig. 23.4) (2). Moreover, many of them can also be stimulated by carbon dioxide (fig. 23.3) (3).

Reflex responses should therefore be expected to depend on a variety of factors rather than a unique stimulus. For instance, the excitatory influence on upper airway muscles elicited by collapsing pressure could be modified by changes in osmolality and/or concentration of hydrogen ions of the laryngeal surface liquid. Similarly, the reflex reactions to irritants in the larynx could be accentuated by a decrease in chloride ion concentration or an increase in hydrogen ion concentration of the surface liquid.

Since the composition of the airway surface liquid can be modified by the relative humidity of the inspired air, mouth breathing versus nose breathing (7), airway secretions and various pharmacological agents (8), we may envisage the possibility that various interventions will enhance or suppress reflex responses mediated by laryngeal receptors. Very recently it was shown that furosemide, a blocker of the sodium/chloride cotransport, reduces the tussigenic effect of inhaled distilled water (21). This antitussigenic action of furosemide could possibly be due to its effect on airway epithelial ion transport (22); this would modify the composition of the interstitial fluid surrounding the receptors responsible for the cough reflex and therefore interfere with their activation.

ACKNOWLEDGMENTS

This work was supported by NIH Grant HL-20122.

REFERENCES

1. Agostoni, E., J.E. Chinnock, M. De Burgh Daly, and J.G. Murray. Functional and histological studies of the vagus nerve and its branches to the heart, lungs and abdominal viscera in the cat. *J. Physiol.* (London) 135:182-205, 1957.

2. Anderson, J.W., F.B. Sant'Ambrogio, O.P. Mathew, and G. Sant'Ambrogio. Water-responsive laryngeal receptors in the dog are not specialized endings. *Resp. Physiol.* 79:33-44, 1990.

3. Anderson, J.W., F.B. Sant'Ambrogio, G.P. Orani, G. Sant'Ambrogio, and O.P. Mathew. Carbon dioxide responsive laryngeal receptors in the dog. *Resp. Physiol.*, 82:217-226, 1990.

4. DuBois, F.S., and J.O. Foley. Experimental studies on the vagus and spinal accessory nerves in the cat. *Anat. Rec.* 64:285-307, 1936.

5. Jammes, Y., P. Barthelemy, and S. Delpierre. Respiratory effects of cold air breathing in anesthetized cats. *Resp. Physiol.* 54:41-54, 1983.

6. Karlsson, J.-A., G. Sant'Ambrogio, and J. Widdicombe. Afferent neural pathways in cough and reflex bronchoconstriction. *J. Appl. Physiol.* 65:1007-1023, 1988.

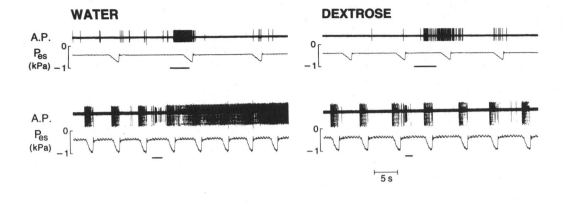

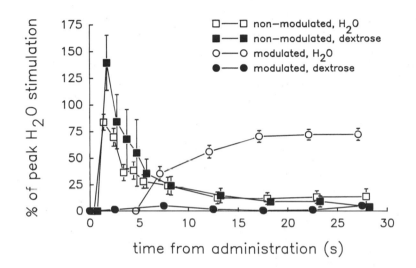

FIG. 23.4 The upper panels illustrate the behavior of two different types of water-responsive receptors. In each panel the traces are of action potentials (A.P.) and esophageal pressure (P$_{es}$). Application of the test solution is indicated by the thick horizontal lines. The nonmodulated "irritant" receptor (upper traces) was stimulated by both water and isotonic dextrose, while the respiratory modulated receptor (lower traces) was only stimulated by water. The average time course of the response of the two types of laryngeal receptors is represented in the lower panel. Note that the "irritant" receptors (n = 12) responded with a short-delay, short-duration discharge to both water and dextrose, while the modulated receptors (n = 21) responded only to water with a long-delay, long-duration discharge.

7. Man, S.F.P., G.K. Adams, III, and D.F. Proctor. Effects of temperature, relative humidity, and mode of breathing on canine airway secretions. *J. Appl. Physiol.* 46:205-210, 1979.

8. Marin, M.G. Pharmacology of airway secretion. *Pharmacol. Rev.* 38:273-289, 1986.

9. Mathew, O.P. Upper airway negative-pressure effects on respiratory activity of upper airway muscles. *J. Appl. Physiol.* 56:500-505, 1984.

10. Mathew, O.P., Y.K. Abu-Osba, and B.T. Thach. Influence of upper airway pressure changes in respiratory frequency. *Resp. Physiol.* 49:223-233, 1982.

11. Mathew, O.P., Y.K. Abu-Osba, and B.T. Thach. Genioglossus muscle responses to upper airway pressure changes: Afferent pathways. *J. Appl. Physiol.* 52:445-450, 1982.

12. Mathew, O.P., J.W. Anderson, G.P. Orani, F.B. Sant'Ambrogio, and G. Sant'Ambrogio. Cooling mediates the ventilatory

depression associated with airflow through the larynx. *Resp. Physiol.*, 82:359-368, 1990.

13. Orani, G.P., J.W. Anderson, G. Sant'Ambrogio, and F.B. Sant'Ambrogio. Upper airway cooling and 1-menthol reduce ventilation in the guinea pig. *J. Appl. Physiol.* 70:2080-2086, 1991.

14. Sant'Ambrogio, F.B., J.W. Anderson, and G. Sant'Ambrogio. Effect of 1-menthol on laryngeal receptors. *J. Appl. Physiol.* 70:788-793, 1991.

15. Sant'Ambrogio, F.B., O.P. Mathew, W.D. Clark, and G. Sant'Ambrogio. Laryngeal influences on breathing pattern and posterior cricoarytenoid muscle activity. *J. Appl. Physiol.* 58:1298-1304, 1985.

16. Sant'Ambrogio, G., O.P. Mathew, J.T. Fisher, and F.B. Sant'Ambrogio. Laryngeal receptors responding to transmural pressure, airflow and local muscle activity. *Resp. Physiol.* 54:317-330, 1983.

17. Sant'Ambrogio, G., O.P. Mathew, and F.B. Sant'Ambrogio. Laryngeal cold receptors. *Resp. Physiol.* 59:35-44, 1985.

18. Sant'Ambrogio, G., O.P. Mathew, and F.B. Sant'Ambrogio. Role of intrinsic muscle and tracheal motion in modulating laryngeal receptors. *Resp. Physiol.* 61:289-300, 1985.

19. Sant'Ambrogio, G., F.B. Sant'Ambrogio, and O.P. Mathew. Effect of cold air on laryngeal mechanoreceptors in the dog. *Resp. Physiol.* 64:45-56, 1986.

20. Van Lunteren, E., K.P. Strohl, D.M. Parker, E.N. Bruce, W.B. Van de Graaff, and N.S. Cherniack. Phasic volume-related feedback on upper airway muscle activity. *J. Appl. Physiol.* 56:730-736, 1984.

21. Ventresca, P.G., G.M. Nichol, P.J. Barnes, and K.F. Chung. Inhaled furosemide inhibits cough induced by low chloride content solutions but not by capsaicin. *Am. Rev. Respir. Dis.* 142:143-146, 1990.

22. Welsh, M.J. Mechanism of airway epithelial transport. *Clin. Chest Med.* 7:273-283, 1986.

24
Diaphragmatic Afferents

Yves Jammes and Emmanuel Balzamo

DIAPHRAGMATIC RECEPTORS AND AFFERENT FIBERS

Dogiel (5) first identified muscle spindles and Golgi tendon organs in the diaphragmatic cupolae in humans, monkeys, dogs, cats, and rabbits. From these initial histological observations, the existence of a sensory component in the phrenic nerve has been accepted. This gave rise to numerous structural and neurophysiological investigations. Few histological studies on diaphragmatic receptors have been performed, and they were mostly done in cats, in which Duron (7) has identified only muscle spindles in the crural portion of this muscle. However, Winckler and Delaloye (30) and Winckler (31) reported the existence of muscle spindles in the diaphragmatic cupolae in humans. The histological evidence of free sensory endings such as those described in skeletal muscles by Mense (22) has never been demonstrated in the diaphragm.

The composition of the phrenic nerve has been studied only in cats. After degenerating the motor component in this nerve, Hinsey et al. (10), using light microscopy, found a ratio of three unmyelinated fibers (Group IV) for each myelinated one in the sensory component. Histograms of fiber diameters in the sensory phrenic nerve revealed two peaks at 3–4 and 13 μm, which correspond to thin (Group III) and large (Groups I and II) myelinated fibers, respectively. Using electron micrographs of the whole phrenic trunk, Duron (7) has shown that the number of the unmyelinated fibers in this nerve is more than twice that of myelinated ones, with a diameter ranging between 0.3 and 1.4 μm.

SPONTANEOUS ACTIVITY AND PHYSIOLOGICAL STIMULI

When recording afferents from the cut peripheral end of a phrenic nerve or from nerve filaments dissected from the intact nerve trunk, two general types of discharge patterns are identified. Some fibers discharge phasically during either diaphragmatic contraction (Corda et al. [3]: 54 phasic units / 85 total units; Jammes et al. [12]: 42/50; Graham et al. [9]: 19/25) or relaxation (Corda: 10/85; Jammes: 8/50; Graham: 6/25). These fibers have a relatively high firing rate (137 ± 3 sec^{-1}). Measurement of conduction velocity from the pauci-fiber preparation showed that it ranged between 20 m/sec (Group III fibers) and 50 m/sec (Group I/II fibers) (9). The other type of phrenic sensory fiber displays a near tonic, low-frequency discharge (2 ± 0.5 sec^{-1}), never modulated by diaphragmatic contractions. The conduction velocity of afferent phrenic fibers carrying tonic activity ranged between 0.8 and 1.3 m/sec (Group IV phrenic fibers) (9).

Based on the activation of their spontaneous discharge by succinylcholine, muscle spindles were identified in the crural part of the diaphragm but not the cupolae or its sternal part (3). They displayed rhythmic activity in phase either with diaphragmatic relaxation ("passive" muscle spindles) or contraction ("active" spindles). Golgi tendon organs discharge in phase with spontaneous diaphragmatic contractions and thus have a low excitation threshold (3, 7, 12). Increasing the strength of diaphragmatic contraction by tracheal occlusion performed at the end-expiratory level enhances markedly the spontaneous afferent discharge of Golgi tendon organs (12).

Tonic sensory fibers in the diaphragm are activated mostly by extracellular metabolic changes, as produced by lowering muscle pH (injection of lactic acid into the phrenic artery) or muscle ischemia, increased osmolarity (injection of hypertonic NaCl solution) or by injection of phenyldiguanide, a drug well known to stimulate unmyelinated sensory fibers (9, 11, 12). The average latency period to the point of maximal change in firing rate after retrograde injection of test agents in the left carotid artery varied between 5 sec (lactic acid) and 13 sec (NaCl), and the activation of these receptors began 18 sec after the onset of total muscle ischemia (9). On the other hand, the above changes in extracellular fluid composition elicit in parallel a marked decline (-34 to -61%) in the phasic discharge of diaphragmatic afferent fibers. Thus, when diaphragm fatigue occurs with accompanying metabolic changes in this muscle, the peripheral sensory pathway to the respiratory centers should be modified, with increased chemosensory information on the metabolic state of muscle fibers and a decline in proprioceptive paths.

VENTILATORY CONTROL

In rabbits, Dolivo (6) reported that blockade of large phrenic fibers using anodal block induced a lengthening of the inspiratory time, but this was studied in animals breathing spontaneously and the observed effect may be a mechanical and/or a metabolic consequence of diaphragm paralysis. In cats with spinal cords sectioned at C8 level,

FIG. 24.1 Quantitative analysis of phrenic neurograms performed before and after distal section of the phrenic trunks. On the ordinate is impulse frequency of phrenic motoneurons and on the abscissa is the integrated raw signal (arbitrary units). Both variables were measured for consecutive 100-msec periods during phrenic discharges. Examples of power spectra with values of centroid frequency are given for each situation.

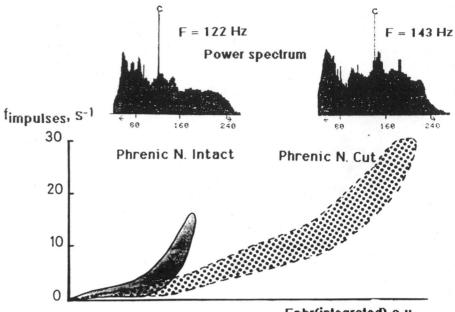

under artificial ventilation (12), cold block of large phrenic fibers during spontaneous diaphragmatic contractions prolonged the inspiratory time and reduced the respiratory frequency, whereas procaine block of thin fibers did not induce any change in phrenic motor discharge. In five other animals (16), we observed under the same experimental conditions that section of both phrenic trunks exerted significant changes in ventilatory timing (ΔT_I = + 13%, ΔT_{tot} = + 16%) and also modified the power spectrum density function of the phrenic neurogram, increasing the high-frequency power toward the end of inspiration (fig. 24.1). Thus, sensory activity in the phrenic nerves during unloaded breathing seems to play a role in the control of ventilatory timing and to govern also the discharge pattern of phrenic motoneurons. This influence seems to be mainly produced by the phasic activity of diaphragmatic proprioceptors.

RESPIRATORY EFFECTS OF PHRENIC AFFERENT STIMULATION

Gill and Kuno (8) first recorded inhibitory postsynaptic potentials in phrenic motoneurons in response to dorsal root stimulation in cats. In a recent work Speck (26) has elegantly demonstrated in decerebrated or C2 spinalized cats that the inhibitory ipsilateral phrenic response is due to spinal cord circuits (short latency: 5 msec), whereas the contralateral inhibitory phrenic response is abolished after C2 spinal section, thus involving supraspinal connections (long latency: 20 msec). Speck (28) has also shown that neural pathways important in producing the phrenic-to-phrenic inhibitory reflex pass through the region of the Bötzinger Complex. Phrenic nerve afferents, identified in the dorsal column (17), project also to other brainstem

sites, including the dorsal respiratory group neurons (27), the external cuneate (17), the lateral reticular nuclei (18), and also the cerebellum (19). In all the above studies the stimulus consisted of single or double electric pulses. When repetitive phrenic nerve stimulation was applied for a few consecutive inspiratory discharges or a 1 min period, the ventilatory effects of phrenic afferent fiber stimulation are more complex. An inspiratory triggering effect ("on-switch" mechanism) by phrenic afferents is elicited when brief (2 sec) repetitive phrenic nerve stimulation is delivered early in the expiratory period (14, 20). Trains of square wave shocks delivered for 30 sec to one or both phrenic nerves induced immediate changes in breathing pattern, characterized by tachypnea, a marked shortening in the firing time of phrenic motor discharge (T_{phr}) with a decline in the T_{phr}/T_{tot} ratio, and a reduced peak firing rate of motoneurons (12). When repetitive stimulation of the phrenic nerve was maintained for 1 min, Marlot et al. (20) reported a biphasic response: a short-term inhibitory response for a few breaths, which was suppressed in animals pretreated with bicuculline (a blockade agent of GABA neurotransmission), followed by a long-term excitation beginning after 15 to 20 sec of nerve stimulation.

Infinite inspiratory loads, such as those produced by tracheal occlusion at end-expiration (TO), prolong the diaphragmatic contraction in vagotomized cats with intact spinal cords (13). Spinal cord section at the C8 level abolished the changes in inspiratory duration in response to TO, but TO was then associated with a reduction in the amplitude of the integrated diaphragmatic EMG (14). This inhibitory response is attributed to the markedly increased activity of diaphragmatic Golgi tendon organs with TO (12). On the other hand, the ventilatory response to submaximal ventilatory loading, such as produced by breathing against external resistive loads for few breaths, does not seem to involve the participation of phrenic afferents. Indeed, in vagotomized cats, spinal section at C8 level abolished all the load-induced changes in breathing pattern (21).

Revelette et al. (24) have reported that capsaicin injection into the phrenic artery of the dog induced tonic diaphragmatic contractions within 1 or 2 sec. This response, interpreted as an excitatory effect on phrenic motoneurons exerted by the activation of Group III and/or IV phrenic sensory fibers, was abolished after surgical destruction of the cervical spinal cord but persisted after cervical dorsal rhizotomy or C2 spinal cord transection. There is a marked contradiction, however, between the very short latency of the capsaicin-induced diaphragmatic response and the minimal 5 sec delay needed to activate free muscle endings in the diaphragm.

When inspiratory loading is prolonged for minutes or hours diaphragm fatigue may occur. Diaphragm failure can be produced also by stimulating the phrenic nerves or the diaphragm itself with trains of electric pulses (15). Under these situations of increased strength of contraction, changes in extracellular fluid composition could occur in the diaphragm, activating chemosensory nerve endings. Aubier et al. (1) reported changes in ventilatory timing in dogs during the response to breathing against a fatiguing load or in a state of reduced diaphragmatic blood flow (as in shock). Tachypnea was followed by bradypnea. Because this response was not affected by vagotomy or cross perfusion of the head (eliminating the stimulation of arterial and central chemoreceptors), it was tempting to speculate that the activation of some diaphragmatic receptors, such as Groups III and IV fibers, may play a major role in the observed changes in ventilatory timing during diaphragm fatigue.

Recently, Supinski et al. (29) have shown in the same species that fatigue of *in situ* muscle strips from the left diaphragm elicited a significant increase in integrated right hemidiaphragm EMG with a slight increase in respiratory frequency. Phrenic nerve section during fatigue was followed by an immediate increase in the peak height of phrenic neurogram, suggesting that activation of some diaphragmatic receptors during the development of fatigue may reflexly inhibit the phrenic motor drive. In all above studies, however, there was never simultaneous recordings of both sensory and motor phrenic pathways in the same situation.

In anesthetized, artificially ventilated cats, we tried to verify that changes in breathing pattern during diaphragm fatigue were concomitant with the activation of chemosensory nerve endings in this muscle (16). Diaphragm fatigue, obtained by supramaximal direct electrical stimulation of both cupolae with trains of pulses for 30 min periods, was assessed from declined maximal relaxation rate of twitches and a left shift in the diaphragmatic EMG power spectrum,

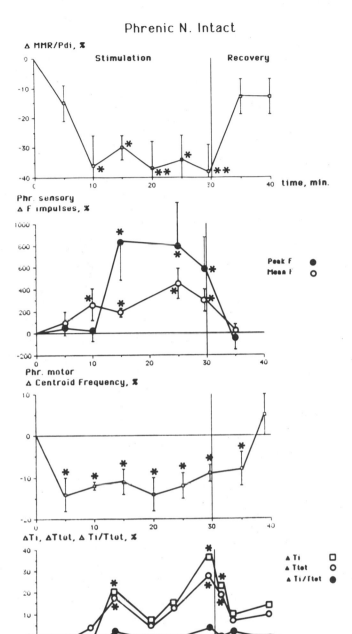

FIG. 24.2 Changes in spontaneous phrenic afferent discharge (Phr. sensory), recruitment of phrenic motoneurons (Phr. motor), inspiratory duration (ΔT_I), total breath duration(ΔT_{tot}), and duty cycle ($\Delta T_I/T_{tot}$) were measured during electrically induced fatiguing contractions of the diaphragm in cats. Fatigue was assessed from a decreased relaxation rate of twitches (MMR/Pdi). (* $P<0.05$; ** $P<0.01$)

as shown previously in rabbits (15). Action potentials of phrenic sensory fibers were recorded from nerve slips, and Group III and IV afferents were identified by their early activation by the retrograde injection of lactic acid solution

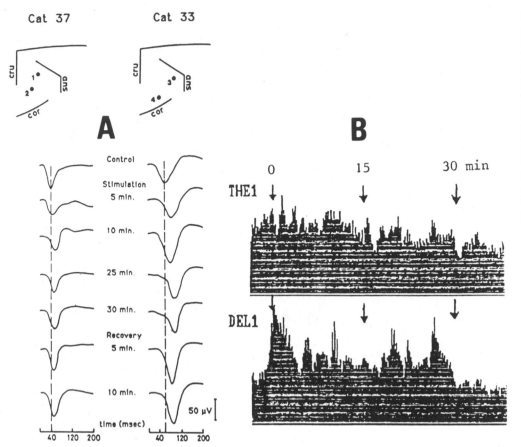

FIG. 24.3 (A) Phrenic evoked potentials recorded on the sensorimotor cortex of cats 37 and 33 before and during fatiguing diaphragmatic contractions maintained for 30 min, then during a 10-min recovery period. Dashed lines indicate the mean value of control peak. (B) Fast Fourier transform analysis of EEG rhythms in theta (top) and delta (bottom) frequency bands performed in cat 37 before and during 30 min of fatiguing diaphragmatic contractions, then during recovery.

into the left common carotid artery. When muscle failure occurred after 10 to 15 min of stimulation, the peak firing rate of phrenic afferent discharge was enhanced eight to nine times (fig. 24.2). At the same moment, the durations of both phrenic motor discharge (T_I) and total cycle duration (T_{tot}) increased progressively, and these changes tended to persist for 10 min after the stimulation stopped. The recruitment of phrenic motoneurons, as assessed by power spectrum analysis of the phrenic discharge, was modified within less than 5 min of the onset of stimulation, but no more changes were observed when fatigue occurred. Section of both phrenic nerves abolished the ventilatory response to diaphragm fatigue, suggesting that Group III and/or IV phrenic afferents exert specific influence on supraspinal structures which govern the breathing rhythm.

CORTICAL INTEGRATION OF DIAPHRAGMATIC AFFERENTS AND THE "SENSE OF BREATHING"

Except for the studies of Marquez and Barillot (unpublished data, cited in 2) and of Davenport et al. (4) in cats, there are no reports of phrenic nerve afferents projecting to the sensorimotor cortex. The last authors found that the mean value of onset latency of phrenic afferent evoked potentials was 9.7 msec and that peak latency was 23 msec. In five anesthetized cats we observed that peripheral stimulation

of the phrenic nerves evoked cortical potential waveforms roughly on the same zones. Phrenic evoked potentials were also recorded during the development of diaphragm fatigue produced by trains of electrical stimulation of this muscle for a 30-min period. Figure 24.3A reveals that there was an increase in peak latency of waveforms after 10 to 15 min of muscle stimulation and recovery occurred 5 min after the fatigue run stopped.

Using fast Fourier transform (FFT) analysis of spontaneous cortical activity recorded on the sensorimotor cortex, we observed also that the energy in the delta frequency band increased markedly a few seconds after the onset of the fatigue run (fig. 24.3B). Then, these changes in the EEG rhythm seem to adapt and, when muscle fatigue occurred (after 10 to 15 min), there was a reinforcement of energy in the delta frequency band and decreased energy in the theta band. All these EEG changes in response to diaphragm fatigue were abolished by bilateral phrenic nerve section. At present, it seems difficult to discuss the possible mechanisms of such modifications in the cortical integration of phrenic sensory paths with the development of diaphragm fatigue. However, some recent observations by Scardella et al. (25) and Petrozzino et al. (23) demonstrate the role of endogenous opioids in the ventilatory response to diaphragm fatigue induced by acute flow-resistive loads in awake goats. Marlot et al. (20) have also shown that the phrenic motor response to prolonged stimulation of phrenic afferents involves the participation of several different neurotransmitters.

REFERENCES

1. Aubier, M., T. Trippenbach, and C. Roussos. Respiratory muscle fatigue during cardiogenic shock. *J. Appl. Physiol.* 51:499-508, 1981.

2. Bassal, M., and A.L. Bianchi. Effets de la stimulation des structures nerveuses centrales sur les activités respiratoires éfferentes chez le Chat. I. Réponses à la stimulation corticale. *J. Physiol.* (Paris) 77:741-757, 1981.

3. Corda, M., C. von Euler, and G. Lennerstrand. Proprioceptive innervation of the diaphragm. *J. Physiol.* (London) 178:161-177, 1965.

4. Davenport, P.W., F.J. Thompson, R.L. Reep, and A.N. Freed. Projection of phrenic nerve afferents to the cat sensorimotor cortex. *Brain Res.* 328:150-153, 1985.

5. Dogiel, A.S. Die Nervenendigungen in Bauchfell in den Sehnen der Musckespindels und dem Centrum Tendineum des Diaphragms beim Menschen und bei Saugethieren. *Arch. Mikroskop. Anat. Entwicklungsmech.* 59:1-31, 1902.

6. Dolivo, M. Effet de l'interruption de la conduction nerveuse dans un nerf phrénique sur la fréquence respiratoire. *Helv. Physiol. Acta* 10:366-371, 1952.

7. Duron, B. Intercostal and diaphragmatic muscle endings and afferents. In *Regulation of breathing,* part 1, ed. T.F. Hornbein, 473-540. New York: Marcell Dekker, 1981.

8. Gill, P.Y., and M. Kuno. Excitatory and inhibitory actions on phrenic motoneurons. *J. Physiol.* (London) 168:274-289, 1963.

9. Graham, R., Y. Jammes, S. Delpierre, C. Grimaud, and C. Roussos. The effects of ischemia, lactic acid and hypertonic sodium chloride on phrenic afferent discharge during spontaneous diaphragmatic contractions. *Neurosci. Lett.* 67:257-262, 1986.

10. Hinsey, J.C., K. Hare, and R.A. Phillips. Sensory components of the phrenic nerve of the cat. *Proc. Soc. Exp. Biol.* 41:411-414, 1939.

11. Jammes, Y., B. Buchler, S. Delpierre, C. Grimaud, A. Rassidakis, and C. Roussos. Investigation of the presence of small afferent fibers in the cat phrenic nerve and their possible functional role. *Clin. Resp. Physiol.* 20:4A, 1984.

12. Jammes, Y., B. Buchler, S. Delpierre, A. Rassidakis, C. Grimaud, and C. Roussos. Phrenic afferents and their role in inspiratory control. *J. Appl. Physiol.* 60:854-860, 1986.

13. Jammes, Y., M.J. Mathiot, S. Delpierre, and C. Grimaud. Role of vagal and spinal sensory pathways on eupneic diaphragmatic activity. *J. Appl. Physiol.* 60:479-485, 1986.

14. Jammes, Y. Chest wall and diaphragmatic afferents: Their role during external mechanical loading and respiratory muscle ischemia. In *Respiratory muscles in chronic obstructive pulmonary disease,* ed. A. Grassino et al., 49-57. London: Springer Verlag, 1988.

15. Jammes, Y., P. Collett, P. Lenoir, A. Lama, F. Berthelin, and C. Roussos. Diaphragmatic fatigue produced by constant or modulated electric currents. *Muscle and Nerve* 14:27-34, 1991.

16. Jammes, Y., E. Balzamo, M.C. Gardette, and C. Tomei. Electrically-induced diaphragm fatigue and reflex changes in the ventilatory control in cats. *Proceedings of the International Conference. Modulation of Respiratory Pattern: Peripheral and Central Mechanisms,* 94, 1990.

17. Larnicol, N., D. Rose, and B. Duron. Identification of phrenic afferents in the dorsal columns: A fluorescent double-labelling study in the cat. *Neurosci. Lett.* 52:49-53, 1984.

18. Macron, J.M., D. Marlot, and B. Duron. Phrenic afferent input to the lateral medullary reticular formation of the cat. *Resp. Physiol.* 59:155-167, 1985.

19. Marlot, D., J.M. Macron, and B. Duron. Projections of phrenic afferents to the cat cerebellar cortex. *Neurosci. Lett.* 44:95-98, 1984.

20. Marlot, D., J.M. Macron, and B. Duron. Inhibitory and excitatory effects on respiration by phrenic nerve afferent stimulation in cats. *Resp. Physiol.* 69:321-333, 1987.

21. Mathiot, M.J., Y. Jammes, and C. Grimaud. Role of vagal and spinal sensory pathways in diaphragmatic response to resistive loads. *Neurosci. Lett.* 73:131-136, 1987.

22. Mense, S. Slowly conducting afferent fibers from deep tissues: Neurobiological properties and central nervous actions. In *Progress in sensory physiology 6,* ed. D. Ottoson, 149-219. New York: Springer Verlag, 1986.

23. Petrozzino, J.J., A.T. Scardella, J.K.J. Li, N. Krawciw, N.H. Edelman, and T.V. Santiago. Effect of naloxone on spectral shifts of the diaphragm EMG during inspiratory loading. *J. Appl. Physiol.* 68:1376-1385, 1990.

24. Revelette, W.R., L.A. Jewell, and D.T. Frazier. Effect of diaphragm small fiber afferent stimulation on ventilation in dogs. *J. Appl. Physiol.* 65:2097-2106, 1988.

25. Scardella, A.T., R.A. Parisi, D.K. Phair, T.V. Santiago, and N.H. Edelman. The role of endogenous opioids in the ventilatory response to acute flow-resistive loads. *Am. Rev. Respir. Dis.* 133:26-31, 1986.

26. Speck, D.F. Supraspinal involvement in the phrenic-to-phrenic inhibitory reflex. *Brain Res.* 414:169-172, 1987.

27. Speck, D.F., and W.R. Revelette. Excitation of neurons in the dorsal respiratory group by phrenic nerve afferents. *J. Appl. Physiol.* 62:946-952, 1987.

28. Speck, D.F. Bötzinger complex region role in phrenic-to-phrenic inhibitory reflex of cat. *J. Appl. Physiol.* 67:1364-1370, 1989.

29. Supinski, G.S., A.F. DiMarco, F. Hussein, and M.D. Altose. Alterations in respiratory muscles activation in the ischemic fatigued canine diaphragm. *J. Appl. Physiol.* 67:720-729, 1989.

30. Winckler, G., and B. Delaloye. A propos de la présence de fuseaux neuro-musculaires dans le diaphragme humain. *Acta Anat.* 29:114-116, 1957.

31. Winckler, G. Caractéristiques des fuseaux neuro-tendineux du diaphragme humain. *J. Anat. Entwicklungsgesch.* 123:180-183, 1962.

25

Responses of Group III and IV Muscle Afferents to Mechanical and Metabolic Stimuli Likely to Occur during Exercise

Marc P. Kaufman, Janeen M. Hill, Joel G. Pickar, and Diane M. Rotto

Static exercise has been firmly established to increase arterial pressure, myocardial contractility, heart rate, and ventilation. The mechanism causing these increases is not known. Three theories have been postulated to explain the increases in cardiovascular and ventilatory function evoked by exercise. The first theory proposes that the increases are due to a reflex originating in the contracting skeletal muscle (2), while the second theory, called "central command," proposes that the increases are caused by direct action of central locomotor circuits on the medullary and spinal neuronal pools controlling ventilatory and cardiovascular function (5, 7). The third theory proposes that the increases are caused by a contraction-induced metabolite that travels to either the cardiopulmonary region, the carotid body, or the brain to exert its excitatory action (1, 19). The three theories are not mutually exclusive. There is substantial evidence that the neural mechanisms postulated by each play at least some role in causing the cardiovascular or ventilatory increases evoked by static exercise (17). We have focused our efforts on understanding one of these theories, namely, that exercise increases cardiovascular and ventilatory function by a reflex originating in contracting skeletal muscle.

The reflex theory was first suggested by Zuntz and Geppert (21), who proposed that sensory nerves in the exercising muscles were stimulated by the accumulation of metabolic by-products of contraction. Subsequently, the reflex theory received its first experimental support from the work of Alam and Smirk (2), who reported in humans that postexercise ischemia of working muscles increased arterial pressure. Nonpainful electrically induced static contractions, believed to eliminate central command, evoked increases in heart rate and arterial pressure that had time courses and magnitudes almost identical to those evoked by voluntary static contractions of equal force (4, 9). Finally, attempts to perform static handgrip in humans whose forearms were paralyzed by either lidocaine or succinylcholine evoked pressor responses (presumably because of central command) that were only half of those evoked by this maneuver when the subjects could contract their forearm muscles (6, 8).

Strong support for the hypothesis that static contraction reflexly increases cardiovascular and ventilatory function has come from experiments performed on anesthetized animals. For example, Coote et al. (3) statically contracted the triceps surae muscles of cats by electrically stimulating the ventral roots, a maneuver that increased arterial pressure, heart rate, and ventilation. After cutting the L_6–S_1 dorsal roots, the responses to contraction were abolished. The magnitude of the contraction-induced pressor response was found to be related linearly to the magnitude of the peak tension developed by the contracting triceps surae. Finally, occlusion of the arterial supply to the contracting muscles evoked a greater pressor reflex than that evoked when the arterial supply to the muscle was not occluded.

McCloskey and Mitchell (12) also found that static contraction of the hindlimb muscles of anesthetized cats increased ventilation, arterial pressure, and heart rate. In addition, these investigators found that anodal blockade of the L_7–S_1 dorsal roots prevented impulses from Group I and II afferents from reaching the spinal cord but did not prevent the contraction-induced increases in ventilatory and cardiovascular function. However, topical application of a local anesthetic to the dorsal roots did not block impulse conduction in Group I and II afferents but did block the contraction-induced cardiovascular increases and reduced the ventilatory increases. McCloskey and Mitchell (12) concluded that the reflex ventilatory and cardiovascular increases evoked by contraction were caused by the stimulation of Group III and IV muscle afferents.

In the experiments to be described, we have attempted to determine the discharge properties of these Group III and IV afferents and have paid particular attention to mechanical and metabolic stimuli that are likely to discharge these thin fiber afferents during muscular contraction. Only a brief description of the methods will be given because they have been given in detail elsewhere (10, 11). Cats were anesthetized with sodium pentobarbital (35 mg/kg, iv). The right common carotid artery, left femoral artery, right external jugular vein, and cervical trachea were cannulated. Additional doses of anesthetic were given intravenously as needed. The lungs were ventilated with room air by a Harvard pump. Arterial PO_2 and PCO_2 and pH were sampled periodically (Radiometer ABL-3) and maintained within normal limits.

Afferent impulses were recorded from the L_7–S_1 dorsal roots. For filaments containing either silent or spontaneously active fibers, their receptive fields were located in the triceps surae muscles using both noxious and non-noxious stimuli. Noxious stimulation consisted of vigorously pinching the receptive fields with the fingers or a blunted forceps. When performed on the forearm of the investigators, both maneuvers were considered painful. Non-noxious stimulation consisted of either probing the receptive field with a cotton-tipped applicator or gently squeezing the receptive field with a blunted forceps; neither of the two maneuvers, when performed on the investigators, were considered painful. We discarded any fiber whose receptive field could not be located in the triceps surae muscles. Conduction velocities were measured using methods described previously (10). Afferents conducting impulses between 2.6 and 30.0 m/sec were classified as Group III fibers, and those conducting impulses at 2.5 m/sec or less were classified as Group IV fibers.

In the first series of studies, we characterized the responses of Group III and IV muscle afferents to static contraction of the triceps surae muscles. This type of contraction stimulated 76% of the Group III afferents tested and 59% of the Group IV afferents tested. Even though contraction stimulated the majority of group III and IV afferents, their patterns of discharge in response to this maneuver were often dissimilar. For example, Group III afferents frequently discharged a burst of impulses at the onset of contraction and then decreased their firing rate as the muscle fatigued during the contraction period. In contrast, Group IV afferents often responded to contraction after a 5–30 sec latent period, with activity increasing or being maintained above control levels even as the triceps surae muscles fatigued (10).

Ischemia, caused by tightening a snare placed around the abdominal aorta, increased the responses to static contraction of 13% of the Group III afferents and 47% of the Group IV afferents. Ischemia caused afferents that were stimulated by contraction under freely perfused conditions to be stimulated even more by contraction with the aorta occluded. Likewise, ischemia caused afferents that were not stimulated by contraction to be stimulated by this maneuver when the aorta was occluded (11).

Our finding that muscle ischemia increased the responses of thin fiber afferents to contraction provided evidence for the hypothesis that these afferents responded to a mismatch between blood supply and demand in the exercising muscle. We next sought to determine the effects of various metabolic products of contraction on the discharge of Group III and IV muscle afferents. We found that large doses of sodium or lithium lactate (400 mM; 1 ml) at neutral pH stimulated only two of forty-six Group III and IV afferents. Likewise, large doses of monobasic sodium phosphate (400 mM; 1 ml) at a neutral pH stimulated only eight of forty-seven Group III and IV afferents. Of the eight stimulated, seven were Group III afferents and one was a Group IV afferent. A smaller dose of monobasic sodium phosphate (20 mM; 1 ml) also stimulated only one of twenty-six Group III and IV afferents. Likewise, neither 2-chloroadenosine (100 μg), which is not taken up by red blood cells, nor adenosine (100 μg), which is, had much

effect on the afferents' discharge, stimulating only seven of fifty-nine (13).

In contrast to the lack of effect of lactate, phosphate, and adenosine on the afferents' discharge, lactic acid and arachidonic acid stimulated them. Specifically, lactic acid (400 mM; 1 ml) stimulated thirty-six of the fifty-two afferents tested. A smaller dose of lactic acid (25 mM; 1 ml) given to the same afferents that were given first the large dose (i.e., 400 mM; 1 ml) still stimulated fourteen of thirty-seven afferents even though significant tachyphylaxis was present. In addition, arachidonic acid (2 mg) stimulated twenty-five of fifty Group III and IV afferents tested, an effect that was attenuated by indomethacin, a cyclooxygenase inhibitor. However, the increase in thin fiber afferent discharge evoked by arachidonic acid was long in onset (i.e., about 1–2 min) and usually small in amplitude (13). This work suggests that lactate, phosphate, and adenosine, each of which is a metabolic product of muscular contraction, play little if any role in the stimulation of Group III and IV afferents during exercise. On the other hand, the cyclooxygenase and lipoxygenase products of arachidonic acid as well as lactic acid may play significant roles in the stimulation of these afferents during exercise.

In the next series of experiments, we tested the hypothesis that intraarterial injections of lactic acid and hydrochloric acid, which created levels of these substances in muscle similar to those seen during contraction, reflexly increased cardiovascular and ventilatory function (14). Hydrochloric acid (32 and 57 mM; 1 ml) injected into the arterial supply of the triceps surae muscles decreased intramuscular pH from 7.26 ± 0.05 to 7.17 ± 0.05 ($P<0.01$) and reflexly increased arterial pressure (23 ± 7 mmHg; $P<0.01$), heart rate (11 ± 2 beats/min; $P<0.001$), and ventilation (187 ± 72 ml/min; $P<0.05$). Static contraction of the triceps surae muscles decreased intramuscular pH from 7.28 ± 0.06 to 7.13 ± 0.06 ($P<0.01$). Lactic acid was more potent in causing reflex increases than was equimolar HCl. For example, lactic acid containing 4 mM lactate and 0.87 mM H^+ reflexly increased arterial pressure, heart rate, and ventilation, whereas 0.87 mM HCl did not. Intraarterial sodium lactate (13 and 33 mM) at a neutral pH had no effect on these variables. In addition, carbonic anhydrase inhibition with acetazolamide, which blocks carbonic anhydrase activity in red cells, and with sodium cyanate, which blocks the activity of this enzyme in skeletal muscle, had no effect on the reflex responses evoked by lactic acid injection. These results suggest that CO_2 generated by lactic acid injection is not the metabolic stimulus for the pressor reflex.

We next attempted to evoke a reflex pressor response to injection of arachidonic acid (2 mg) into the arterial supply of the triceps surae muscles of anesthetized cats. The preparation was identical to that used in the experiments which successfully evoked a reflex pressor response to lactic acid injection (14). We performed this experiment in fourteen cats and in only one cat did arachidonic acid injection evoke a pressor effect. The most frequent response was a small decrease in arterial pressure, which was not affected by cutting the dorsal roots and therefore was not a reflex. We speculate that this small depressor effect was caused by the recirculation and conversion of arachidonic acid to vasodilator prostaglandins, such as PGI_2.

Because close arterial injection of exogenous lactic but not arachidonic acid evoked a reflex pressor response, we next attempted to determine if arachidonic acid sensitized rather than stimulated Group III and IV muscle afferents during contraction. Therefore in anesthetized cats we recorded the responses of Group III muscle afferents to static contraction before and after injection of arachidonic acid (1–2 mg; ia) or indomethacin (5 mg/kg; iv). Arachidonic acid increased the responses of group III afferents (n = 11) to contraction by 265% (P<0.025). Indomethacin decreased the responses of group III afferents (n = 9) to contraction by 61% (P<0.025). Arachidonic acid given after indomethacin increased the responses of two of four Group III afferents to contraction. We conclude that both cyclooxygenase and lipoxygenase products of arachidonic acid metabolism sensitize Group III muscle afferents to static contraction (15).

We also examined the effects of indomethacin and aspirin, two cyclooxygenase blocking agents, on the responses to static contraction of thirty-seven Group IV afferents with endings in the triceps surae muscles of anesthetized cats. We found that indomethacin (5 mg/kg; iv) decreased the responses to contraction of each of eight Group IV afferents tested. Likewise, aspirin (50 mg/kg; iv) decreased the responses to contraction of each of four Group IV afferents tested. On the other hand, we found that arachidonic acid (2 mg) injected into the femoral artery did not increase the responses to contraction of Group IV afferents that were stimulated by this maneuver. In addition, arachidonic acid injection did not cause any of seven Group IV afferents not stimulated by static contraction to become responsive to this maneuver. Nevertheless, arachidonic acid injection with the muscle at rest stimulated five of seven contraction-insensitive and two of four contraction-sensitive Group IV afferents. Our data suggest that cyclooxygenase metabolites of endogenous arachidonic acid are needed for the full expression of the responses of Group IV muscle afferents to static contraction. Our data also suggest that exogenous administration of arachidonic acid neither increases the responses to contraction of Group IV afferents stimulated by this maneuver nor affects Group IV afferents that are not stimulated by contraction (16).

When hindlimb skeletal muscle is statically contracted, it often becomes hypoxic. This condition might also serve as a stimulus to thin fiber muscle afferents signaling a mismatch between blood supply and demand in the exercising muscle. To investigate this possibility, we recorded the discharge of Group III and IV afferents in a resting triceps surae muscle, while we ventilated the lungs of anesthetized cats for 3 min with either 3–5% O_2 in N_2 or 10% CO_2 in 90% O_2. The lungs were ventilated with a mixture of room air and oxygen before switching to the hypoxic or hypercapnic gas mixture. We found that hypoxemia, which decreased arterial PO_2 from 132 ± 3 to 23 ± 1 mmHg, stimulated (P<0.05), on average, Group IV afferents (n = 9) that were responsive to contraction, but had no effect (P>0.05) on the discharge of Group IV afferents (n = 6) that were unresponsive to contraction. In addition, hypoxemia with the muscle at rest had no effect (P>0.05) on the mean discharge of either Group III afferents that were responsive to contraction (n = 8) or on the mean discharge of Group III afferents that were unresponsive to contraction (n = 8). Furthermore, the venous PO_2 of blood draining the triceps surae muscle was somewhat lower when the lungs were ventilated with 3% O_2 and the muscle was at rest (20 ± 1 mmHg) than when the lungs were ventilated with room air and oxygen and the muscle was contracting statically (23 ± 1 mmHg; P<0.05). Ventilating the lungs with 10% CO_2 had only weak effects on the discharge of Group III and IV afferents in resting skeletal muscle regardless of whether these afferents were responsive or unresponsive to contraction while the lungs were ventilated with room air.

The data from the hypoxemia study has excited us because we believe it provides further support for the notion that the Group IV afferents responsive to contraction are stimulated by metabolic events occurring in the working muscle. We are not surprised by the small effect of CO_2 on the afferents' discharge because in previous experiments (15) we have shown that HCl infusion was not nearly as effective a stimulus as was equimolar lactic acid infusion. Ventilating the lungs with CO_2 is, we believe, analogous to HCl infusion, a stimulus which we previously have shown evokes only small reflex effects (14).

We have not yet investigated the mechanism whereby hypoxia stimulated these afferents. Two possibilities include the release of either arachidonic acid or lactic acid. In one preliminary experiment, we have obtained some evidence that lactic acid may play a role in the hypoxia-induced stimulation of these afferents. We used sodium dichloroacetate in a large dose (600 mg/kg; iv) to attenuate the production of lactic acid by the triceps surae muscles. We found that dichloroacetate, a substance which increases the activity of the pyruvate dehydrogenase complex, abolished the response of the afferent to hypoxia and greatly attenuated its response to static muscular contraction (fig. 25.1). However, dichloroacetate did not affect the afferent's response to probing its receptive field, a finding which suggests that this substance did not nonspecifically desensitize the afferent.

In summary, our findings raise the possibility that lactic acid plays some role as the metabolic stimulus that activates thin fiber afferents during exercise. Additional support for this possibility has come from studies showing

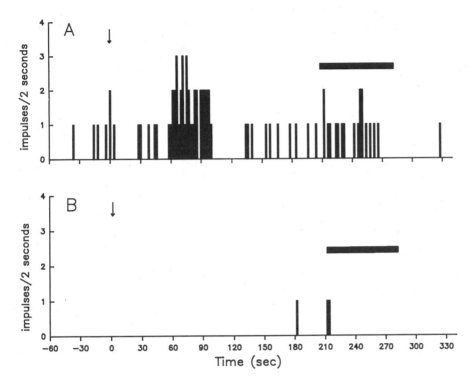

FIG. 25.1 Effect of hypoxemia and static contraction on the discharge of a slowly conducting Group III afferent (conduction velocity = 5.8 m/sec) whose ending was in the triceps surae muscles.
(A) At the arrow, the gas mixture ventilating the cat's lungs was switched from a slightly hyperoxic mixture to a 3% O_2 in N_2 mixture. Note the stimulation of the afferent after a latency of about 60 sec. While still breathing 3% O_2, the triceps surae muscles were statically contracted for 1 min (horizontal bar). (B) 20 min after dichloroacetate (600 mg/kg; iv). The arrow and horizontal bar represent the same maneuvers as those in A. Note that the afferent's response to hypoxemia and contraction were greatly reduced. The femoral venous lactate concentration during contraction was 3.9 mM in A, but was only 2.2 mM in B. In this case dichloroacetate appeared to attenuate the afferent's sensitivity to both mechanical and metabolic factors.

that both the time course and the magnitude of the exercise-induced increases in arterial pressure and sympathetic activity of the peroneal nerve were strongly correlated with the decrease in intracellular pH in the working forearm muscles of humans (18, 20). It is important to point out, however, that this metabolic stimulus may well be multifactorial and, therefore, no one substance will satisfy all the criteria.

REFERENCES

1. Adams, L., J. Garlick, A. Guz, K. Murphy, and S.J.G. Semple. Is the voluntary control of exercise in man necessary for the ventilatory response? *J. Physiol.* (London) 355:71-83, 1984.

2. Alam, M., and F.H. Smirk. Observation in man upon a blood pressure raising reflex arising from the voluntary muscles. *J. Physiol.* (London) 89:372-383, 1937.

3. Coote, J.H., S.M. Hilton, and J.F. Perez-Gonzalez. The reflex nature of the pressor response to muscular exercise. *J. Physiol.* (London) 215:789-804, 1971.

4. Davies, C.T.M., and D.W. Starkie. The pressor response to voluntary and electrically evoked isometric contractions in man. *Euro. J. Appl. Physiol.* 53:359-363, 1985.

5. Eldridge, F.L., D.E. Millhorn, and T.G. Waldrop. Exercise hyperpnea and locomotion: Parallel activation from the hypothalamus. *Science* 211:844-846, 1981.

6. Freyschuss, U. Cardiovascular adjustments to somatomotor activation. *Acta Physiol. Scand.* 342:1-63, 1970.

7. Goodwin, G.M., D.I. McCloskey, and J.H. Mitchell. Cardiovascular and respiratory responses to changes in central command during isometric exercise at constant muscle tension. *J. Physiol.* (London) 226:173-190, 1972.

8. Hobbs, S.F., and S.C. Gandevia. Cardiovascular responses and the sense of effort during attempts to contract paralyzed muscles: Role of the spinal cord. *Neurosci. Lett.* 57:85-90, 1985.

9. Hultman, E., and H. Sjoholm. Blood pressure and heart rate response to voluntary and non-voluntary static exercise in man. *Acta Physiol Scand.* 115:499-501, 1982.

10. Kaufman, M.P., J.C. Longhurst, K.J. Rybicki, J.H. Wallach, and J.H. Mitchell. Effects of static muscular contraction on impulse activity of Group III and IV afferents in cats. *J. Appl. Physiol.* 55:105-112, 1983.

11. Kaufman, M.P., K.J. Rybicki, T.B. Waldrop, and G.A. Ordway. Effect of ischemia on responses of Group III and IV afferents to contraction. *J. Appl. Physiol.* 57:644-650, 1984.

12. McCloskey, D.I., and J.H. Mitchell. Reflex cardiovascular and respiratory responses originating in exercising muscle. *J. Physiol.* (London) 224:173-186, 1972.

13. Rotto, D.M., and M.P. Kaufman. Effect of metabolic products of muscular contraction on the discharge of Group III and IV afferents. *J. Appl. Physiol.* 64:2306-2313, 1988.

14. Rotto, D.M., C.L. Stebbins, and M.P. Kaufman. Reflex cardiovascular and ventilatory responses to increasing H^+ ion activity in cat hindlimb muscle. *J. Appl. Physiol.* 67:256-263, 1989.

15. Rotto, D.M., H.D. Schultz, J.C. Longhurst, and M.P. Kaufman. Sensitization of Group III muscle afferents to static contraction by arachidonic acid. *J. Appl. Physiol.* 68:861-867, 1990.

16. Rotto, D.M., J.M. Hill, H.D. Schultz, and M.P. Kaufman. Cyclooxygenase blockade attenuates responses of Group IV muscle afferents to static contraction. *Am. J. Physiol.* 259:H745–750, 1990.

17. Shepherd, J.T., C.G. Blomquist, A.R. Lind, J.H. Mitchell, and B. Saltin. Static (isometric) exercise. *Circ. Res.* 48:1179-1188, 1981.

18. Sinoway, L., S. Prophet, I. Gorman, T. Mosher, J. Shenberger, M. Dolecki, R. Briggs, and R. Zelis. Muscle acidosis during static exercise is associated with calf vasoconstriction. *J. Appl. Physiol.* 66:429–436, 1988.

19. Van Benthuysen, K.M., G.D. Swanson, and J.V. Weil. Temporal delay of venous blood correlates with onset of exercise hyperpnea. *J. Appl. Physiol.* 57:874–880, 1984.

20. Victor, R.G., L.A. Bertocci, S.L. Pryor, and R.L. Nunnally. Sympathetic nerve discharge is coupled to muscle cell pH during exercise in humans. *J. Clin. Invest.* 82:1301–1305, 1988.

21. Zuntz, N., and J. Geppert. Über die Natur der normalen atermreize und den ort iher wirkung. *Pflügers Arch.* 38:337–338, 1886.

26

Neurotransmitter Mechanisms in the Periphery of Respiratory Afferents

Jan M. Lundberg and Kjell Alving

BACKGROUND

The sensory nerves in the airways represent a first line of defense and alarm system. It is well known that the acute allergic reaction is associated with rapid sensory nerve activation as revealed by irritant sensations in the airway mucosa. Furthermore, additional central protective neural reflexes (sneezing and coughing) contribute to the initial phase of the allergen reaction in the airways. There is now evidence for a close anatomical association between mast cells and peptide containing sensory nerves in the airway mucosa (3, 24). Some of these nerve fibers close to mast cells contain tachykinins (neurokinin A [NKA] and substance P [SP]) and calcitonin gene-related peptide (CGRP) and are most likely of sensory origin, since they are sensitive to capsaicin treatment (see 11). There is also evidence for a functional relationship between mast cells and sensory nerves. Thus, SP evokes histamine release from mast cells in tissues such as the human skin (12).

After capsaicin pretreatment, which causes depletion of sensory neuropeptides like SP and CGRP in the lung due to degeneration of peripheral terminal endings, the allergen-induced bronchoconstrictor and protein extravasation reactions are inhibited in guinea pig lung (19, 26). Furthermore we have recently developed an allergy model using the ascaris-sensitized pig, where systemic capsaicin pretreatment inhibits the allergen-induced vasodilation in the airway mucosa (1), suggesting that local peptide release from sensory nerves is essential for this reaction.

NEUROPEPTIDE RELEASE

It has recently been established that the peptide release induced by capsaicin has two components. At low concentration capsaicin evokes peptide release via a tetrodotoxin-sensitive mechanism suggesting the dependence of Na^+-channel action potential propagation and axon reflexes (14, 16), while at high concentration the capsaicin effect is not influenced by tetrodotoxin and probably due to a direct action on the varicose nerve endings (16) (table 26.1). Resiniferatoxin, which has structural similarities to capsaicin, is even more potent to cause CGRP release from the lung (9). Regarding the type of Ca^{++}-channel which is involved in peptide secretion from sensory nerves, omega-conotoxin

Table 26.1. Experimental and therapeutical agents influencing sensory nerve function[a]

Stimulatory	Inhibitory
Capsaicin	Tetrodotoxin, lidocaine — axon reflex (Na^+)[b]
Resiniferatoxin	Omega-conotoxin (N-type Ca^{++})
Histamine (H_1)	Ruthenium red (capsaicin, Ca^{++})
Bradykinin (B_2)	Nedocromil sodium
Nicotine	α_2-adrenoceptor agonists
Ether	μ-opiate receptor agonists
Formalin	Antihistamines (H_1)
Cigarette smoke, vapor phase	

[a] Stimulation or inhibition of sensory nerves activates or interferes with peptide release from pulmonary afferents.
[b] The mechanisms of stimulation or inhibition are indicated in parenthesis.

but not nifedipine inhibits CGRP release from lung afferents, which suggests that the N-type of Ca^{++}-channels are essential for this process (16) (table 26.1).

Based on pharmacological analysis with receptor antagonists and release experiments, histamine seems to represent a key factor in the functional link between mast cells and sensory nerves at least in the guinea pig, pig, and man (table 26.1) (see 1, 3). Thus activation of H_1-receptors is associated with neuropeptide release (27) from lung afferents, either via a direct action of histamine on the sensory nerves and/or possibly via plasma protein leakage and formation of bradykinin. Sensory nerve activation and neuropeptide release by bradykinin (27) may be a direct effect via bradykinin B_2 receptors (7) and involvement of protein kinase C (6) (table 26.1).

Alpha-2 adrenoceptor agonists have been demonstrated to inhibit neuropeptide release from pulmonary sensory nerves (16, 20). Also opiate agonists inhibit peptide release from pulmonary afferents (4, 20) (table 26.1). Furthermore, whereas the massive peptide release evoked by the irritant agents capsaicin (18) and resiniferatoxin (9) is blocked by ruthenium red, probably by interfering with Ca^{++} entry, histamine- and bradykinin-induced CGRP release from the guinea pig lung is caused by other mechanisms (16). Data from the pig also suggest that nedocromil sodium inhibits bradykinin-evoked activation of sensory nerves (2) (table 26.1).

NEUROPEPTIDE-INDUCED INFLAMMATION

Neuropeptides exert a broad spectrum of biological activities, especially on vascular and bronchial smooth muscle as well as on migration, proliferation, and release of mediators from inflammatory cells. Substance P causes protein extravasation and vasodilatation via activation of neurokinin-1 receptors, whereas the SP-evoked vasodilatation is endothelium-dependent and caused by release of a labile endothelial-derived relaxant factor (EDRF), which most likely is nitric oxide (24). Since the vasodilatation evoked by sensory nerve activation is independent of the endothelium and not influenced by SP tachyphylaxis or tachykinin antagonists (see 8), the accumulated data suggest that CGRP is the key mediator of the vasodilatory component of the allergen-induced response.

A prominent activity of NKA is bronchoconstriction via activation of neurokinin-2 receptors. Tachykinins as well as CGRP stimulate proliferation of various cell types, including endothelial cells and fibroblasts (see 10, 22), suggesting a possible involvement in more long-term structural changes. In addition to being a potent vasodilator agent with very long-lasting actions (25), CGRP also modulates the mitogenic response (5) and cytokine production (15) of mononuclear cells and evokes granulocyte chemotaxis (25).

A final aspect of mast cell-sensory nerve interactions is that repeated, chronic activation of sensory nerves seems to evoke enhanced neuropeptide synthesis as exemplified by aerosol immunization in rats (23). Furthermore, cigarette smoke exposure is a strong stimulus for activation of peptide-containing capsaicin-sensitive nerves, thereby causing neurogenic inflammation in the rat tracheal mucosa (17) and pig nasal mucosa (21). Interestingly, chronic cigarette smoke exposure is associated with hyperresponsive sensory mechanisms (especially cough reflexes) and increased neuropeptide content in tracheal tissue (13).

It is concluded that release of multiple peptides from peripheral branches of capsaicin-sensitive pulmonary afferents is likely to occur upon inhalation of both irritants and allergens. A variety of both acute and long-term local effects can then be elicited by these neuropeptides.

REFERENCES

1. Alving, K., R. Matran, J.S. Lacroix, and J.M. Lundberg. Capsaicin and histamine antagonist-sensitive mechanisms in the immediate allergic reaction of pig airways. *Acta Physiol. Scand.* 138:49-60, 1990.

2. Alving, K., R. Matran, and J.M. Lundberg. Effect of nedocromil sodium in allergen-, PAF-, histamine- and bradykinin-induced airways vasodilatation and pulmonary obstruction in the pig. *Br. J. Pharmacol.* In press, 1991.

3. Alving, K., C. Sundström, R. Matran, T. Hökfelt, and J.M. Lundberg. Association between histamine-containing mast cells and sensory nerves in the skin and airways of control and capsaicin-treated pigs. *Cell Tiss. Res.* 264:529-538, 1991.

4. Bartho, L., R. Amman, A. Saria, J. Szolcsanyi, and F. Lembeck. Peripheral effects of opioid drugs on capsaicin-sensitive neurones of the guinea pig bronchus and rabbit ear. *Naunyn Arch. Pharmacol.* 336:316-321, 1989.

5. Casini, A., P. Geppetti, C.A. Maggi, and C. Surrenti. Effects of calcitonin gene-related peptide (CGRP), neurokinin A and neurokinin A (4–10) on the mitogenic response of human peripheral blood mononuclear cells. *Naunyn Arch. Pharmacol.* 339:354-358, 1989.

6. Dray, A., J. Bettaney, P. Forster, and M.N. Perkins. Bradykinin-induced stimulation of afferent fibers is mediated through protein kinase C. *Neurosci. Lett.* 91:301-307, 1988.

7. Dray, A., and M.N. Perkins. Bradykinin activates peripheral capsaicin-sensitive fibers via a second messenger system. *Agents Actions* 25:214-215, 1988.

8. Franco-Cereceda, A., A. Rudehill, and J.M. Lundberg. Calcitonin gene-related peptide but not substance P mimics capsaicin-induced coronary vasodilation in the pig. *Euro. J. Pharm.* 142:235-243, 1987.

9. Franco-Cereceda, A., Y.-P. Lou, and J.M. Lundberg. Resiniferatoxin-evoked CGRP release and bronchoconstriction in the guinea-induced lung are inhibited by ruthenium red. *Euro. J. Pharm.* 187:291-292, 1990.

10. Haegerstrand, A., C.-J. Dalsgaard, B. Jonzon, O. Larsson, J. Nilsson. Calcitonin gene-related peptide stimulates proliferation of human endothelial cells. *Proc. Natl. Acad. Sci. USA* 87:3299-3303, 1990.

11. Holzer, P. Local effector functions of capsaicin-sensitive sensory nerve endings: Involvement of tachykinins, calcitonin gene-related peptide and other neuropeptides. *Neurosci.* 24:739-768, 1988.

12. Hägermark, Ö, T. Hökfelt, and B. Pernow. Flare and itch induced by substance P in human skin. *J. Invest. Dermatol.* 71:233-235, 1978.

13. Karlsson, J.A., C. Zachrisson, and J.M. Lundberg. Hyperresponsiveness to tussive stimuli in cigarette smoke-exposed guinea-pigs: A role for capsaicin-sensitive calcitonin gene-related peptide-containing nerves. *Acta Physiol. Scand.* 141:445-454, 1990.

14. Kröll, F., J.-A. Karlsson, J.M. Lundberg, C.G.A. Persson. Capsaicin-induced bronchoconstriction and neuropeptide release in guinea pig perfused lungs. *J. Appl. Physiol.* 68:1679-1687, 1990.

15. Lotz, M., J.H. Vaughan, and D.A. Carson. Effect of neuropeptides on production of inflammatory cytokines by human monocytes. *Science* 241:1218-1221, 1988.

16. Lundberg, J.M., A. Franco-Cereceda, J.S. Lacroix, and J. Pernow. Release of vasoactive peptides from autonomic and sensory nerves. *Blood Vessels,* 28:27-34, 1990.

17. Lundberg, J.M., and A. Saria. Capsaicin-induced desensitization of airway mucosa to cigarette smoke, mechanical and chemical irritants. *Nature* 302:251-253, 1983.

18. Maggi, C.A., R. Patacchini, P. Santicioli, S. Giuliani, F. Del Bianco, P. Gepetti, and A. Meli. The efferent function of capsaicin-sensitive nerves: Ruthenium red discriminates between different mechanisms of activation. *Euro. J. Pharm.* 170:167-177, 1989.

19. Manzini, S., C.A. Maggi, P. Gepetti, and C. Bacciarelli. Capsaicin desensitization protects from antigen-induced bronchospasm in conscious guinea-pigs. *Euro. J. Pharm.* 138:307-308, 1987.

20. Matran, R., C.-R. Martling, and J.M. Lundberg. Inhibition of cholinergic and non-adrenergic, non-cholinergic bronchoconstriction in the guinea pig mediated by neuropeptide Y, α_2-adrenoceptors and opiate receptors. *Euro. J. Pharm.* 163:15-23, 1988.

21. Matran, R., K. Alving, and J.M. Lundberg. Cigarette smoke, nicotine and capsaicin aerosol-induced vasodilation in pig respiratory mucosa. *Br. J. Pharmacol.* 100:535-541, 1990.

22. Nilsson, J., C. von Euler, and C.-J. Dahlsgaard. Stimulation of connective tissue cell growth by substance P and substance K. *Nature* 315:61-62, 1985.

23. Nilsson, G., K. Alving, S. Ahlstedt, T. Hökfelt, and J.M. Lundberg. Peptidergic innervation of rat lymphoid tissue and lung: Relation to mast cells and sensitivity to capsaicin and immunization. *Cell Tiss. Res.* 262:125-133, 1990.

24. Palmer, R.M.J., A.G. Ferrige, and S. Moncada. Nitric oxide release accounts for the biological activity of endothelium-derived relaxing factor. *Nature* 327:524-526, 1987.

25. Piotrowski, W., and J.C. Foreman. Some effects of calcitonin gene-related peptide in human skin and on histamine release. *Br. J. Dermatol.* 114:37-46, 1986.

26. Saria, A., J.M. Lundberg, G. Skofitsch, and F. Lembeck. Vascular protein linkage in various tissue induced by substance P, capsaicin, bradykinin, serotonin, histamine and by antigen challenge. *Naunyn Arch. Pharmacol.* 324:212-218, 1983.

27. Saria, A., C.-R. Martling, Z. Yan, E. Theodorsson-Norheim, R. Gamse, and J.M. Lundberg. Release of multiple tachykinins from capsaicin-sensitive sensory nerves in the lung by bradykinin, histamine, dimethylphenyl pipcrazinium, and vagal nerve stimulation. *Am. Rev. Resp. Dis.* 137:1330-1335, 1988.

Part VI

Respiratory Chemoreception:
Peripheral and Central

27

An Overview

Robert S. Fitzgerald and Machiko Shirahata

Fundamental to the existence of an organism is oxygen. This most essential nutrient must be captured from the environment. Whereas for most mammalian species carbohydrate, protein, fat, minerals, and even water can be environmentally unavailable for days, perhaps weeks, the absence of oxygen from the environment for more than a few minutes is lethal. In the course of evolutionary development, organisms ranging in complexity from single to multicell animals have developed highly interactive systems and strategies for capturing oxygen. Simplest, of course, is the diffusion of oxygen from the environment across a membrane into the cytosol of the cell and then to the metabolic machinery.

Insects, on the other hand, have developed fascinating systems of tracheae and spiracles located in the thoracic and abdominal regions which lead the oxygen right into the tissues. Accompanying the system is often a clever strategy such as that used by the aquatic beetle, the water boatman. This beetle is called a "bubble breather" because in its development it spends substantial amounts of time under water. To do so it takes on a gas supply before submerging by trapping an air bubble under its wing next to the spiracles. As oxygen is consumed from the bubble, the partial pressure of oxygen falls below that in the water. Consequently oxygen diffuses from the water into the bubble. Carbon dioxide goes in the opposite direction. However, the bubble grows smaller for a variety of reasons, making it necessary for the boatman to resurface periodically. Other aquatic beetles, however, have learned how to capture bubbles containing oxygen produced by algae, and incorporate this into their bubble while remaining submerged.

For mammals, a successful interaction of the cardiovascular and pulmonary systems is essential to extract oxygen for delivery from the environment to the tissues. Modulation of the pattern of one of these systems can affect the performance of the other (1, 2). For example, increased pressure in the carotid sinus decreases the respiratory rate, while decreases in carotid sinus pressure increase the rate (5). Increases in tidal volume provoke decreases in vascular resistance and tachycardia. In addition, certain anatomical structures are common to the reflex responses of these two interdependent systems. For example, carotid body stimulation promotes not only changes in both static and dynamic lung volumes but also changes in heart rate, stroke volume, and vascular resistance (3).

Before reflecting on the modulation of these systems, it is important to note that several key processes in the initiation of their activities remain poorly understood. The heart, of course, has inherent rhythmicity which is modulated by the autonomic nervous system and circulating catecholamines. Certain vascular beds are autoregulatory but can be modulated by the same two agents. Autoregulation is by no means completely understood. Further, the origin of respiratory rhythmicity is still a mystery. Some maintain there is a pacemaker in the brainstem that is modulated by afferent input. Others present data that suggest that without input from the periphery there is no inspiratory effort, or at best an extremely infrequent one. Consider, finally, exercise. The organism is either at rest or exercising at some level. The hyperpnea of exercise has, as yet, no universally acceptable explanation. Clearly the organism requires more oxygen and manufactures more carbon dioxide as the metabolic rate increases; it is likely that temperature in certain loci increases. Hence it is appropriate that respiration increases. But the current understanding of the components (and their interrelationship) responsible for exercise hyperpnea is quite limited.

When one proposes to explore the modulation of the respiratory pattern due to input from the chemoreceptors, it is a matter of studying the impact of hypoxia and/or hypercapnia on known components of the respiratory control apparatus. Even in this instance there are some enigmas. In a normal subject lowering the partial pressure of oxygen provokes a clear increase in respiration, while the presence of carbon monoxide or anemia decreasing arterial oxygen content to the same extent does not. Subjects suffering from chronic obstructive lung disease frequently have blood gas values which are both hypoxic and hypercapnic, and respiration should be greatly increased. In fact, most frequently it is not elevated proportional to the abnormal levels of oxygen and carbon dioxide.

Contributions in this section address several mechanisms thought to be critical in the modulation of the neural pattern of input (from carotid bodies) or the mechanical pattern of output. Dr. Lahiri and his colleagues report on the role of carbonic anhydrase in the carotid body. They conclude that the chemodetection of decreased oxygen is not mediated by the intracellular pH in Type I cells, but is regulated by hydrogen ion. Carbonic anhydrase is necessary for the rapid response to increases in CO_2. The response to hypercapnia may involve activating the Na^+-H^+ exchanger to eliminate the increased H^+ ion generated by the carbonic anhydrase–assisted hydration of the increased CO_2. This, in turn, reverses the Na^+-Ca^{++} exchanger bringing Ca^{++} into the Type I cell and ridding the cell of the increased Na^+. This leads to the release of dopamine and perhaps norepinephrine.

Dr. Nurse and his colleagues use dissociated Type I cells and neurons from the petrosal ganglion of the rat to characterize the electrophysiological capabilities of these fundamental units of chemotransduction in the carotid body. They conclude that hypoxia does indeed reduce the outward potassium current from the Type I cell by about 15–20%. This would tend to depolarize the cell, promoting the entry of extracellular calcium through voltage-gated channels and the subsequent release of an excitatory neurotransmitter. However, because of the limited size of the inward current and the possibility that spiking in the cells was infrequent, a generalization of the above model to rat Type I cells seemed preliminary. Furthermore, the outward potassium current began only at -20mV. If one assumed that the resting membrane potential was in the -50mV to -60mV range, one would have to propose a mechanism for depolarizing the Type I cell from this range to -20mV.

Most models of carotid body chemotransduction include the release of an excitatory neurotransmitter from the Type I cell where they have been detected by several investigators (3, 4). Our own bias at this point is that, at least in cats, one of the excitatory neurotransmitters is acetylcholine. Our hypothesis is that upon hypoxic or hypercapnic challenge acetylcholine is released from the Type I cell and binds to receptors on the afferent neuron. Depolarization of the neuron follows and an action potential is generated.

Modulation of the respiratory pattern by hypercapnic stimulation of the central chemoreceptors also seems to involve acetylcholine. Dr. Neubauer discusses this as well as the presence of carbonic anhydrase in CO_2-chemosensitive cells in the central nervous system. Anatomic localization of the central chemoreceptors remains a large problem. Central chemosensitivity was originally believed to be confined to the ventrolateral surface of the medulla. Now it appears that cells sensitive to CO_2 may also be found on the dorsal surface of the medulla and in the hypothalamus as well as certain sections of the cortex (this volume).

Whether these cells communicate with each other in controlling respiration remains to be determined.

Dr. Cherniack presents a comprehensive overview of the physiological importance of the central chemoreceptors, both for respiration and for circulation. He reviews the evidence describing their location and the mechanisms involved in their response to CO_2 including studies which suggest a significant role for acetylcholine. Lastly he discusses the interaction of the peripheral and central chemoreceptors in the control of respiration.

This review leaves one wondering if an understanding of the modulation of the respiratory pattern might not better be attained by assuming that there is more than one "respiratory control system." That is, peripheral chemoreceptors, central chemoreceptors, brainstem nuclei, efferent neural pathways, and circulatory input have one interrelationship during rest, a second during sleep, a third during exercise, a fourth during obstructive lung disease, and so on. In a sense, this might not be surprising since it is the cardiopulmonary control system that regulates the ability of the organism to capture its most essential environmental nutrient, oxygen. To do so, a capacity for having the interrelationships among the cardiopulmonary components change easily would be advantageous.

REFERENCES

1. Daly, M. de B., J.L. Hazzledine, and A. Ungar. The reflex effects of alterations in lung volume on systemic vascular resistance in the dog. *J. Physiol.* (London) 188:331-351, 1967.

2. Eckberg, D.L., and C.R. Orshan. Respiratory and baroreceptor reflex interactions in man. *J. Clin. Invest.* 59:780-785, 1977.

3. Eyzaguirre, C., R.S. Fitzgerald, S. Lahiri, and P. Zapata. Arterial chemoreceptors. In *Handbook of Physiology* Section 2, vol. 3, ed. J.T. Shepherd and F.M. Abboud, 557-622. Bethesda, Md.: American Physiological Society, 1983.

4. Fidone, S.J., and C. Gonzalez. Initiation and control of chemoreceptor activity in the carotid body. In *Handbook of Physiology* Section 3, vol. 2, ed. N.S. Cherniack and J.G. Widdicombe, 247-312. Bethesda, Md.: American Physiological Society, 1986.

5. Grunstein, M.M., J.P. Derenne, and J. Milic-Emili. Control of depth and frequency of breathing during baroreceptor stimulation in cats. *J. Appl. Physiol.* 39:395-404, 1975.

28

Carbonic Anhydrase, Cl^--HCO_3^- Exchanger, and Cellular pH in O_2 and CO_2 Chemoreception in the Cat Carotid Body *in Vitro*

S. Lahiri, R. Iturriaga, W.L. Rumsey, D.F. Wilson, and D. Spergel

Glomus cells in the carotid body (CB) serve as the sensor for the neuron in the petrosal ganglion. The levels of PO_2, PCO_2 and pH of the arterial blood are detected by the glomus cells and the chemoreception is expressed as neurotransmitter release and sensory discharge (4). Carbonic anhydrase (CA) is present in the glomus cells of the CB (for review see 9). Knowledge of its subcellular distribution and isoenzyme types would help to understand the role that CA might play in the mechanisms and modulations of chemoreception of CO_2 and O_2. For the purpose of this presentation we will assume that it is present in the cytosol of the glomus cells.

It is now generally known that CB chemosensory fibers in the cat respond to a rapidly delivered CO_2 stimulus by increasing the discharge frequency, but the peak response is not sustained to a maintained stimulus (2, 11). The mechanisms of these responses to CO_2 is not clearly understood, but one proposal suggests that it parallels intracellular pH (pH_i) regulation following acid load. According to the more current version of the acid hypothesis of chemotransduction in the CB, a bicarbonate "pump" presumably located in the glomus cell membrane regulates pH at the receptor site and the function of the pump is PO_2-dependent: high PO_2 maximizes the pump activity, which lowers the cellular $[H^+]$, while hypoxia raises it (6, 15). Accordingly, the effect of hypercapnia and hypoxia could be explained in terms of cellular pH regulation alone.

Another hypothesis proposes that hypercapnia and hypoxia are sensed by separate mechanisms (see for example 11, 12) but that the hypercapnic stimulus "interacts" with or "converges" on the hypoxic chemoreception. In either case CA could contribute significantly by determining the net $[H^+]$ in the cell or in a specific cellular compartment in response to CO_2. A change in the $[H^+]$ could mobilize Ca^{++} raising its cytosolic concentration, leading to neurotransmitter release and chemosensory excitation. Also, studies of the role of CA in the CB could potentially lead to an understanding of the O_2-CO_2 stimulus interaction in the response of the chemoreceptor. According to the acid hypothesis of Torrance (6, 15), blockade of CA activity in the CB would eliminate the catalyzed hydration and dehydration of CO_2 and consequently the hypoxic effects. Indeed several *in vivo* studies reported that CA inhibition decreased both hypercapnic and hypoxic chemosensory and chemoreflex responses (1, 6, 10).

Disequilibrium of CO_2-HCO_3^- in the circulating blood after CA inhibition, however, makes it difficult to accurately measure the stimulus level in the arterial blood at the CB. The reaction of the sampled blood goes to completion only slowly, raising PCO_2 and $[H^+]$, and hence the measured values provide a falsely higher stimulus level, leading to an underestimation of the response. This disequilibrium effect could be overcome by using a pre-equilibrated cell-free solution in CB studies *in situ* or *in vitro*. The purpose of the study was to measure the role of the carotid body CA and CO_2-HCO_3^- in the chemoreceptor response to hypercapnia and hypoxia in the transient and physiological steady-states.

METHODS

We used a recently developed *in vitro* cat carotid body preparation perfused and superfused with the same Tyrode solution (7). The CB maintained its chemosensory responses to natural stimuli for several hours. Briefly, the vascularly isolated carotid bifurcation, including CB and the carotid sinus nerve (CSN), was excised from anesthetized cats (sodium pentobarbitone 35 mg/kg ip followed by 10 mg when necessary) and placed in a chamber for simultaneous perfusion and superfusion at 36.5 ± 0.5 °C. The CB was perfused (at a hydrostatic pressure of 80 torr) with a modified Tyrode equilibrated at a PO_2 of 120 torr (normoxia), or >450 torr (hyperoxia) or <20 torr (hypoxia). The superfusate was equilibrated at PO_2 <20 torr. The composition of the Tyrode solution was the following (mM): Na^+, 154; K^+, 4.7; Ca^{++}, 2.2; Mg^{++}, 1.1; Cl^-, 110; glutamate, 42.0; and glucose, 5.0. It was buffered with 5 mM HEPES to pH 7.40 with 1M NaOH. To study the effects of CO_2-HCO_3^-, the Tyrode was modified by adding $NaHCO_3$ in place of 21.4 mM NaCl.

Chemosensory discharges were recorded from the whole CSN, which was placed on bipolar platinum electrodes and lifted into paraffin oil. The neural signals were amplified, displayed on an oscilloscope, selected with an amplitude discriminator, and counted electronically. To study the effects of CA inhibition, methazolamide (10–20 mg/l) was dissolved in the Tyrode and perfused for 30 min. For measurement of changes in intracellular pH (pH_i) the carotid body was loaded for 5–10 min with Tyrode containing the fluorescent pH indicator 2',7'-bis(2-carboxyethyl)-5(6)-

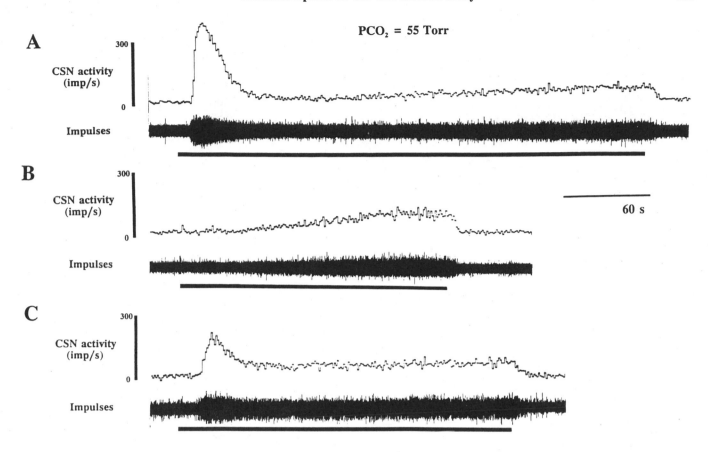

FIG. 28.1 Effects of methazolamide (10 mg/l) on carotid chemosensory responses to perfusion of Tyrode equilibrated with CO_2 in O_2 ($PCO_2 = 55$ torr, $HCO_3^- = 21.4$ mM, pH 7.25). (A) Chemosensory response without methazolamide. (B) After 30 min of perfusion with Tyrode containing methazolamide. (C) After 30 min of washing out methazolamide. Bars indicate duration of perfusion of Tyrode with CO_2-HCO_3^-.

carboxyfluorescein (BCECF/AM) at a concentration of 5 µM. After dye loading the CB was perfused with Tyrode for 10 min to wash out the excess dye. The fluorescent signal was monitored using a macroscope with an epifluorescence attachment (excitation 420–490 nm, emission >515 nm). The fluorescent signal was detected by a light-sensitive video camera and stored in a VCR.

RESULTS AND DISCUSSION

The results illustrate the following: (1) methazolamide (10–20 mg/l, pH 7.40) reversibly blocked the initial but not the late chemosensory response to CO_2-HCO_3^- administration (fig. 28.1); (2) methazolamide delayed the response to perfusate flow interruption and to hypoxia but did not diminish the maximal response in the nominal absence of CO_2-HCO_3^- (fig. 28.2); (3) the carotid body did not show a pH_i decrease corresponding to the chemosensory response to flow interruption (fig. 28.3); (4) the carotid body showed predictable pH_i changes with the administration of NH_4Cl (fig. 28.4); (5) equilibration of CB with CO_2-HCO_3^- in the external medium greatly modified the hypoxic response; and (6) the nominal absence of CO_2-HCO_3^- did not prevent O_2 chemoreception.

Figure 28.1 shows that switching from hyperoxic Tyrode buffer alone ($PCO_2 < 1$ torr, pH 7.40) to Tyrode equilibrated at $PCO_2 = 55$ torr in O_2 (HEPES-HCO_3^- 21.4 mM, pH 7.25) was followed by a large overshoot in the chemosensory response. The decline of the peak response was presumably due to regulation of pH_i after the acid load. It is reasonable that acid extrusion by the chemoreceptor cells was responsible for what is known as adaptation. The Na^+-H^+ exchanger present in the glomus cell (3), presumably activated by the acid load, contributed to the pH_i regulation. Accordingly blockade of the exchanger would arrest adaptation and maintain the activity provided that other exchanger mechanisms do not obliterate the effect.

Methazolamide (fig. 28.1B) diminished the rapid initial rise of the chemosensory response because the rapidly catalyzed formation of acid did not take place and hence did not activate the mechanisms for adaptation. However, methazolamide did not prevent the gradual rise of chemosensory activity due to hypercapnia. After removal of methazolamide the initial response began to reappear with a slight delay (fig. 28.1C).

Figure 28.2 illustrates the chemosensory response to hypercapnia and hypoxia. The CB was initially perfused

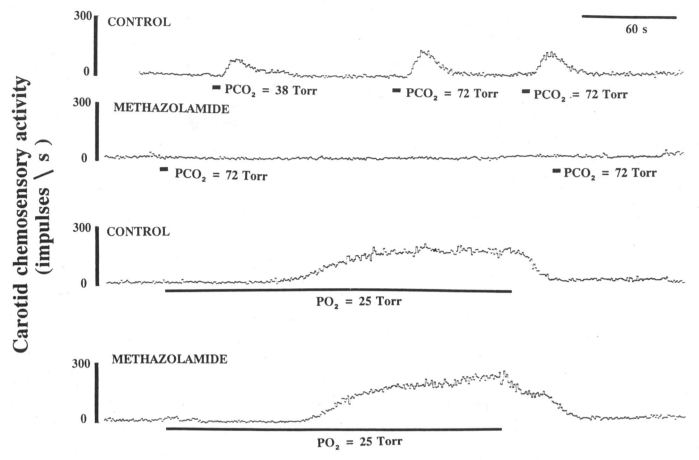

FIG. 28.2 Effects of methazolamide (20 mg/l) on carotid chemosensory response to bolus injections of Tyrode (0.5 ml) equilibrated at PCO_2 of 38 and 72 torr in O_2 (*upper two panels*) and to hypoxic ($PO_2 = 25$ torr) Tyrode (*lower two panels*). The carotid body was initially perfused in hyperoxia. Note that methazolamide eliminated the immediate response to CO_2 but did not diminish the maximal response to low PO_2. Bars mark the duration of hypoxic perfusion of Tyrode containing CO_2-HCO_3^- injections.

with hyperoxic Tyrode. Injections of Tyrode (0.5 ml), equilibrated at a PCO_2 of 38 torr or 72 torr, elicited immediate responses which were blocked during perfusion with methazolamide (upper two panels). The response to hypoxia was delayed but the maximal response did not diminish. In fact, the maximal response was slightly increased. Thus the hypoxic response occurred despite nominal absence of CO_2-HCO_3^-. These results do not support the conclusion of Shirahata and Fitzgerald that CO_2-HCO_3^- is essential for hypoxic chemotransduction (this volume). They probably missed the hypoxic effect because the duration of the test was short for the effect to develop in the absence of CO_2-HCO_3^-.

The hypothesis that the hypoxic response was not due to acidosis is supported by the observations presented in figures 28.3 and 28.4. Ischemic hypoxia caused by perfusate flow interruption in the nominal absence of CO_2-HCO_3^- sharply increased chemosensory activity without any detectable increase in the intracellular acidity. Note that the Tyrode was free of CO_2-HCO_3^-, which delayed the response to ischemia. A similar CB preparation, however, predictably (see 13) responded to the NH_4Cl administration

(fig. 28.4). An initial pH_i increase was followed by a decrease in the chemosensory activity, and with the decrease of pH_i the chemoreceptor activity increased. Thus, the chemosensory response to ischemic hypoxia without a significant change in the fluorescent signal indicates that O_2 chemosensory response was not due to a concomitant intracellular acidification.

The observation that oligomycin, which augmented the chemosensory response to acidosis concomitantly suppressing those to hypoxia (12), is consistent with the conclusion that the hypoxic response is not mediated by cellular acidosis in the CB. Any acidosis during hypoxia after oligomycin should have increased the sensory discharge.

We also studied the effects of hypoxia on chemosensory discharge with and without CO_2-HCO_3^- in the medium. A set of experimental results is shown in figure 28.5. The presence of 5% CO_2 in the extracellular medium augmented the speed and the maximal chemosensory response to hypoxia even when the external pH was similar. The effect of CO_2-HCO_3^- in the external medium on the hypoxic response could be explained by pH_i regulation; an increased acidity would augment the hypoxic response.

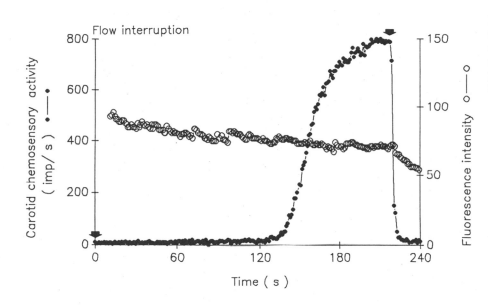

FIG. 28.3 Effects of perfusate flow interruption on carotid chemosensory and carotid body intracellular pH (fluorescent signal) responses during hyperoxic perfusion. Arrows indicate beginning and end of the flow interruption.

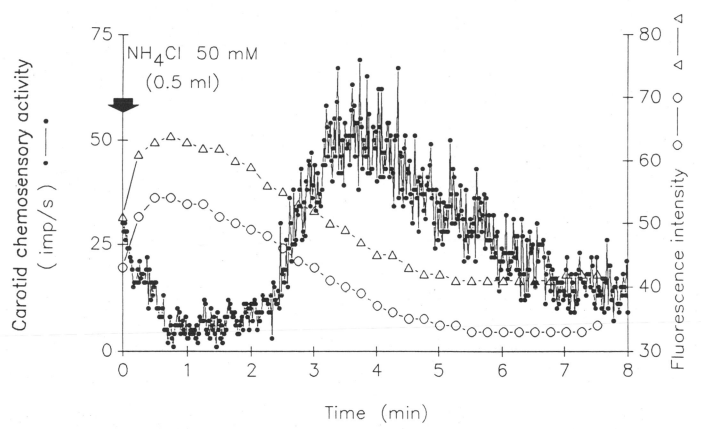

FIG. 28.4 Carotid chemosensory and carotid body intracellular pH (fluorescent signals from two different areas) responses to bolus (0.5 ml) injection of Tyrode containing 50 mM NH_4Cl. Arrow indicates injection into the perfusion line.

These results show that the hypoxic response occurred in the nominal absence of CO_2-HCO_3^- in the extracellular medium. Since the function of the Cl^--HCO_3^- exchanger depends on the presence of external HCO_3^- (13, 14), the results suggest that the response to hypoxia does not require the function of the exchanger in the plasma membrane. However, the blockade of the exchanger modified the re-

sponse to hypoxia presumably mostly due to an initial baseline increase in the pH_i.

In separate experiments we found that methazolamide attenuated the hypercapnic response in the presence of CO_2-HCO_3^- in the external medium and reduced the speed and maximal response to hypoxia. In terms of pH_i, these results suggest that CA is needed to generate and maintain

FIG. 28.5 Effects of CO_2-HCO_3^- on carotid chemosensory responses to hypoxia (PO_2 = 30 torr). The carotid body was first perfused-superfused with Tyrode free of CO_2-HCO_3^- (open circles) and then with Tyrode equilibrated with PCO_2 at 38 torr (closed circles). In both cases the Tyrode pH was 7.37 throughout and the PO_2 was 125 torr. Arrows indicate duration of hypoxic perfusion.

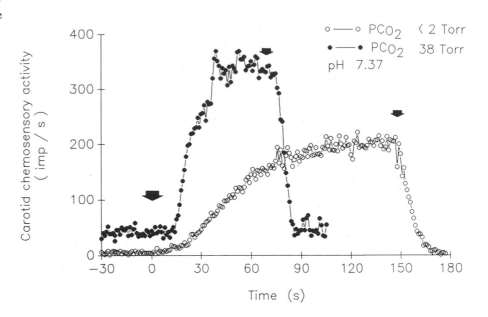

$[H^+]_i$ at a higher level in the chemoreceptor compartment, which is in a dynamic physiological steady state and which is independent of the membrane exchanger function.

The mechanism coupling $[H^+]_i$ rise and the parallel increase in the sensory discharge has not been established. However, a plausible mechanism is that a rise in $[H^+]_i$ is followed by activation of the Na^+-H^+ exchanger and a subsequent rise in $[Na^+]i$, which in turn reverses the Na^+-Ca^{++} exchanger function, accumulating cellular Ca^{++}. This increase in Ca^{++} leads to exocytosis and release of dopamine and perhaps norepinephrine. Gonzalez et al. (5) advanced such a mechanism. The neurochemicals acting at synapses between glomus cells and nerve endings could generate neural discharge. There are several ways the scheme can be verified, one of which is a direct measurement of intracellular Ca^{++}, pH_i and catecholamine release.

In summary, the results show that hypoxic chemoreception is greatly modified by the Cl^--HCO_3^- exchanger. External CO_2-HCO_3^- and the Cl^--HCO_3^- exchanger are critical for the rapid responses. The hypoxic response is not mediated by cellular acidosis but is regulated by the pH_i. Carbonic anhydrase is necessary for the rapid as well as the steady-state response to CO_2, and consequently to hypoxia. Accordingly, CA in the CB make chemoreception and chemosensory responses physiologically rapid and meaningful *in vivo*.

ACKNOWLEDGMENTS

This work was supported by NIH Grants HL-19737-15 and HL-43413-02.

REFERENCES

1. Ahmad, H.R., N.S. Cherniack, and N. Prabhakar. Effect of carbonic anhydrase inhibitor on hypoxic and hypercapnic responses of aortic and carotid chemoreceptor in the anaesthetized cat. *J. Physiol.* (London) 417:109P, 1990.

2. Black, A.M.S., D.I. McCloskey, and R.W. Torrance. The responses of carotid body chemoreceptor in the cat to sudden changes in hypercapnic and hypoxic stimuli. *Resp. Physiol.* 13:36-49, 1971.

3. Buckler, K.J., P.C.G. Nye, C. Peers, and R.D. Vaughan-Jones. Regulation of intracellular pH in single type I carotid body cells isolated from the neonatal rat. *J. Physiol.* (London) 423:65P, 1990.

4. Eyzaguirre, C., R.S. Fitzgerald, S. Lahiri, and P. Zapata. Arterial chemoreceptor. In *Handbook of Physiology*, Section 2, vol. 3, ed. J.T. Shepherd and F.M. Abboud, 557-621. Baltimore, Md.: American Physiological Society, 1983.

5. Gonzalez, C., A. Rocher, A. Obeso, J.R. López-López, J. López-Barneo, and B. Herreros. Ionic mechanisms of the chemoreception process in type I cells of the carotid body. In *Arterial chemoreception*, ed. C. Eyzaguirre, S. Fidone, R.S. Fitzgerald, S. Lahiri, and D. McDonald, 44-57. New York: Springer-Verlag, 1990.

6. Hanson, M.A., P.C.G. Nye, and R.W. Torrance. The exodus of an extracellular bicarbonate theory of chemoreception and the genesis of an intracellular one. In *Arterial chemoreceptor*, ed. C. Belmonte, D. Pallot, H. Acker, and S. Fidone, 403-416. Leicester: University Press, 1981.

7. Iturriaga, R., W.L. Rumsey, A. Mokashi, D. Spergel, D.F. Wilson, and S. Lahiri. *In vitro* perfused-superfused cat carotid body for physiological and pharmacological studies. *J. Appl. Physiol.* 70:1393-1400, 1991.

8. Iturriaga, R., S. Lahiri, and A. Mokashi. Carbonic anhydrase and chemoreception in the cat carotid body. *Am. J. Physiol.* (*Cell Physiol.*) 261:C565-C573, 1991.

9. Lahiri, S. Carbonic anhydrase and chemoreception in carotid and aortic bodies. In *The carbonic anhydrases. Cellular physiology and molecular genetics,* ed. S.J. Dodgson, R.F. Tashian, G. Gros, and N.D. Carter. New York: Plenum. In press, 1991.

10. Lahiri, S., R.G. DeLaney, and A.P. Fishman. Peripheral and central effects of acetazolamide in the control of ventilation. *The Physiol.* 19:261, 1976.

11. Lahiri, S., E. Mulligan, and A. Mokashi. Adaptive response of carotid body chemoreceptor to CO_2. *Brain Res.* 234:367-382, 1982.

12. Mulligan, E., and S. Lahiri. Separation of carotid body chemoreceptor response to O_2 and CO_2 by oligomycin and by antimycin. *Am. J. Physiol.* 242:C200-C206, 1982.

13. Roos, A., and W.F. Boron. Intracellular pH. *Physiol. Rev.* 61:296-434, 1981.

14. Thomas, R.C. The role of bicarbonate, chloride and sodium ions in the regulation of pH in snail neurones. *J. Physiol.* (London) 273:317-338, 1977.

15. Torrance, R.W. A new version of the acid receptor hypothesis of carotid chemoreceptor. In *Morphology and mechanisms of chemoreceptor,* ed. A.S. Paintal, 131-135. Delhi: Vallabhbhai Patel Chest Institute, 1976.

29

Physiological Roles of the Central Chemoreceptors

Neil S. Cherniack

A key feature of the respiratory system is its ability to significantly limit the changes in arterial PCO_2 (P_aCO_2) caused by varying activity or residence at different altitudes (15, 37). This near constancy of P_aCO_2 together with the impressive ventilatory effects produced by inhaled CO_2 demonstrates the presence in the body of important receptors that respond either directly to PCO_2 changes or the acid-base alterations induced by CO_2 (6, 10, 11, 34, 36, 39).

Several types of CO_2-sensitive receptors have been identified. The arterial chemoreceptors (the carotid body and to a lesser extent the aortic body) increase their discharge and ventilation when PCO_2 or hydrogen ion concentration rises (23, 32). Receptors in the airways (probably the stretch receptors which also respond to lung expansion) reduce their activity when PCO_2 is raised (15, 37). In addition there may be receptors in the pulmonary arteries which hypercapnia excites (15, 37, 39). But even after experimental interventions have eliminated all of these peripheral CO_2 receptors, a pronounced rise in ventilation still occurs when CO_2 is breathed (6, 34). This finding indicates that there must be other receptors that are extremely sensitive to CO_2 within the central nervous system (6, 34, 39).

Recent studies show that some of these central chemoreceptors are located in the ventral portion of the medulla, close to the surface where they are intermingled with neurons that regulate blood pressure, tracheal tone, and airway secretions (6, 11, 34, 39). The physiological role of these central receptors and their location and modes of operation are reviewed below.

METHODS

To study the effects of central chemoreceptor stimulation in isolation, experiments are frequently carried out in animals in which the central nervous system connections of arterial chemoreceptors have been severed (5, 24). Since arterial chemoreceptors affect more than respiration, their denervation distorts to a certain extent normal physiology (24). Hence, a number of investigators have attempted to study central chemoreceptors in the intact subject, taking advantage of the differences in the time course of the response of peripheral and central chemoreceptors to CO_2 stimulation (2, 18). Although peripheral chemoreceptor discharge closely mimics the temporal profile of changes in P_aCO_2 when CO_2 is inhaled, ventilation increases for a much

longer period of time (often for more than 10 min) after P_aCO_2 reaches a constant level (25). This temporal dissociation of changes in P_aCO_2 and ventilation has been believed to reflect the time required for P_aCO_2 to equilibrate with the PCO_2 at the central chemoreceptors in the brain. More recent studies suggest that changes in medullary PCO_2 can occur quite rapidly and have led to the proposal that the slower increase in ventilation is due to the time required to process signals from central chemoreceptors by respiratory circuits (2). The finding that central chemoreceptors contribute 70–80% of the total ventilatory response to CO_2 has been confirmed by experiments using other techniques, such as injections of CO_2 or acids into the vertebral arteries or cerebrospinal fluid, and by studies employing isolated perfusion of the brain *in vivo* to stimulate only the central chemoreceptors (6, 24, 36, 37).

In vivo, CO_2 can influence respiration indirectly by its direct effects on the circulation and smooth and skeletal muscle, and by altering rates of catecholamine secretion (e.g., 33, 66). Hence a number of *in vitro* methods have been developed to better elucidate mechanisms of CO_2 stimulation. These methods include preparations of the isolated brain and spinal cord of the newborn rat and slices of tissue from different regions of the medulla (28, 54). These preparations allow extracellular and intracellular nerve recordings to be made in situations where the neuronal environment can be controlled with much greater precision than *in vivo*. However, interconnections among neurons are disrupted in slice preparations, and it may be difficult to discern the usual respiratory function of a given nerve cell. Although these problems are less severe where neuronal recordings can be correlated to recordings made from the proximal stubs of the phrenic nerve, results may be distorted because this preparation depends on the use of immature animals (54).

CHARACTERISTICS OF THE CO_2 RESPONSE

The afferent discharge of arterial chemoreceptors increases linearly as P_aCO_2 is raised (18, 23, 32). Since the activity of the central chemoreceptors has not yet been directly measured because their location remains uncertain, inferences have been made about the characteristics of the afferent response from studies of respiratory motor output. In both intact and peripherally chemodenervated anesthetized animals, there is no ventilation and no phasic respiratory

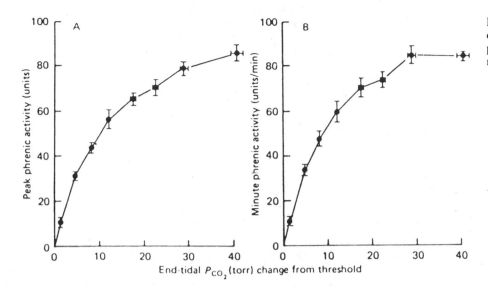

FIG. 29.1 Increases over apneic threshold of end-tidal CO_2. (*A*) Peak tidal phrenic nerve activity and (*B*) neural minute phrenic nerve activity. (22)

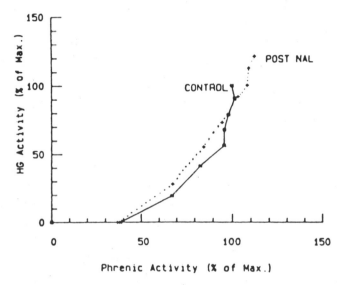

FIG. 29.2 Average data from eight cats showing the relationship between phrenic nerve activity and hypoglossal (HG) activity before and after naloxone (NAL) infusion. Note hypoglossal activity starts after phrenic activity but plateaus later. (56)

nerve or neuronal activity until P_aCO_2 reaches some minimum level (the apneic threshold) (22, 36, 37, 46, 56). Thereafter phrenic motor responses are linearly related to changes in P_aCO_2 until levels reach a very high value. Ultimately no further increases occur, and there may be a decline in response with additional hypercapnia (56) (see fig. 29.1). Cranial and cervical nerves innervating upper airway muscles and accessory muscles like the sternohyoid show a similar pattern with a threshold, a linear portion, and then a plateau, but the exact PCO_2 values for the threshold and the plateau differ among nerves, as shown in figure 29.2 (46, 56).

Rather than there being a distinct threshold, some investigators believe PCO_2 responses are better represented by

S-shaped curves. In awake subjects it may be difficult to demonstrate an apneic threshold for CO_2, since minimal ventilation continues in many conscious subjects as PCO_2 is lowered because of nonspecific drives coincident with voluntary activity. With passive hyperventilation obvious respiratory activity is rather easily eliminated even during wakefulness (36). However, CO_2 may have respiratory actions even when there is no clearly demonstrable respiratory activity. For instance, anesthetized animals made apneic by hyperventilation can be made to respire spontaneously by the administration of hypoxic gases to lower P_aO_2 (37). Hyperventilation of these now hypoxic animals allows apnea to reoccur. This suggests that even very low levels of PCO_2 can stimulate central chemoreceptors, but whether this discharge produces respiratory activity depends on the level of other excitatory chemical and less specific inputs to the respiratory neurons.

The increased ventilation produced by inhaled CO_2 varies considerably in conscious humans (10, 11, 36, 37). Reported responses have varied from 1 to 8 l/min/torr PCO_2, which may reflect the effects of other internal and external stimuli on respiratory neurons rather than an actual variability in the sensitivity of central chemoreceptors (36, 37). Anesthesia and sleep depress the increase in phrenic nerve activity caused by hypercapnia but not as much as they reduce the responses to CO_2 of cranial nerves or motor nerves supplying the accessory respiratory muscles (10). In REM sleep, the effect of stimuli originating in the brain may become sufficiently large to mask the effects of central chemoreceptor stimulation and eliminate any consistent hypercapnic effect on ventilation (10).

Lack of certainty concerning the exact stimulus to the central chemoreceptors may also contribute to the apparent variability of CO_2 responses. For example, changes in cerebral blood flow may alter the CO_2 stimulus to the central chemoreceptors so that venous PCO_2 of the brain or PCO_2

in the cerebrospinal fluid may better reflect the actual stimulus to the central chemoreceptors (52).

In intact animals, it is clear that the respiratory responses to PCO_2 depend on the presence or absence of other respiratory inputs (19, 21, 36, 37, 52). The apneic threshold, but not CO_2 responsivity (defined here as the change in ventilation divided by the change in P_aCO_2), is affected by acidosis and alkalosis (36). In conscious humans with acidosis the ventilation achieved at any given PCO_2 is greater than it is normally, while with alkalosis it is less (36, 37). Hypoxia, on the other hand, in awake humans alters CO_2 responsivity but has smaller effects on apneic threshold as shown in figure 29.3 (12, 36). Hypoxia increases CO_2 sensitivity, and the effect is magnified until PO_2 is lowered to about 30 to 40 torr as shown in figure 29.3. This effect requires the presence of peripheral chemoreceptors. Most studies report that exercise has no effect on CO_2 responsivity (36). All observers agree that exercise behaves as if it lowers the apneic threshold (58).

LOCATION OF CENTRAL CHEMORECEPTORS

Studies carried out in the past thirty years have established that the pH of the cerebrospinal fluid can significantly alter respiration (6, 34, 39, 40, 44, 64). Acid pH levels excite breathing, while alkaline pH levels inhibit breathing (6, 36, 39, 40, 44). These findings seemed to indicate that central chemoreceptors can receive information from cerebrospinal fluid and thus some or all are placed superficially in the medulla. Experiments from different groups of investigators have provided evidence indicating that the cells in the medulla which are responsive to CO_2 are located in its ventrolateral portion within a millimeter of the surface (6, 34, 39, 44, 64). Application of acidic solutions or respiratory stimulants like lobeline to the ventral medullary surface (VMS) augmented breathing and excited respiratory responses to CO_2, while topical applications of local anesthetics abolished respiratory responses to inhaled CO_2 (6, 44, 64).

Three areas within 1 mm of the VMS seem to be important in central chemoreceptor sensitivity (13, 34, 64). The rostral area (which extends from the pontine-medullary border to the rostral hypoglossal rootlets) and the caudal area (which spans the distance from the caudal hypoglossal rootlets to the medullary spinal junction) were believed to be regions in which central chemoreceptors or their endings were located. The two chemosensitive regions were separated by an intervening intermediate area through which chemoreceptor fibers traveled into the interior of the medulla. Acids applied on the intermediate area in these studies did not stimulate respiration (64). These observations were supported by subsequent studies that demonstrated strong effects of bilateral focal cooling in discrete VMS areas on the CO_2 apneic threshold (13). Using thermodes with cooling plates 1–2 mm^2 to lower surface temperature

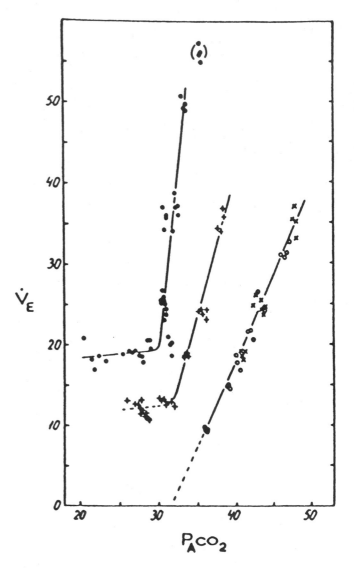

FIG. 29.3 Ventilation ($\dot{V}_E$) as a function of P_aCO_2 at a steady-state P_aO_2 of 37 (•), 47(+) and 169 (x) torr in conscious humans. (53)

from 37°C to 20°C produced a progressive increase in the PCO_2 required to initiate respiration in anesthetized cats. This degree of cooling was enough to interfere with synaptic transmission but not with conduction along nerve fibers or with cell function (fig. 29.4). The most prominent depressant effects of cooling on breathing were observed in the intermediate area. Greater cooling could produce apnea, but even then breathing could be reinstituted by raising P_aCO_2 levels.

Different respiratory effects have been observed on cooling rostral and caudal areas (13, 29). Cooling the caudal area tended to diminish the amplitude of phrenic nerve excursion but often increased respiratory rate. In the rostral area, the rate slowed as surface temperature was lowered. Changes like those produced by cooling occurred with the topical application of local anesthetics. Areas close to the

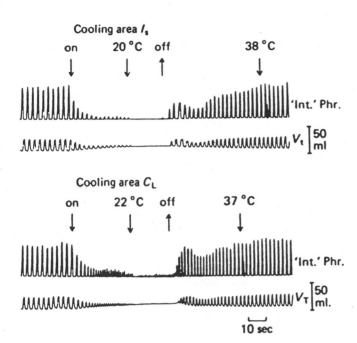

FIG. 29.4 Effects of focal cooling of intermediate areas (I_S, upper trace) and caudal areas (C_L, lower trace) of ventral medullary surface on tidal phrenic activity (Int Phr) and tidal volume (V_T) in spontaneously breathing cat after bilateral vagotomy. (13)

surface where temperature reduction causes apnea have also been reported in dogs (1). Unilateral intramedullary cooling of the nucleus paragigantocellularis lateralis in cats abolished all respiratory responses to CO_2 even if P_aCO_2 were raised considerably (8). This suggested that afferent signals from the central chemoreceptors converge on neurons in this nucleus (8). In chronic cats, coagulation of the VMS elevated P_aCO_2 and markedly depressed responses to inhaled CO_2 and to hypoxia (65). Intermediate area cooling also modifies the effects of discharge of vagally supplied receptors in the airways and decreases the sympathetic nerve activity induced by CO_2 inhalation (41, 45).

EFFECTS OF VENTRAL MEDULLA ON NON-RESPIRATORY FUNCTION

Interventions at the VMS that affect the response to CO_2 also depress the formation of tracheal secretion elicited by irritant receptor stimulation at the carina and prevent the tracheal constriction arising from mechanical probing of the carina (17). Systemic blood pressure is frequently reduced by intermediate area cooling (14, 26, 63, 69). Independent studies have demonstrated that the region near the VMS is populated by a group of neurons which are largely responsible for resting vasomotor tone (26, 63). These vasomotor neurons have been divided into rostral (epinephrine-producing) pressor neurons, and caudal (norepinephrine-producing) depressor neurons (14, 26, 63). The VMS vasomotor neurons receive connections from many areas of the brain, including regions which contain

high concentrations of respiratory-related neurons, like the nucleus tractus solitarius (63). Surface areas from which the rostral pressor neurons can be affected by neuroamines and peptides overlap the rostral and intermediate respiratory chemosensitive areas, while the caudal depressor area overlaps the caudal respiratory chemosensitive area (35, 63). The possibility that these vasomotor neurons might be responsible in some way for the respiratory effects observed from the VMS has occurred to many investigators (e.g., 39). More recent experiments have shown a clear separation of the locations in the ventral medulla from which respiratory and vasomotor effects can be elicited by NMDA and other glutamate agonists in cats (38, 47).

Neurons in the ventral medulla may act on breathing and blood pressure by producing an excitatory input that is necessary for both vasomotor and respiratory activity (39, 42, 43, 61). This does not seem to be entirely correct since areas of the ventral medulla cause either pressor or depressor responses, and cooling of the VMS does not prevent the respiratory excitation produced by stimulation of somatic afferents or the tachypnea caused by heating the hypothalamus or the whole body (43, 68). Nonetheless, many neurons in the VMS seem to respond to multiple inputs, including hypercapnia, peripheral chemoreceptor stimulation, and input from the hypothalamus and somatic afferents.

While neurons near the VMS respond to CO_2 and can be considered central chemoreceptors, it is uncertain whether there are CO_2 neurons in other areas of the brain (3, 30). Arita and coworkers have shown that intravertebral artery injections of solutions equilibrated with 100% CO_2 can excite neurons in both the ventral and dorsal medulla (3, 30). In many instances this excitation correlates with local decreases in extracellular pH and increases in phrenic nerve activity. Studies with brain slices indicate that even after synaptic transmission is prevented by altering the bathing fluids, high levels of CO_2 or acid solutions can depolarize neurons in slices of dorsal and ventral medulla, even though the number of neurons stimulated in dorsal locations is usually less (28, 31). These studies usually involve the use of severely acidic and/or hypercapnic solutions, and their relationship to normal physiology is problematic. Also, in slices it is difficult to know whether the neurons excited have a respiratory function. At the present time it seems reasonable to conclude that the ventral medulla contains central chemoreceptors but so may other areas of the brain.

MECHANISMS IN THE RESPONSE OF THE CENTRAL CHEMORECEPTORS

It has been argued for many years whether CO_2 and H^+ act independently as respiratory stimulants or whether all of the effects of CO_2 on breathing are secondary to pH changes induced by CO_2 either intra- or extracellularly (6, 34, 39, 67). Many studies have assumed that there is some site corresponding to the location of the central chemoreceptors where changes in pH account for all the ventilation changes whether they were caused by CO_2 inhalation or systemic acid infusion. No such extracellular site has as yet been identified. It is clear that pH changes in the arterial blood do not entirely explain the respiratory changes caused by inhaling CO_2. The cerebrospinal fluid (CSF) or brain extracellular fluid (ECF) may be more similar to the environment of central chemoreceptors than the blood (6, 34, 39). The pH of brain ECF and the CSF is actively regulated and varies considerably from pH values in the blood (19, 34). Generally, CO_2 inhalation produces greater effects on brain fluid pH than does the infusion of acid into the blood stream. Studies which have measured pH changes in both blood and bulk CSF find that neither pH change by itself accounts for breathing changes brought about by inhaled CO_2 (19, 34). These studies have suggested that central chemoreceptors were at some site which could be influenced both by the CSF and by the blood (19).

Studies by Ahmad and by Millhorn et al. show that pH near the VMS changes far more rapidly than pH in the bulk CSF (away from the surface) (2, 40). When pH changes are measured at the VMS, however, inhaled CO_2 seems to have a much greater effect on breathing than acids infused into the blood or applied to the exterior of the brain (67). Since CO_2 crosses cell membranes with much greater ease than hydrogen ions, these observations have led to the revival of the hypothesis that intracellular pH is the actual stimulus to central chemoreceptors. Cell structure is, however, quite complex and pH in the cell interior is not uniform. Even if internal pH does specify respiratory responses, we will need to know the crucial intracellular site(s).

It is probable that pH changes by themselves do not generate action potentials but rather trigger a series of intermediate steps which involve neurotransmitters. Many neurotransmitters exert excitatory effects on respiration when applied to or microinjected into the VMS, and may in addition alter respiratory responses to CO_2 (6, 9, 20, 38, 39, 47–50, 60, 70). These agents include glutamate, tachykinins, and serotonin. It is not clear, however, whether the agents act at the central chemoreceptors or at sites upstream or downstream from them. Neurons containing these substances are present in the medulla, as are cells containing the appropriate receptors.

Dev and Loeschcke have proposed that H^+ alters respiratory discharge by inhibiting the metabolism of acetylcholine in the synapse (20). Like many other enzymes, the activity of acetylcholine esterase is pH sensitive. Cholinergic agents stimulate breathing when applied to the VMS, as do antagonists to acetylcholine esterase (e.g., physostigmine). Dev et al. found that atropine, a muscarinic receptor antagonist, blocked the response to CO_2 (20). This has recently been confirmed by Nattie, who used more specific antagonists to show that the M2 muscarinic binding site was the pertinent receptor (20, 50, 51). It is of interest that

Loeschcke attributed the weaker effects of infused acid on breathing to the greater difficulty in accessibility of H^+ to the synapse (34).

Studies of cold-blooded animals provide clues that may be useful in understanding the principles of central receptor operation. At 37°C, respiration seems to be regulated so that blood pH is maintained at about 7.4. In cold-blooded animals, however, the pH at rest becomes more alkaline as the animal is cooled and more acidic when temperature is raised above 37°C (9). But because of temperature-dependent changes in dissociation constants, the ratio of H^+/OH^- remains the same. If breathing is in fact adjusted to keep this ratio fixed, then it is conceivable that pH changes affect breathing by altering the degree of dissociation of a moiety present in some crucial proteins. As the pH changes, electrostatic forces might alter, for example, the configuration of some receptor protein, thus initiating intracellular events that lead ultimately to increased respiratory activity. Reeves has proposed that pH alters the dissociation of imidazole-histidine groups in key proteins in CO_2 chemoreceptors thereby eliciting physiological effects (60). On the other hand, temperature effects on the pH of the imidazole-histidine moiety are similar to that of the fluid with which it is in contact. Nattie, in an intriguing series of experiments, has examined the effects of diethylpyrocarbonate (DEPC), which alters the dissociation of imidazole on the respiratory responses to inhaled CO_2 in cats and rabbits (48, 49). He demonstrated in both species that DEPC depressed respiratory response to CO_2 but did not alter the response to hypoxia (fig. 29.5). In cats, DEPC effects were greatest when applied to the rostral chemosensitive area of the VMS and were reversed by a specific antagonist. Although the cellular processes which allow respiratory responses to CO_2 to occur remain unclear, a number of different neurochemicals including acetylcholine appear to be involved.

RELATIONSHIP OF CENTRAL TO PERIPHERAL CHEMORECEPTORS

The carotid bodies are excited both by hypoxia and by hypercapnia (16, 18, 23, 24, 32). When CO_2 is inhaled under hypoxic conditions, the change in respiratory activity for a given change in PCO_2 is considerably more than it is under hyperoxic conditions (32, 34). This greater than additive response occurs by substantial effects at the carotid body itself since the increment in carotid body discharge produced by hypercapnia is also considerably enhanced by hypoxia (23, 32). In fact, under hyperoxic conditions, the carotid body response to CO_2 is virtually nil (32).

Some studies suggest that carotid body stimulation potentiates the responses of the central chemoreceptors to CO_2 (24, 62). These studies have used techniques that allow independent manipulation of the CO_2 stimulus peripherally and centrally. Results may have been inconsistent

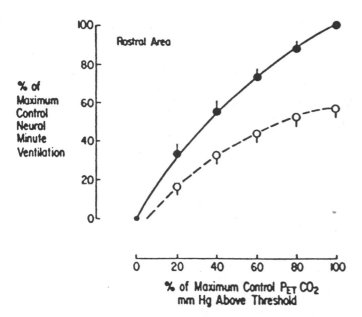

FIG. 29.5 Average responses to CO_2 before (•) and after (o) application of diethylpyrocarbonate to the rostral ventrolateral medulla in 6 cats. (48)

because they have required extensive surgical interventions and/or because of the complex actions of CO_2 centrally. Brain PCO_2 increases cerebral blood flow and can excite vasomotor as well as respiratory neurons (33, 61, 63). Hypercapnia may cause the release of both excitatory and inhibitory neuroactive substances in supramedullary regions which can indirectly alter respiratory responses to hypercapnia. For example, decerebration enhances the hypoglossal motor response to CO_2 while decortication inhibits it (46).

A number of studies suggest that VMS interventions which affect CO_2 response can alter responses to peripheral chemoreceptor stimulation (13, 39). Selected neurons in the ventral medulla in vivo can respond to both CO_2 and to peripheral chemoreceptor stimulation. While most of the central projections of the carotid body synapse in the nucleus tractus solitarius, some pathways bypass this nucleus and proceed more directly to central medullary neurons (24). Cooling or procaine application to the VMS or superficial coagulation of that area has been reported to reduce respiratory responses to hypoxia and to electrical stimulation of the central end of the carotid sinus nerve (42, 65). Alkalosis confined to the brain decreases carotid body afferent discharge by augmenting inhibitory signals which travel from the brain to the carotid body (24).

The effect of hypercapnia on central and peripheral chemoreceptors may differ. It has been proposed that hypercapnia by a central action enhances the discharge of expiratory neurons while carotid body stimulation has an inspiratory augmenting effect (62). The relative excitatory effects of CO_2 on peripheral versus central chemoreceptors seem to be greater on cranial nerves like the hypoglossal than on the phrenic (7).

Reduction in VMS temperature depresses the excitatory effects on breathing of irritant receptor stimulation and enhances the apnea produced by stimulation of receptors in the lung (which are supplied by unmyelinated fibers of the vagus nerve) (13, 41, 45). However, responses to stretch receptor stimulation are not affected by VMS manipulations (13). It is not certain whether any of these effects arise directly from the central chemoreceptor or from some interconnected structure.

CENTRAL CHEMORECEPTORS IN THE RESPONSE TO INCREASED METABOLIC RATE

While peripheral chemoreceptors and especially central chemoreceptors are responsible for preventing excessive P_aCO_2 changes when CO_2 is inhaled, the receptors or other mechanisms which account for maintenance of P_aCO_2 when metabolism is increased remain unknown (4, 27, 43, 55, 57–59). Stimulation of limb proprioceptors excites respiration during exercise (43). This is unlikely to precisely preserve P_aCO_2 because of the inconsistent relationship between limb motion and metabolic CO_2 production. Other ideas to explain PCO_2 maintenance with increased metabolic rate include an elevation in mixed venous PCO_2, which stimulates possible venous CO_2 receptors, and oscillations in PCO_2 occurring with inspiration and expiration, which produce swings in peripheral and/or central chemoreceptor output that are proportional to metabolic rate (55, 57, 59).

While venous PCO_2 rises as metabolism is increased, venous CO_2 receptors have not been convincingly demonstrated, despite the many studies that have examined this possibility (55). Oscillations in both P_aCO_2 and pH at the VMS have been observed with breathing, although the medullary pH swings are minute. The arterial swings are larger, augmenting with increased metabolic rate (27, 40, 57). Carotid body discharge is also greater as the PCO_2 swings enlarge even when mean levels are unchanged (24). While such a metabolically related signal at the carotid body could underlie a rather tight regulation of P_aCO_2, experiments have been reported in which there is little effect on the regulation of PCO_2 with metabolism changes even in the absence of the carotid bodies (4, 59).

Recent exercise studies also indicate that P_aCO_2 may not be as closely maintained during exercise as previously believed, rising in some species and falling in others (4). This has led to the proposal that when metabolism is raised, a number of stimuli excite respiration, though probably not in a very precise manner (4). These may include slight temperature changes and changes in the chemical composition of the blood (not just changes in CO_2 or H^+). This rather gross excitation is then finely tuned by the peripheral and central chemoreceptors.

This idea is supported by the studies of Prabhakar et al. (59), which showed much greater changes in P_aCO_2 when metabolic rate was increased by the infusion of a mitochondrial uncoupler in peripherally chemodenervated and vagotomized cats if central CO_2 responsivity was also eliminated by coagulation of the VMS. Confirming previous studies, Prabhakar et al. showed that VMS coagulation did not prevent the respiratory stimulation caused by muscle receptor stimulation. This shows that CO_2 receptors are necessary to limit changes in PCO_2 but that signals from exercising limbs can stimulate breathing even in the absence of CO_2 receptors.

In addition to the ability to limit CO_2 changes, central chemoreceptors have an additional stabilizing effect arising from their relatively slow response to respiratory stimuli. This is shown by observations of periodic breathing and cyclic changes in P_aCO_2 when the VMS is cooled in animals with intact peripheral chemoreceptors (12, 37).

In summary, central chemoreceptors play an important role in limiting PCO_2 changes during increases in metabolic rate or CO_2 inhalation. They also have a major stabilizing effect on respiration. They seem to be designed to produce a steady level of respiratory activity rather than to initiate abrupt responses. Because of their intricate coupling to many other neurons in the body (e.g., vascular neurons) they seem to allow stable and coordinated cardiorespiratory responses to stresses that threaten CO_2 or H^+ homeostasis.

REFERENCES

1. Adams, E.M., T. Chonan, N.S. Cherniack, and C. von Euler. Effects on respiratory pattern of focal cooling in the medulla of the dog. *J. Appl. Physiol.* 65:2004-2010, 1988.

2. Ahmad, H.R., and H.H. Loeschcke. Fast bicarbonate-chloride exchange between brain cells and brain extracellular fluid in respiratory acidosis. *Pflügers. Arch.* 395:293-299, 1982.

3. Arita, H., W. Kogo, and K. Ichikawa. Rapid and transient excitation of respiration mediated by central chemoreceptors. *J. Appl. Physiol.* 64:1369-1375, 1988.

4. Bennett, F.M., and W.E. Fordyce. Gain of the ventilatory exercise stimulus: Definition and meaning. *J. Appl. Physiol.* 65:2011-2017, 1988.

5. Berkenbosch, A., J. Heeringa, C.N. Olievier, and E.W. Kruyt. Artificial perfusion of the ponto-medullary region of cats: A method for separation of central and peripheral effects of chemical stimulation of ventilation. *Respir. Physiol.* 37:347-364, 1979.

6. Bruce, E.N., and N.S. Cherniack. Central chemoreceptors. *J. Appl. Physiol.* 62:389-402, 1987.

7. Bruce, E.N., J. Mitra, and N.S. Cherniack. Central and peripheral chemoreceptor inputs to phrenic and hypoglossal motoneurons. *J. Appl. Physiol.* 53:1504-1511, 1982.

8. Budzinska, K., C. von Euler, F.F. Kao, T. Pantaleo, and Y. Yamamoto. Effects of graded focal cold block in rostral areas of medulla. *Acta Physiol. Scand.* 124:329-340, 1985.

9. Burton, R.F. The role of imidazole ionizations in the control of breathing. *Comp. Biochem. Physiol.* 83A:333-336, 1986.

10. Cherniack, N.S. Respiratory dysrhythmias during sleep. *N. Engl. J. Med.* 305:325-330, 1981.

11. Cherniack, N.S. The central nervous system and respiratory muscle coordination. *Chest* 97:52S-57S, 1990.

12. Cherniack, N.S., and G.S. Longobardo. Cheyne-Stokes breathing: An instability in physiological control. *N. Engl. J. Med.* 288:952-957, 1973.

13. Cherniack, N.S., C. von Euler, I. Homma, and F.F. Kao. Graded changes in central chemoreceptor input by local temperature changes on the ventral surface of medulla. *J. Physiol.* (London) 287:191-211, 1979.

14. Ciriello, J., M.M. Caverson, and C. Polosa. Function of the ventrolateral medulla in the control of the circulation. *Brain Res. Rev.* 11:359-391, 1986.

15. Cunningham, D.J.C. The control system regulating breathing in man. *Rev. Biophys.* 6:433-483, 1974.

16. Daristotle, L., and G.E. Bisgard. Central-peripheral chemoreceptor ventilatory interaction in awake goats. *Resp. Physiol.* 76:383-392, 1989.

17. Deal, E.C., Jr, M.A. Haxhiu, M.P. Norcia, E. van Lunteren, and N.S. Cherniack. Cooling the intermediate area of the ventral medullary surface affects tracheal responses to hypoxia. *Resp. Physiol.* 69:335-345, 1987.

18. Dejours, P. Approaches to the study of arterial chemoreceptors. In *Arterial Chemoreceptors,* ed. R.W. Torrance, 41-48. Oxford, U.K.: Blackwell, 1968.

19. Dempsey, J.A., and H.V. Forster. Mediation of ventilatory adaptations. *Physiol. Rev.* 62:262-308, 1982.

20. Dev, N.B., and H.H. Loeschcke. Topography of the respiratory and circulatory responses to acetylcholine and nicotine of the ventral surface of the medulla oblongata. *Pflügers Arch.* 379:19-27, 1979.

21. Edelman, N.H., P.E. Epstein, S. Lahiri, and N.S. Cherniack. Ventilatory responses to transient hypoxia and hypercapnia in man. *Resp. Physiol.* 17:302-314, 1973.

22. Eldridge, F.L., P. Gill-Kumar, and D.E. Millhorn. Input-output relationships of central neural circuits involved in respiration in cats. *J. Physiol.* (London) 311:81-95, 1981.

23. Fitzgerald, R.S., and G.A. Dehyhani. Neural responses of the cat carotid and aortic bodies to hypercapnia and hypoxia. *J. Appl. Physiol.* 52:596-601, 1982.

24. Fitzgerald, R.S., and S. Lahiri. Reflex responses to chemoreceptor stimulation. In *Handbook of Physiology,* Section 3, vol. 2, ed. N.S. Cherniack and J. Widdicombe, 313-362. Bethesda, Md.: American Physiological Society, 1986.

25. Gelfand, R., and C.J. Lambertsen. CO_2-related ventilatory response dynamics: How many components. In *Modelling and the control of breathing,* ed. B.J. Whip and D.M. Wiberg, 301-308. New York: Elsevier, 1983.

26. Granata, A.R., M. Kumada, and D.J. Reis. Sympatho-inhibition by noradrenergic neurons is mediated by neurons in the C1 area of the rostral medulla. *J. Autonom. Nerv. Sys.* 14:387-395, 1988.

27. Grant, B.J.B., R.P. Stidwill, B.A. Cross, and S.J.C. Semple. Ventilatory response to inhaled and infused CO_2: Relationship to the oscillating signal. *Resp. Physiol.* 44:365-380, 1981.

28. Harada, Y., M. Kuno, and Y.Z. Wang. Differential effects of carbon dioxide and pH in central chemoreceptors in the rat respiratory center *in vitro. J. Physiol.* (London) 368:679-693, 1985.

29. Homma, I., A. Isobe, M. Iwase, A. Kanamaru, and M. Sibuya. Two different types of apnea induced by focal cold block of ventral medulla in rabbits. *Neurosci. Lett.* 87:41-45, 1988.

30. Ichikawa, K., S. Kuwana, and H. Arita. ECF pH dynamics with the ventrolateral medulla: A microelectrode study. *J. Appl. Physiol.* 64:193-198, 1989.

31. Jarolimek, W., U. Migeld, and H.D. Lux. Neurosensitivity to pH in slices of the rat ventral medulla oblongata. *Euro. J. Physiol.* 416:247-253, 1990.

32. Lahiri, S., and R.G. Delaney. Stimulus interaction in the responses of carotid body chemoreceptor single afferent fibers. *Resp. Physiol.* 24:249-266, 1975.

33. Lambertsen, C.J., J.G. Semple, M.S. Symth, and R. Gelfand. H^+ and PCO_2 as chemical factors in respiratory and circulatory control. *J. Appl. Physiol.* 16:473-484, 1961.

34. Loeschcke, H.H. Review lecture: Central chemosensitivity and the reaction theory. *J. Physiol.* (London) 332:1-24, 1982.

35. Loeschcke, H.H., J.D. Lattre, M.E. Schlaefke, and C.O. Trouth. Effects on respiration and circulation of electrically stimulating the ventral surface of the medulla oblongata. *Resp. Physiol.* 10:184-197, 1970.

36. Lloyd, B.B., M.G.M. Jukes, and D.J.C. Cunningham. The relation between alveolar oxygen pressure and the respiratory response to carbon dioxide in man. *Quart. J. Exp. Physiol.* 43:214-227, 1958.

37. Longobardo, G.S., N.S. Cherniack, and B. Gothe. Factors affecting respiratory system stability. *Ann. Biomed. Engrg.* 17:377-396, 1989.

38. McAllen, R.M. Location of neurons with cardiovascular and respiratory function at the ventral surface of the cat's medulla. *Neurosci.* 18:43-49, 1986.

39. Millhorn, D.E. and F.L. Eldridge. Role of ventrolateral medulla in regulation of respiratory and cardiovascular systems. *J. Appl. Physiol.* 61:1249-1263, 1986.

40. Millhorn, D.E., F.L. Eldridge, and J.P. Kiley. Oscillation of medullary extracellular fluid pH caused by breathing. *Resp. Physiol.* 55:193-203, 1984.

41. Millhorn, D.E., and J.P. Kiley. Effect of graded cooling of intermediate areas on respiratory response to vagal input. *Resp. Physiol.* 58:51-64, 1984.

42. Millhorn, D.E., F.L. Eldridge, and T.G. Waldrop. Effects of medullary area I(s) cooling on respiratory response to chemoreceptor inputs. *Resp. Physiol.* 49:23-39, 1982.

43. Millhorn, D.E., F.L. Eldridge, and T.G. Waldrop. Effects of medullary area I(s) cooling on respiratory response to muscle stimulation. *Resp. Physiol.* 49:41-48, 1982.

44. Mitchell, R.A., H.H. Loeschcke, J.W. Severinghaus, B.W. Richardson, and W.H. Massion. Regions of respiratory chemosensitivity on the surface of the medulla. *Ann. NY Acad. Sci.* 109:661-681, 1963.

45. Mitra, J., N.R. Prabhakar, M.A. Haxhiu, and N.S. Cherniack. The effects of hypercapnia and cooling of the ventral medullary surface on capsaicin induced respiratory reflexes. *Resp. Physiol.* 60:377-385, 1985.

46. Mitra, J., N.R. Prabhakar, M.A. Haxhiu, and N.S. Cherniack. Comparison of the effects of hypercapnia on phrenic and hypoglossal activity in anesthetized decerebrate and decorticate animals. *Brain Res. Bull.* 17:181-187, 1986.

47. Mitra, J., N.R. Prabhakar, J. Overholt, and N.S. Cherniack. Respiratory and vasomotor effects of excitatory amino acids on ventral medullary surface. *Brain Res. Bull.* 18:681-684, 1987.

48. Nattie, E.E. Diethylpyrocarbonate (an imidazole binding substance) inhibits rostral VLM CO_2 sensitivity. *J. Appl. Physiol.* 61:843-850, 1986.

49. Nattie, E.E. Diethylpyrocarbonate inhibits rostral ventrolateral medullary H^+ sensitivity. *J. Appl. Physiol.* 64:1600-1609, 1988.

50. Nattie, E., and L. Aihua. Fluorescent microbead localization and 4-d AMP microinjection that decrease baseline and CO_2 sensitive phrenic output. *Neurosci. Abstr.* 15:1192, 1989.

51. Nattie, E.E., J.W. Mills, and L.C. Ou. Pirenzepine prevents diethylpyrocarbonate inhibition of cerebral CO_2 sensitivity. *J. Appl. Physiol.* 65:1962-1966, 1988.

52. Neubauer, J.A., D.A. Strumpf, and N.H. Edelman. Regional medullary blood flow during isocapnic hyperpnea in anesthetized cats. *J. Appl. Physiol.* 55:447-452, 1983.

53. Nielsen, M. and H. Smith. Studies on the regulation of respiration in acute hypoxia. *Acta Physiol. Scand.* 24:293-313, 1952.

54. Onimaru, H., and I. Homma. Respiratory rhythm generator neurons in medulla of brainstem-spinal cord preparation from newborn rat. *Brain Res.* 403:380-384, 1987.

55. Orr, J.A., R.M. Fedde, H. Shams, H. Röskenbleck, and P. Scheid. Absence of CO_2-sensitive venous chemoreceptors in the cat. *Resp. Physiol.* 73:211-224, 1988.

56. Overholt, J.L., J. Mitra, E. van Lunteren, N.R. Prabhakar, and N.S. Cherniack. Naloxone enhances the response to hypercapnia of spinal and cranial respiratory nerves. *Resp. Physiol.* 74:299-310, 1988.

57. Phillipson, E.A., G. Bowes, E.R. Townsend, J. Puffin, and T.D. Cooper. Carotid chemoreceptors ventilatory response to changes in venous CO_2 load. *J. Appl. Physiol.* 51:1398-1403, 1981.

58. Poon, C.S. Ventilatory control in hypercapnia and exercise: Optimization hypothesis. *J. Appl. Physiol.* 64:1481-1491, 1986.

59. Prabhakar, N.R., J. Mitra, E.M. Adams, and N.S. Cherniack. Involvement of ventral medullary surface in respiratory responses induced by 2,4-dinitrophenol. *J. Appl. Physiol.* 66:598-605, 1989.

60. Reeves, R.B. An imidazole alphastat hypothesis for vertebrate acid-base regulation: Tissue carbon dioxide content and body temperature in bullfrogs. *Resp. Physiol.* 14:219-236, 1972.

61. Reis, D.J. Central neural control of cerebral circulation and metabolism. In *LERS Monograph Series.* Vol. 2, ed. E.T. Mackenzie, J. Seylaz, and A. Bes, 91-119. New York: Raven Press, 1984.

62. Robbins, P.A. Evidence for interaction between the contributions to ventilation from central and peripheral chemoreceptors in man. *J. Physiol.* 401:503-518, 1988.

63. Ross, C.A., D.A. Ruggiero, D.H. Park, T.H. Jon, A.F. Sved, J. Fernandez-Pardal, J.M. Saavedra, and D.J. Reis. Tonic vasomotor control by the rostral ventral medulla: Effect of electrical or chemical stimulation of the area containing L1 adrenaline neurons on arterial pressure, heart rate, and plasma catecholamines and vasopressin. *J. Neurosci.* 4:274-294, 1984.

64. Schlaefke, M.E. Central chemosensitivity: A respiratory drive. *Rev. Physiol. Biochem. Pharmacol.* 90:171-249, 1981.

65. Schlaefke, M.E., W.R. See, A. Herker-See, and H.H. Loeschcke. Respiratory response to hypoxia and hypercapnia after elimination of central chemosensitivity. *Pflügers Arch.* 381:241-248, 1979.

66. Schnader, J.Y., G. Juan, S. Howell, R. Fitzgerald, and C. Roussos. Arterial CO_2 partial pressure affects diaphragmatic function. *J. Appl. Physiol.* 58:823-829, 1985.

67. Shams, H. Differential effects of CO_2 and H^+ as central stimuli of respiration in the cat. *J. Appl. Physiol.* 58:357-364, 1985.

68. See, W.R., M.E. Schlaefke, and H.H. Loeschcke. Role of chemical afferents in the maintenance of rhythmic respiratory movements. *J. Appl. Physiol.* 54:453-459, 1983.

69. van Lunteren, E., J. Mitra, N.R. Prabhakar, M.A. Haxhiu, and N.S. Cherniack. Ventral medullary surface inputs to cervical sympathetic respiratory oscillations. *Am. J. Physiol.* 252:R1032-R1038, 1987.

70. Woof, J., A. Mega, and W. Goritski. Rostral ventrolateral medulla muscarinic receptor involvement in central ventilatory chemosensitivity. *J. Appl. Physiol.* 66:1462-1470, 1989.

30

Studies on Chemosensory Mechanisms in Rat Carotid Body Using Dissociated Cell Cultures

C.A. Nurse, A. Stea and C. Vollmer

The mammalian carotid body is an arterial chemosensory organ located near the carotid bifurcation and is intimately associated with the pulmonary and cardiovascular systems (1, 4, 11). It is sensitive to natural changes in the chemical composition of arterial blood. Low PO_2 (hypoxia), elevated PCO_2 (hypercapnia), and low pH (acidity) excite the organ and reflexly stimulate respiration. The biophysical and neural mechanisms by which this single sensory organ responds to such varied stimuli have remained elusive for many years (4) and only recently did clues on possible transduction mechanisms emerge (2, 7, 10). Progress in this area was hampered by difficulties in (1) visualizing and obtaining reliable recordings *in situ* from the small (10 μm) parenchymal glomus or Type I cells, and (2) separating effects due secondarily to circulatory changes. These difficulties prompted us 4–5 years ago to adopt an *in vitro* strategy using a previously developed system for culturing rat Type I cells (5). This strategy also favored the application of high-resolution patch-clamp/whole-cell recording techniques (6), which for these small cells were likely to be more reliable than conventional intracellular recording. Our studies have utilized cultures derived from neonatal, juvenile, and adult rat carotid bodies to address various aspects of Type I cell differentiation and function with a view to understanding the mechanisms associated with their putative chemosensory role (12, 13, 14, 15). More recently we have begun studies using co-cultures of Type I cells and sensory (petrosal) neurons (16) with the ultimate goal of producing *in vitro* a functional chemosensory complex capable of afferent signaling.

METHODS

Carotid bodies from 1-day-old to adult rats (Wistar: Charles River, Quebec) were dissected, cleaned, and dissociated into single cells and small-cell clusters by combined enzymatic and mechanical methods as previously described (12). The dispersed cells were plated on a thin layer of collagen and grown in nutrient medium at 37°C in a humidified atmosphere of 95% air: 5% CO_2 for varying periods between 1 day and 12 weeks (12). For neuronal cultures, dissociated sensory neurons from petrosal ganglia, or the complex of the petrosal and jugular ganglia were obtained by similar procedures and cultured in the presence or absence of carotid body cells.

Identification and characterization of Type I cells in these cultures were carried out using glyoxylic acid-induced amine fluorescence (5, 12) and immunoreactivity against tyrosine hydroxylase (TH), neuron specific enolase, NSE (13), and dopamine-β-hydroxylase (DBH). Rabbit antibodies (TH, DBH: Chemicon, CA) were applied to fixed, permeabilized cell cultures at dilutions 1/500 to 1/1000 in phosphate buffer and visualized by immunofluorescence using fluorescein-conjugated goat anti-rabbit IgG (1/50 dilution) as previously described (13). Carbonic anhydrase (CAH) activity was detected using a modification of Hansson's cobalt-precipitation technique (13).

Before recording the cultures were rinsed, bathed with a physiological salt solution, and mounted on the stage of an inverted phase contrast microscope. The bathing solution was grounded via an agar bridge and Ag:AgCl electrode and contained typically (mM) the following: NaCl, 140; $CaCl_2$, 1; $MgCl_2$, 2; glucose, 10; and HEPES, 10, at pH 7.2. Patch pipettes (5–10 MΩ resistance) were fabricated from Corning 7052 glass, fire polished and used to form gigaohm seals with Type I cells or sensory neurons. For conventional whole-cell recording (6), pipettes were filled with a nominal intracellular fluid containing (mM) the following: KCl, 140; $CaCl_2$, 1; EGTA, 11 ($Ca_i \approx 10^{-8}$M); HEPES, 10, at pH 7.2. In experiments where minimal disruption of the cell's cytoplasm was desirable during whole-cell recording, the perforated-patch technique (8) was used, and this required the addition of the pore-forming antibiotic, nystatin, to the pipette. Whole-cell currents were recorded with a WPI S7050A or Dagan 8900 patch-clamp/whole-cell clamp amplifier equipped with a 1 GΩ headstage feedback resistor, digitized with an AXOLAB 1100 computer interface (Axon Instruments, CA), stored on disk in an AT compatible computer, and analyzed using PCLAMP (5.0) software (Axon Instruments).

Cultures were fixed in 1% glutaraldehyde and 2% paraformaldehyde, postfixed in 2% OsO_4 and stained *en bloc* with uranyl acetate. Ultrathin sections were cut through selected Type I cell clusters parallel to the plane of the coverslip, stained with uranyl acetate and Reynold's lead citrate, and examined in a Philips EM 300 electron microscope (12). Diameters of the large dense-cored granules in Type I cells were measured with the aid of a digitizing tablet.

FIG. 30.1 Appearance and properties of cultured Type I cells. (A) Phase micrograph of three isolated Type I cell clusters, (B) type I cell cluster (black arrow) and two adjacent sensory (petrosal) neurons (white arrows), (C) TH-immunoreactivity (fluorescein) of cluster and, (D) isolated Type I cells, (E) DBH-immunoreactivity of cluster, and (F) selective CAH-activity in two clusters. Culture age (days): A (33); B (16); C, D (13); E (19); F (25).

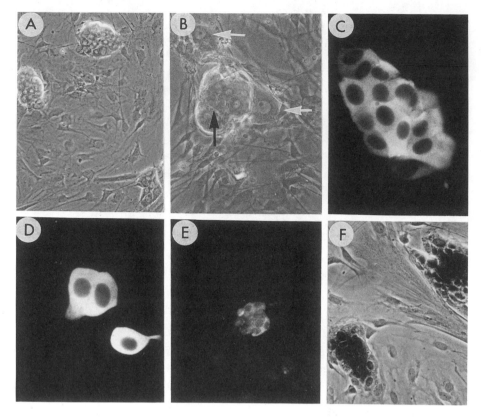

RESULTS

In these cultures glomus or Type I cells survived for many weeks and grew typically in clusters or islands surrounded by various background cells (fig. 30.1A), which in co-culture included sensory neurons (arrows; fig. 30.1B). As expected for Type I cells, most or all of the cells in a cluster were positive for catecholamine fluorescence (5, 12), and immunoreactivity against TH (fig. 30.1C and 13). Single, TH-positive Type I cells (and smaller groups of 2 cells), also survived (fig. 30.1D), but these were more difficult to identify reliably in living, unstained cultures. Many Type I cell clusters were also immunoreactive against DBH, but as *in situ* (3), the staining was variable with some brightly stained cells in the cluster surrounding weakly or negatively stained ones (fig. 30.1E). Most important to the mechanisms of CO_2-chemotransduction, carbonic anhydrase (CAH) was selectively localized in Type I cells (fig. 30.1F) and was predominantly intracellular (13).

Under whole-cell voltage clamp, cultured (rat) Type I cells contained voltage-gated Na^+, K^+ (and Ca^{++}) currents and had large input resistances of circa 2 GΩ (15). Generally the maximum (TTX-sensitive) inward Na^+ currents were small (<50 pA) though action potentials were evoked in a few cells. Voltage-gated outward K^+ currents were elicited with depolarizing steps from −60 mV (fig. 30.2A) and were activated at potentials above −30 mV (fig. 30.2B). More than 75% of this outward current was abolished by 10 mM tetraethylammonium. On exposure to hypoxia (PO_2 in the bathing solution reduced from 160 to 20 torr), the outward K^+ current decreased reversibly by about 15% with both conventional whole cell (n = 20; figs. 30.2A, B) and the perforated-patch recording technique (15). This O_2-sensitive K^+ current was not detected in closely related cells (e.g., cultured small, intensely flourescent [SIF] cells from sympathetic ganglia) and persisted in Type I cells over several weeks in culture (15).

Cultured petrosal neurons also contained voltage-gated Na^+ and K^+ currents (fig. 30.3), though at least two populations were identified based on differential sensitivity of the inward Na^+ currents to TTX (16).

Electron microscopic examination of sections through clusters of cultured Type I cells revealed large cytoplasmic dense-cored vesicles (DCV), membrane densities at contacts between adjacent Type I cells, and other synapse like specializations, including coated vesicles (fig. 30.4A). A typical distribution of DCV in one Type I cell of a cluster cultured for 35 days is shown in figure 30.4B. Occasional profiles of Type I cells contained both large DCV and smaller clear vesicles about 50 nm (fig. 30.4D), not unlike those present in cholinergic terminals. Since acetylcholine (ACh) is a putative neurotransmitter in the carotid body (4) and similar profiles have been seen in other neural crest derivatives with dual adrenergic/cholinergic functions (9), we speculate that in the rat at least some Type I cells, which we have shown contain acetylcholinesterase (12), may release both dopamine and ACh. Experiments using antibodies against choline acetyltransferase (CAT) are now in progress to test this idea further.

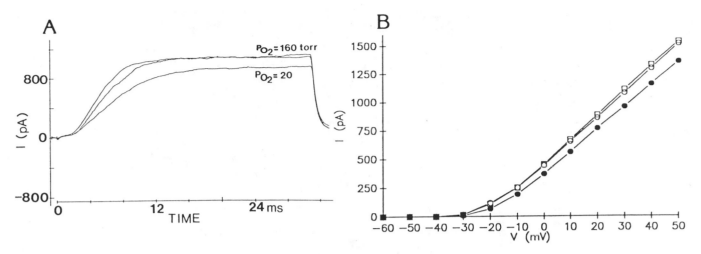

FIG. 30.2 Effect of hypoxia on whole-cell currents in Type I cells. (*A*) Outward K$^+$ currents during voltage step from -60 mV to $+20$ mV, recorded before (160 torr) and after exposure to hypoxia (20 torr). (*B*) Plot of steady-state outward current following various voltage steps from initial potential of -60 mV, before (open circles; 160 torr), after (open squares, 160 torr), and during exposure to hypoxia (closed circles; 20 torr).

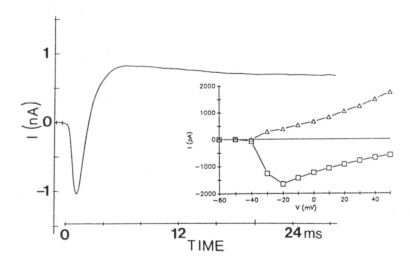

FIG. 30.3 Whole-cell currents in cultured petrosal neuron following a voltage step from -60 mV to $+10$ mV. (*Inset*) I-V plot of peak inward (squares) and outward (triangles) currents versus membrane potential.

Exposure of several cultures to hypoxia (5% O$_2$) for 2–6 hr resulted in the accumulation of numerous vesicle-like structures in Type I cells (fig. 30.4*C*). These profiles (including coated-vesicles) suggest increased membrane recycling and likely reflects stimulation of transmitter release by hypoxia (11).

DISCUSSION

We have developed a successful *in vitro* system that permits the investigation of chemosensory mechanisms in the rat carotid body using combined electrophysiological, morphological, and biochemical techniques. The parenchymal glomus or Type I cells survive in long-term culture and retain several adrenergic properties, including TH and a variable DBH-immunoreactivity and large cytoplasmic DCV. Relevant to the question of O$_2$-chemotransduction we have found that hypoxia causes a 15–20% decrease in outward K$^+$ current in cultured Type I cells of the rat carotid body, supporting recent reports on freshly isolated rabbit Type I cells (7, 10). This effect persisted over several weeks in culture and was not detected in a closely related cell type, namely, SIF cells from sympathetic ganglia (15). Moreover, similar results were obtained with both conventional whole-cell recording (6) and the more recent perforated-patch technique (8), which minimizes disruption of the cell's cytoplasm. The closing of a special class of K$^+$ channels by hypoxia could result in prolonged depolarization followed by calcium entry through voltage—gated channels and release of an excitatory neurotransmitter from Type I cells onto the chemosensory afferent terminals (10). However, since this current appears to be activated at potentials above -20 mV, a preceding depolarization is necessary for this mechanism to be operative, assuming a resting potential of about -50 mV. López-López et al. (10) suggest that the K$^+$ current modulated by PO$_2$ regulates firing frequency and

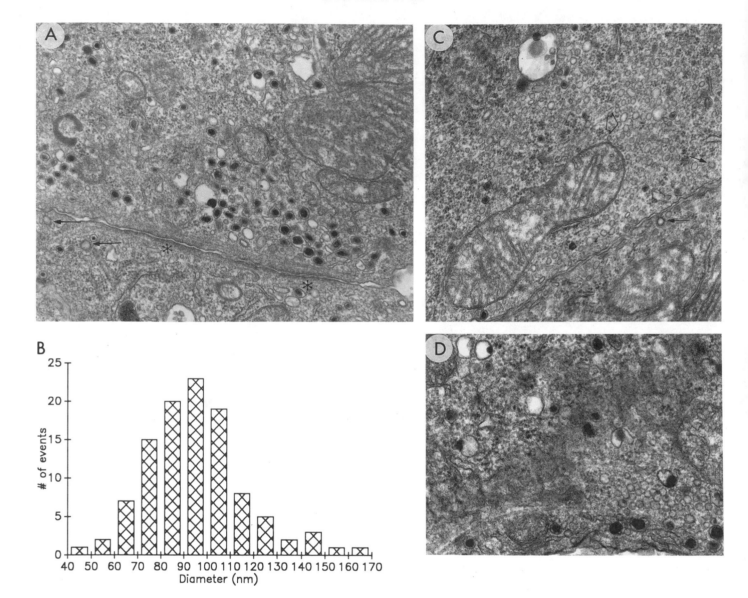

FIG. 30.4 Electron micrographs of cultured Type I cells. (*A*) Junction between two adjacent Type I cells; note dense-cored vesicles (DCV), membrane densities (*), and coated vesicles (arrows). (*B*) Distribution of DCV in one Type I cell cultured for 35 days; mean diameter ± S.D. = 95.1 ± 20.5 nm, n = 107. (*C*) Type I cells following exposure to hypoxia (5% O_2 for 2 hr); note numerous vesicle-like structures (arrowhead) and coated vesicles (arrows). (*D*) Profile of Type I cell containing both DCV and small clear vesicles (lower right).

therefore transmitter release from rabbit Type I cells. We question the generality of this mechanism since in rat Type I cells the inward current was usually small and spiking may well be infrequent in these cells. An alternative mechanism proposed is that the rise in intracellular calcium preceding transmitter release during hypoxia occurs via calcium release from intracellular stores (2). It is of interest to determine which of these potential mechanisms is the primary event during O_2-chemotransduction.

Though we have not yet demonstrated a physiological role in the intact Type I cell for the HCO_3^--permeable anion channels we first described in inside-out patches (14), our data also point to a central role of Type I cells in CO_2-chemotransduction. The demonstration that carbonic anhydrase activity is mainly intracellular and selectively localized to Type I cells (13) favors the hypothesis that intracellular acidification may precede a rise in Ca_i and transmitter release following a CO_2 stimulus.

ACKNOWLEDGMENTS

This work was supported by grants from the Heart and Stroke Foundation of Ontario and the NIH # 1 R01 HL 43412.

REFERENCES

1. Biscoe, T.J. Carotid body: Structure and function. *Physiol. Rev.* 51:437-491, 1971.

2. Biscoe, T.J., and M.R. Duchen. Electrophysiological responses of dissociated Type I cells of the rabbit carotid body to cyanide. *J. Physiol.* 413:447-468, 1989.

3. Chen, I.-L., J.T. Hansen, and R.D. Yates. Dopamine-β-hydroxylase-like immunoreactivity in the cat and rat carotid body: A light and electron microscopic study. *J. Neurocytol.* 14:131-144, 1985.

4. Eyzaguirre, C., and P. Zapata. Perspectives in carotid body research. *J. Appl. Physiol.* 57:931-957, 1984.

5. Fishman, M.C., and A.E. Schaffner. Carotid body cell culture and selective growth of glomus cells. *Am. J. Physiol.* 246:C106-C113, 1984.

6. Hamill, O.P., A. Marty, E. Neher, B. Sackmann, and E.J. Sigworth. Improved patch-clamp techniques for high-resolution current recordings from cells and cell-free membrane patches. *Pflügers Arch.* 391:85-100, 1981.

7. Hescheler, J., M.A. Delpiano, H. Acker, and F. Pietruschka. Ionic currents in Type I cells of the rabbit carotid body measured by voltage-clamp experiments and the effects of hypoxia. *Brain Res.* 486:79-88, 1989.

8. Horn, R., and A. Marty. Muscarinic activation of ionic currents measured by a new whole-cell recording method. *J. Gen. Physiol.* 92:145-159, 1988.

9. Landis, S.C. Rat sympathetic neurons and cardiac myocytes developing in microcultures: Correlation of the fine structure of endings with neurotransmitter function in single neurons. *Proc. Natl. Acad. Sci.* USA 73:4220-4224, 1976.

10. López-López, J., C. Gonzalez, J. Urena, and J. López-Barneo. Low PO$_2$ selectively inhibits K channel activity in chemoreceptor cells of the mammalian carotid body. *J. Gen. Physiol.* 93:1001-1015, 1989.

11. McDonald, D.M. Peripheral chemoreceptors. In *Regulation of Breathing*. Part 1, ed. T. F. Hornbein, 105-319. New York: Marcel Dekker, Inc., 1981.

12. Nurse, C.A. Localization of acetylcholinesterase in dissociated cell cultures of the carotid body of the rat. *Cell Tiss. Res.* 250:21-27, 1987.

13. Nurse, C.A. Carbonic anhydrase and neuronal enzymes in cultured glomus cells of the carotid body of the rat. *Cell Tiss. Res.* 261:65-71, 1990.

14. Stea, A., and C.A. Nurse. Chloride channels in cultured glomus cells of the rat carotid body. *Am. J. Physiol.* 257:C174-C181, 1989.

15. Stea, A., and C.A Nurse. Chemotransduction mechanisms determined by two methods of whole-cell recording. *Biophys. J. Abstr.* 57:312a, 1990.

16. Stea, A., and C.A. Nurse. Physiological studies on cultured rat sensory neurons from the petrosal and jugular ganglia. *Soc. Neurosci. Abstr.* 16:868, 1990.

31

Cellular Mechanisms of Central Chemosensitivity

Judith A. Neubauer

The majority of central nervous system neurons respond to extracellular acidosis with membrane hyperpolarization and a reduction in excitability (14, 19, 21). Classical respiratory physiology has shown, however, that there exists a unique subset of neurons which are excited by hypercapnia and which participate in exciting the central respiratory neurons. These chemosensitive cells are located bilaterally in superficial regions of the ventrolateral medulla. Relatively little is understood regarding the mechanisms involved in the CO_2 transduction process. *In vivo* studies indicate that CO_2 is a much better stimulus of chemosensitive cells than fixed acid (9, 30, 33) suggesting that signal transduction occurs at an intracellular site; that carbonic anhydrase is important in determining the dynamics of the response to CO_2 (13, 20); and that acid chemosensitivity involves some aspect of cholinergic synaptic transmission which may include an acid sensitivity of the muscarinic receptor (3, 8, 25). The exact nature of chemosensitivity, however, has not been elucidated.

Putative chemosensory areas have no anatomical features which might be indicative of chemosensitivity, with the possible exception of a thicker marginal glial layer and marked vascularity (6, 34). Furthermore, electrophysiological recordings from neurons in these areas show that only 25% are chemosensitive and these are dispersed among other nonchemosensitive neurons (27). This lack of anatomical and functional separation has made it difficult to determine the exact nature of chemosensitivity *in vivo*. Thus, the major objective of our work has been to develop *in vitro* preparations of the chemosensitive regions of the medulla that retain the function of chemosensitivity and to use these to evaluate the unique cellular characteristics which provide these neurons with a CO_2 excitability. This work has established that spontaneously active neurons in both organotypic and dissociated cell cultures retain the function of chemosensitivity (5, 26), that these cells only respond to changes in pH induced with CO_2, that CO_2-chemosensitive neurons are present in regions other than the ventral medulla, and that a small population of neurons in dissociated cultures from chemosensitive regions of the medulla can be immunocytochemically stained for carbonic anhydrase II (31).

CHEMOSENSITIVITY OF NEURONS *IN VITRO*

Organotypic cultures were prepared from medullary explants of neonatal rats using the flying coverslip–roller tube method (1). After 2–3 weeks extracellular recordings were made on spontaneously active neurons and their response to CO_2 or HCO_3^- induced changes in extracellular pH were determined. Ventral medullary neurons exhibited a regular baseline firing frequency of 4 ± 0.8 Hz. In contrast, dorsal medullary neurons showed two different patterns of spontaneous activity; half fired regularly (7.2 ± 1.4 Hz) while half fired with a bursting pattern (burst duration 0.8 ± 0.14 min, cycle time 1.74 ± 0.43 min). Decreasing pH with CO_2 caused an increase in the activity of 30% of ventral medullary neurons (fig. 31.1A) and dorsal medullary neurons (fig. 31.1B) with a mean response of 7.5 Hz/$-$pH unit. In contrast, varying pH by changing HCO_3^- had no effect on the firing frequency of neurons in either dorsal or ventral medullary cultures (fig. 31.1C). Thus, we found that neurons in organotypic cultures retain the function of chemosensitivity, that chemosensitive neurons are present in both ventral and dorsal medulla, and that these cells only respond to changes in pH induced with CO_2.

Dissociated cell cultures were prepared by gentle enzymatic and mechanical treatment of tissue dissected from the medulla and hypothalamus of neonatal rats. Extracellular recordings using the loose-cell patch-recording technique (12) revealed neurons with demonstrable spontaneous activity beginning with one day *in vitro* with a mean firing frequency of 2 Hz (range from <1 to 4 Hz). The percentage of neurons displaying spontaneous activity increased with time in culture from 15% at one week *in vitro* to 60% by 6 weeks. Since ion channels are present 2–3 days *in vitro* (16), the increase in activity with time in culture is likely due to neurite outgrowth and synaptic network formation resulting in excitation of quiescent cells. Preliminary studies on medullary neurons 1–4 weeks *in vitro* showed that dissociated neurons retain the sensory property of chemosensitivity. Similar to explant cultures, approximately 25% of the spontaneously active medullary neurons increased their firing rate when pH was decreased by varying PCO_2 (fig. 31.2) while 50% of the medullary neurons decreased their firing rate when pH was decreased. The function of CO_2 excitability was also found among neurons cultured from the hypothalamus (fig. 31.3), with 25% of hypothalamic neurons exhibiting CO_2 chemosensitivity. Thus, CO_2 chemosensitivity of neurons is functionally retained in isolated neurons in culture.

CO_2 chemosensitivity of medullary neurons *in vitro* has also been shown in tissue-slice preparations of the medulla (7, 10). In addition, this chemosensitivity appears to be an intrinsic property of neurons since CO_2 continues to excite

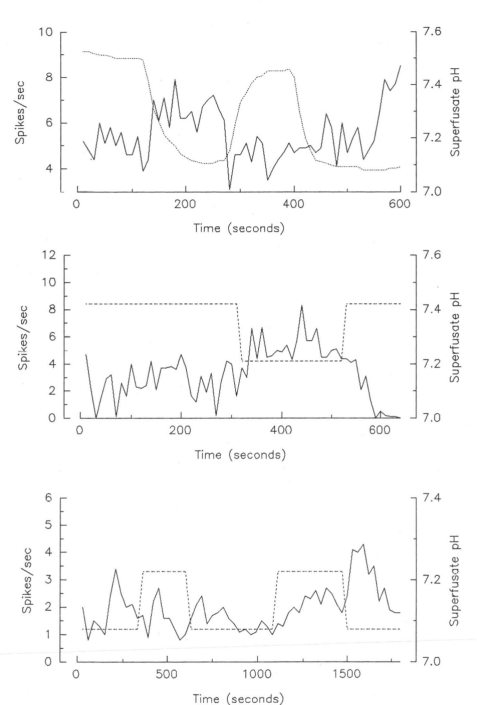

FIG. 31.1 Responses of spontaneously active medullary neurons in organotypic cultures to changes in superfusate pH. Traces illustrate examples of a ventral medullary neuron (A) and a dorsal medullary neuron (B) excited by hypercapnic acidosis and a neuron (C) whose spontaneous activity was unaffected by changing pH with HCO_3^-. Note that only hypercapnic acidosis was effective in doubling firing frequency.

neurons even after synaptic blockade (7). Furthermore, neuronal chemosensitivity in tissue slices is also not restricted to the ventral medulla, with an equal number of dorsal medullary neurons exhibiting chemosensitivity as well. Thus, it appears as though intrinsic neuronal CO_2 excitability may well be a distributed function within the medulla as well as other brain regions. However, whether all or just a subpopulation of these CO_2-sensitive neurons are part of the respiratory neuronal circuitry remains to be determined. Certainly, the bulk of *in vivo* studies employing conventional approaches utilizing techniques of cooling,

coagulation, and neurotoxic chemicals have convincingly demonstrated a ventrolateral medullary site for chemosensitivity (4, 24, 29). Thus, the physiological importance of nonventral medullary chemosensitive neurons is yet to be determined.

IMMUNOCYTOCHEMICAL LOCALIZATION OF CARBONIC ANHYDRASE

While carbonic anhydrase (CA-II isozyme form) is present in high concentrations in oligodendrocytes, it has generally

FIG. 31.2 Response of a spontaneously active ventral medullary neuron in dissociated cell culture. This neuron was excited by hypercapnic acidosis. The solid line depicts the changes in firing frequency (spikes/sec), and the dashed line indicates when the superfusate pH was changed between 7.0 and 7.4. Note that the firing frequency was greatest when the superfusate pH was more acidic.

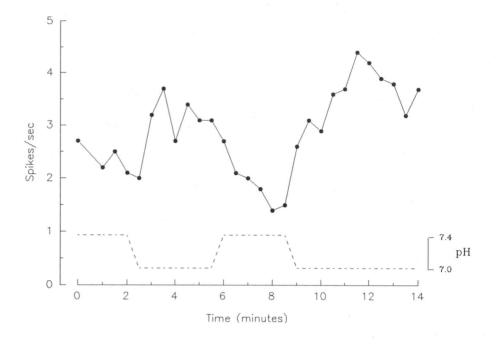

FIG. 31.3 Response of a spontaneously active hypothalamic neuron in dissociated cell culture which was excited by hypercapnic acidosis. The solid line depicts the changes in firing frequency (spikes/sec) and the dashed line indicates when the superfusate pH was changed from 7.2 to 7.6. Note that the firing frequency was greatest when the superfusate pH was more acidic.

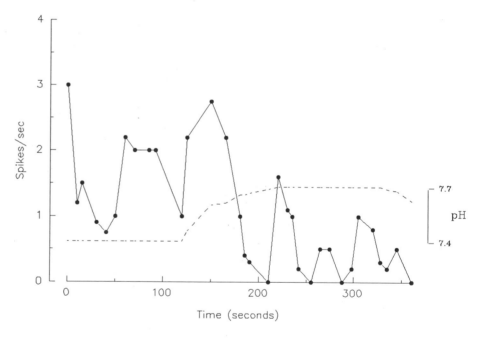

been thought to be absent in neurons. Several recent reports, however, suggest its presence in neurons in retinal amacrine cells (18), in chicken optic tectum (17), in peripheral sensory ganglia, and in the central nervous system (CNS) (15, 28, 35). To test whether sensory neurons involved with central chemosensitivity contain carbonic anhydrase (CA), we used immunocytochemistry to identify CA-II in neurons in dissociated cultures of the ventral medulla chemosensitive regions. To assess whether this was specific to the ventral medulla, cultures of dorsal medulla, pre-motor cortex, and hypothalamus were also prepared. After 5–7 days, cultures were fixed and permeabilized and incubated with a primary antiserum directed against CA-II.

Specific binding of CA-II was visualized using the avidin-biotin peroxidase technique with a diaminobenzidine (DAB) reaction product.

We found that 25% of neurons cultured from the ventral medulla were immunoreactive (a number consistent with the number of neurons from this region suspected as having chemosensitive function). Neuronal CA-II immunoreactivity, however, was not restricted to the ventral medulla. CA-II-containing neurons were also found in the dorsal medulla and the cortex, although the intensity of staining in the latter was significantly weaker. In the hypothalamus 58% of the neurons were positive for CA-II, which may be consistent with its multiple sensory functions including CO_2 sensitivity (32). The presence of CA in sub-populations of neurons in CNS regions other than the ventral medulla suggests that this enzyme may be important in maintaining pH gradients in neurons distributed throughout the CNS and again suggests that CO_2 sensitivity may be a distributed function. The specific functional response of these neurons, however, is probably dependent upon the neural connections of these chemosensitive cells.

Although we have found that about 25% of neurons in ventral medullary cultures contain CA, whether these CA-containing neurons are the chemosensitive neurons is yet to be determined. If one assumes that the proximal signal for chemosensitivity is intracellular pH, then one can hypothesize that such changes could be dynamically controlled by CA since this enzyme would greatly accelerate the pH change and hence the signal transduction process. This hypothesis is tenable for several reasons: first, this function of CA has already been demonstrated in the peripheral chemoreceptor response to CO_2 (2); second, CA inhibitors have been shown to affect the respiratory response to CO_2 (13, 20). For example, we have shown that inhibition of CA with acetazolamide significantly increases the time constant of the transfer function between the phrenic neurogram and ventral medullary extracellular fluid pH responses to CO_2 forcing (20). Hanson et al. (13) found that the respiratory response to vertebral artery injections of CO_2-saturated saline was affected by acetazolamide (but not by benzolamide), suggesting that the location of the CA modulation is beyond the blood-brain barrier. Furthermore, application of these inhibitors directly to the ventral medulla localized the physiologically important compartment to the intracellular medium (13). Finally, since electrophysiological studies both *in vivo* (27) and *in vitro* (5, 26) have demonstrated that about 25% of the neurons in the ventrolateral medullary regions are chemosensitive, this observation is quantitatively consistent with a chemosensitive function for the CA-II immunoreactive neurons.

CHOLINERGIC MECHANISMS

There is substantial experimental support for the involvement of a cholinergic mechanism in acid chemosensitivity. Several groups have shown that atropine depresses the respiratory response to CO_2 (3, 8, 25). In medullary slices, neurons responsive to acid have been shown to also be excited by acetylcholine (Ach), while serotonin and norepinephrine had opposite effects (11). Atropine, hexamethonium, and mecamylamine all depressed acid stimulation of these neurons, while eserine, a cholinesterase inhibitor, increased neuronal activity. This finding suggests that intact cholinergic transmission is necessary for acid excitation. The exact mechanism for this cholinergic response to acid is unclear and may involve the usual factors which control neuronal response of Ach, including increased release of Ach, decreased activity of acetylcholinesterase

(AchE), or an increased postsynaptic sensitivity to Ach. In addition, recent work (23, 25) suggests that the cholinergic involvement is muscarinic and, further, that it may be specific for the M1 receptor. The muscarinic receptor has an intracellular domain that is rich in histidine residues. These residues contain a large number of imidazole groups sensitive to pH changes in the physiological range. Changes in pH can induce alterations in the structure and function of the histidine-containing protein. Based on this pH effect, Nattie (25) has suggested that intracellular acidosis may substantially affect the conformation of the muscarinic receptor in a manner which may increase its sensitivity to Ach. Consistent with this proposal is the observation that diethyl pyrocarbonate (DEPC), an imidazole binding substance, when applied to the ventral medullary surface, inhibits the respiratory response to CO_2 (22). In addition, the M1 receptor blocker pirenzepine prevents the inhibition of the respiratory response to CO_2 by DEPC (23). Although cholinergic transmission appears to be integrally involved in chemosensitivity, it still remains to be resolved whether chemosensitivity is an intrinsic response of cholinergic neurons, or whether it is a phenomenon of cholinergic synaptic transmission due to an acid sensitivity of the muscarinic receptor or some other aspect of the cholinergic synapse.

REFERENCES

1. Baldino, F., Jr. and H.M. Geller. Electrophysiological analysis of neuronal thermosensitivity in rat preoptic and hypothalamic tissue cultures. *J. Physiol.* (London) 327:173-184, 1982.

2. Black, A.M.S., D.I. McCloskey, and R.W. Torrance. The response of carotid body chemoreceptors in the cat to sudden changes of hypercapnic and hypoxic stimuli. *Resp. Physiol.* 13:36-49, 1971.

3. Burton, M.D., and H. Kazemi. Effect of atropine on acetylcholine and acidic CSF augmentation of ventilation. *FASEB J.* 2:A512, 1988.

4. Cherniack, N.S., C. von Euler, I. Homma, and F.F. Kao. Graded changes in central chemoreceptor input by local temperature changes on the ventral surface of medulla. *J. Physiol.* (London) 287:191-211, 1979.

5. Chou, W., J.A. Neubauer, H.M. Geller, and N.H. Edelman. Chemosensitivity of medullary and hypothalamic neurons in cell culture. *Soc. Neurosci. Abstr.*, 16:1061, 1990.

6. Cragg, P., L. Patterson, and M.J. Purves. The pH of brain extracellular fluid in the cat. *J. Physiol.* (London) 272:137-166, 1977.

7. Dean, J.B., D.A. Bayliss, J.T. Erickson, W.L. Lawing, and D.E. Millhorn. Depolarization and stimulation of neurons in nucleus tractus solitarii by carbon dioxide does not require chemical synaptic input. *Neuroscience* 36:207-216, 1990.

8. Dev, N.B., and H.H. Loeschcke. A cholinergic mechanism involved in the respiratory chemosensitivity of the medulla oblongata in the cat. *Pflügers Arch.* 379:29-36, 1979.

9. Eldridge, F.L., J.P. Kiley, and D.E. Millhorn. Respiratory responses to medullary hydrogen ion in cats: Different effects of respiratory and metabolic acidosis. *J. Physiol.* (London) 358:258-297, 1985.

10. Fukuda, Y. Difference between actions of high PCO_2 and low HCO_3 on neurons in the rat medullary chemosensitive areas *in vitro*. *Pflügers Arch.* 398:324-330, 1983.

11. Fukuda, Y., and H.H. Loeschcke. A cholinergic mechanism involved in the neuronal excitation by H+ in the respiratory chemosensitive structures of the ventral medulla oblongata of rats *in vitro*. *Pflügers Arch.* 379:125-135, 1979.

12. Hamill, O.P., A. Marty, E. Neher, B. Sakmann, and F.J. Sigworth. Improved patch-clamp techniques for high-resolution current recordings from cells and cell-free membrane patches. *Pflügers Arch.* 391:85-100, 1981.

13. Hanson, M.A., P.C.G. Nye, and R.W. Torrance. The location of carbonic anhydrase in relation to the blood-brain barrier at the medullary chemoreceptors of the cat. *J. Physiol.* 320:113-125, 1981.

14. Jodkowski, J.S., and J. Lipski. Decreased excitability of respiratory motoneurons during hypercapnia in the acute spinal cat. *Brain Res.* 386:296-304, 1986.

15. Kazimierczak, J., E.W. Sommer, E. Philippe, and B. Droz. Carbonic anhydrase activity in primary sensory neurons. I. Requirements for the cytochemical localization in the dorsal root ganglion of chicken and mouse by light and electron microscopy. *Cell Tiss. Res.* 245:487-495, 1986.

16. Legendre, P., J.L. Brigant, and J.D. Vincent. Développement de l'activite electrique des cellules hypothalamiques en culture. *Ann. Endocrinal.* (Paris) 48:356-362, 1987.

17. Linser, P.J. Multiple marker analysis in the avian optic tectum reveals three classes of neuroglia and carbonic anhydrase-containing neurons. *J. Neurosci.* 5:2388-2396, 1985.

18. Linser, P.J., M. Sorrentino, and A.A. Moscona. Cellular compartmentalization of carbonic anhydrase-c and glutamine synthetase in developing and mature mouse neuronal retina. *Dev. Brain Res.* 13:65-71, 1984.

19. Marshall, K.C., and I. Engberg. The effects of hydrogen ion on spinal neurons. *Can. J. Physiol. Pharmacol.* 58:650-655, 1980.

20. Mishra, J., J.A. Neubauer, J.K.-J. Li, and N.H. Edelman. Relationship of the dynamic characteristics of ventral medullary (V_m) pH and respiratory center output during CO_2 forcing. *Fed. Proc.* 44:1583, 1985.

21. Mitchell, R.A., and D.A. Herbert. The effect of carbon dioxide on the membrane potential of medullary respiratory neurons. *Brain Res.* 75:345-349, 1974.

22. Nattie, E.E. Diethyl pyrocarbonate (an imidazole binding substance) inhibits rostral VLM CO_2 sensitivity. *J. Appl. Physiol.* 61:843-850, 1986.

23. Nattie, E.E., J.W. Mills, and L.C. Ou. Pirenzepine prevents diethyl pyrocarbonate inhibition of central CO_2 sensitivity. *J. Appl. Physiol.* 65:1962-1966, 1988.

24. Nattie, E.E., J.W. Mills, L.C. Ou, and W.M. St. John. Kainic acid on the rostral ventrolateral medulla inhibits phrenic output and CO_2 sensitivity. *J. Appl. Physiol.* 65:1525-1534, 1988.

25. Nattie, E.E., J. Wood, A. Mega, and W. Goritski. Rostral ventrolateral medulla muscarinic receptor involvement in central ventilatory chemosensitivity. *J. Appl. Physiol.* 66:1462-1470, 1989.

26. Neubauer, J.A., W. Chou, S.F. Gonsalves, A.M. Martin, H.M. Geller, and N.H. Edelman. Chemosensitivity of medullary neurons in tissue explant cultures. *FASEB J.* 2(5):A1295, 1988.

27. Pokorski, M. Neurophysiological studies on central chemosensor in medullary ventrolateral areas. *Am. J. Physiol.* 230:1288-1295, 1976.

28. Riley, D.A., S. Ellis, and J.L.W. Bain. Ultrastructural cytochemical localization of carbonic anhydrase activity in rat peripheral sensory and motor nerves, dorsal root ganglia and dorsal column nuclei. *Neuroscience* 13:189-206, 1984.

29. Schlaefke, M.E., W.R. See, A. Herker-See, and H.H. Loeschcke. Respiratory response to hypoxia and hypercapnia after elimination of central chemosensitivity. *Pflügers Arch.* 381:241-248, 1979.

30. Shams, H. Differential effects of CO_2 and H^+ as central stimuli of respiration in the cat. *J. Appl. Physiol.* 58:357-364, 1985.

31. Sterbenz, G.C., J.A. Neubauer, H.M. Geller, and N.H. Edelman. Carbonic anhydrase immunocytochemically localized in chemosensitive regions of the medulla. *FASEB J.* 2:1295, 1988.

32. Tamaki, Y., T. Nakayama, and K. Matsumura. Effects of carbon dioxide inhalation on preoptic thermosensitive neurons. *Pflügers Arch.* 407:8-13, 1986.

33. Teppema, L.J., P.W.J.A. Barts, H.T. Folgering, and J.A.M. Evers. Effects of respiratory and (isocapnic) metabolic arterial acid-base disturbances on medullary extracellular fluid pH and ventilation in cats. *Resp. Physiol.* 53:379-395, 1983.

34. Trouth, C.O., M. Odek-Ogunde, and J.A. Holloway. Morphological observations on superficial medullary CO_2–chemosensitive areas. *Brain Res.* 246:35-45, 1982.

35. Wong, V., C.P. Barrett, E.J. Donati, L.F. Eng, and L. Guth. Carbonic anhydrase activity in first-order sensory neurons of the rat. *J. Histochem. Cytochem.* 31:293-300, 1983.

Part VII

Development of Respiratory Control

32

An Overview

William E. Cameron

This introduction provides an overview of some issues regarding the development of the neural control of respiration in mammals. This chapter will divide the discussion of the development of respiratory control into three parts: (1) the maturation of sensory inputs that influence respiration, (2) the evolution of the central circuits that generate the breath and (3) the alterations of the efferent outputs that transmit this rhythm to the respiratory muscles. More specifically, the changes occurring in the sensory transduction of some respiratory afferents, the synaptic efficacy of their central projections, and the changes in the properties of central neurons or circuits that determine the timing and intensity of the descending respiratory drive will be discussed. Finally, recent data will be reviewed concerning the alterations in the properties of the respiratory motoneurons that occur during postnatal development.

A variety of animal models has been used to study the development of respiratory control. The maturational stage of the nervous system at birth varies dramatically depending on the species selected for study. Figure 32.1 presents a time line that approximates the relative maturity of different mammals at birth. According to this scheme, the least mature at birth is the opossum and the most mature is the primate. If the frame of reference is the human infant, then the opossum is the animal of choice for studying the processes occurring early in gestation, while the neonatal rat is better suited for studies of the latter stages of human gestation. In contrast, the central nervous systems of the piglet, the rabbit pup, and the kitten are more mature at birth than that of the rat and therefore, provide better models for studying postnatal development.

SENSORY COMPONENT

In general, the development of respiratory afferents can be characterized by an increase in the diameter and myelination of the sensory axon, a change in the sensitivity of the peripheral receptors, and a resetting of the gain in some sensory reflexes. The time course of myelination of the vagus nerve has been described in the opossum (25), the rabbit (13), and the cat (29). Based on the number of myelinated fibers in the vagus nerve, it takes the opossum until postnatal day 50 (P50) to achieve the same proportions of myelinated fibers as are found in the rabbit and the cat at birth (22). This difference between species at birth has been designated in figure 32.1 by a broken vertical line

aligning birth in the cat/rabbit with P50 in the opossum. The role that vagal feedback can play in the newborn opossum with such slowly conducting afferents is discussed in detail in the paper by J. Farber (this volume). The state of myelination of the vagus nerve does not reduce, *a priori*, the efficacy of vagal reflexes in some newborn mammals. Even though there are fewer than one-fifth of the adult number of myelinated fibers in the kitten at birth, the gain of the Breuer-Hering inflation reflex in kittens is much more pronounced than in adults (30).

The functional role of myelination has also been examined in the superior laryngeal (31), the phrenic, and the intercostal nerves (29) of postnatal kittens. Stimulation of the superior laryngeal nerve in 5-day-old kitten produced apnea during a period when fewer than half the adult number of myelinated fibers were present. Such stimulation failed, however, to produce a swallowing reflex until later in development (28–30 days). The process of myelination found in the vagus, phrenic, and intercostal nerves of the cat demonstrate a cephalo-caudal progression to the maturation of the respiratory peripheral nerves.

Slowly adapting pulmonary stretch receptors (SARs) of the trachea and lower airways are believed to mediate the Breuer-Hering inflation reflex (20). These receptors have been shown to increase their firing rate and/or sensitivity with postnatal age in the opossum (19), the cat (36), and the dog (21). In dogs (23), similar changes in receptor sensitivity have been noted for positive and negative pressure afferents in the upper airways that travel in the superior laryngeal nerve (SLN). Alterations in the sensitivity of SARs are also indicated by the number of afferents active at functional residual capacity (FRC). There are few SARs active at FRC in the newborn rabbit (36), cat (30, 36), and dog, while over 60% of SARs are active in the adult dog (21). One strategy available to the newborn to increase SAR activity is to maintain an elevated FRC and/or increase the tone of airway smooth muscle which surrounds the receptors (16, 18). The number of spontaneously active rapidly adapting receptors (RARs; irritant receptors) was found to be less in the newborn than in the adult for dogs (21) and for opossums (19). The change in RAR sensitivity with age may account for the increase in reflex response to inhaled dust noted during the first week of postnatal life in the rabbit pup (42).

Changes in receptor sensitivity are not always associated with increases in reflex responses and vice versa, changes

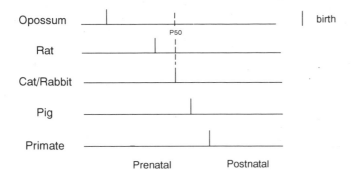

FIG. 32.1 Time line comparing the relative maturity of the various mammals used in studies of neural control of respiration. Birth in the kitten has been aligned with postnatal day 50 (P50) in the opossum, based on Krous et al. (25) and P10 in the rat with the third trimester in the primate, based on Miller and Kalia (32).

in reflex responses are not always paralleled by changes in receptor sensitivity. On the one hand, there is a decrease in the strength of the Breuer-Hering reflex with postnatal age in rats (38), cats (15), and humans (3) during a period when SARs are increasing their sensitivity (see above). On the other hand, the subclass of laryngeal receptors that respond to water and ionic solutions, which exhibit similar receptor behavior in both adult and newborn (1), mediate a markedly larger reflex in newborns than in adults for a variety of animals including the cat (28), the dog (5), and the pig (14, 27). The strength of a respiratory afferent input can be quantified by measuring the amplitude and time course of the postsynaptic potentials produced by its central terminations. Intracellular recording in the ventral respiratory group of piglets (Lawson et al., this volume) has been used to study the postsynaptic potentials evoked by stimulation of the SLN.

For the peripheral chemoreceptor reflex, the increase in receptor sensitivity is paralleled by an increased efficacy of the reflex. In response to moderate hypoxia, the human neonate exhibits a biphasic response in which minute ventilation is initially elevated, followed by return of ventilation to base-line levels or lower (34, 35). The neonate's inability to sustain ventilation in response to moderate hypoxia is believed to be a function of immaturity of the carotid chemoreceptors (33) and/or their central synaptic terminals. The mechanisms of the change in both peripheral transduction and central synaptic efficacy of peripheral chemoreceptors are discussed by Lagercrantz et al. (this volume). Like SAR and RAR afferents, peripheral carotid chemoreceptors have also been demonstrated in sheep to have a lower sensitivity to PO_2 early in development than at more mature stages (2, 24).

It is interesting that in at least one instance the decrease in gain of one reflex is matched by an increase in the gain of another subserving a similar function. It has been noted in kittens (36) and human infants (4) that there is an increase in the response to an added respiratory load (medi-

ated via intercostal muscle spindle receptors) at a time when the strength of the Breuer-Hering inflation reflex is decreasing. The increase in response to added load is believed to be due to the maturation of the gamma innervation of the intercostal muscle spindles (36).

CENTRAL COMPONENT

The central processing of input from respiratory afferents may depend upon the state of the central neurons involved in the generation of respiration. The dependence of the responses to central hypoxia on the level of central respiratory drive in piglets is discussed by England (this volume). Unlike the response to acute hypoxia, the response to chronic hypoxia is not solely manifest as an alteration in neural output to the respiratory muscles but can be expressed as a change in the overall metabolism of the animal. The long-term adaptation to hypoxia in newborn rats is described by Mortola et al. (this volume).

In early development, respiratory bulbospinal neurons show much less activity than that found in the adult. In suckling opossums, the inspiratory bulbospinal neurons fire approximately two spikes per breath (17) and most expiratory bulbospinal neurons become active only under conditions of positive pressure breathing (18). For both populations the firing frequency of these medullary neurons increased with age. A similar increase in discharge frequency has been noted for the medullary neurons in the dorsal respiratory group of anesthetized or decerebrate kittens (37). With so few spikes, it is difficult to imagine that sensory feedback would play a role in shaping motor output at this age (see Farber, this volume).

The impact that sensory feedback has on shaping the descending drive to respiratory motor pools is also evident in work on fetal lambs (12). These authors concluded that the rhythm module of the central pattern generator matured at an earlier stage than the form module in fetal lambs, as evidenced by the shape of the phrenic neurogram. The decrementing pattern of the diaphragmatic EMG found at midgestation in the lamb is converted to an augmenting adult pattern by late gestation. It is interesting to note the similarity in the pattern of the mid-gestation lamb with that found in the phrenic nerve of the *in vitro* neonatal rat brainstem-spinal cord preparation (39, 41). It was beautifully demonstrated by Smith et al. (this volume) that an augmenting pattern in the phrenic nerve (C4 rootlet) of the *in vivo* neonatal rat was converted to a decrementing pattern when both vagi were sectioned. This observation underscores the importance of vagal feedback in shaping the motor output of the newborn rat.

A three-phase organization (inspiratory, postinspiratory, and expiratory neurons) of medullary neurons is found in the newborn piglet, similar to that found in the adult cat (26). Although postinspiratory activity in the phrenic nerve is rarely observed in the anesthetized piglet, it is a

FIG. 32.2 Distribution of phrenic motoneurons at 2 weeks and 1 month based
on their spontaneous discharge recorded
intracellularly in kittens with end-tidal
CO_2 of approximately 5%. Early cells
were active in the first third of the inspiratory cycle, while late cells were activated in the latter two-thirds of the
cycle (11).

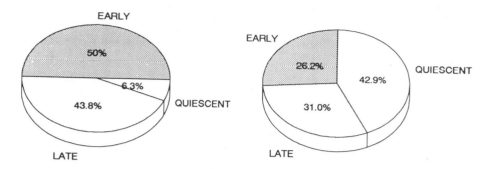

consistent phenomenon in the chloralose-urethane anesthetized kitten (11). In the kitten, it is the early recruited
phrenic motoneurons that exhibit the additional burst of activity during the postinspiratory period. Postinspiratory activity in the diaphragm and expiratory laryngeal braking
contributes to the maintenance of an elevated end-
expiratory lung volume in conscious dog pups (16). Therefore, besides playing a critical function in the termination
of inspiration, postinspiratory neurons provide a mechanism for altering the time constant of expiratory mechanics
in the newborn.

The discharge characteristics of medullary neurons that
shape the descending central respiratory drive to phrenic
motoneurons have been shown to change during postnatal
development (7, 40). One recent study using power spectral
analysis in the anesthetized or decerebrate kitten (37)
showed that the phrenic neurogram in young kittens (24–35
days) had the largest amplitude in a medium frequency
range (20–50 Hz) while in older animals (39 days and
older) the largest spectral peak occurred in the high-
frequency range (50–100 Hz). These authors concluded
that there is an age-related transition to high-frequency oscillations (HFOs) that represents alterations in the brainstem central pattern generator.

MOTOR COMPONENT

In general, there is a spatial sequence in the maturation of
respiratory motoneurons along the neuraxis. In kittens, it
has been demonstrated that the cell bodies of genioglossal
motoneurons of the hypoglossal nucleus reach their adult
size two months before the cell bodies of phrenic motoneurons achieve their mature size (8). However, within the
brainstem, there is some controversy concerning whether
neurons in the nucleus ambiguus develop and/or establish
their adult organization before or after those motoneurons
in the hypoglossal nucleus in the human fetus (see 6). During postnatal maturation in the kitten, there is a dissociation between the growth of the cell body and the dendritic
tree of phrenic motoneurons (9). Between the second and
fourth weeks of postnatal life, the surface area of the
phrenic cell bodies increased by 30% (10) while the total
dendritic surface area was unchanged. During this period,
there was also a reduction in the complexity of dendritic ar-

borization of phrenic motoneurons from an average of 60 to
46 dendritic terminals per cell. A similar reduction of the
dendritic fields has been reported for neurons of the nucleus ambiguus of the postnatal rat (32). This dendritic
simplification of respiratory motor and premotor neurons in
postnatal development may indicate a reorganization of the
synaptic inputs that shape the behavior in these neuron populations.

In addition, there are several interesting physiological
changes that occur during postnatal development (fig.
32.2). In the 2-week-old kitten, most phrenic motoneurons
(94%) are activated during slightly hypercapnic breathing
(5% end-tidal CO_2). By postnatal week 4–5, less than 57%
of these neurons are active during comparable inspiratory
efforts (11). Therefore, the newborn kitten is using most of
its phrenic motor units to generate a breath and must rely
predominantly on frequency modulation to achieve greater
transdiaphragmatic pressures while the older kitten has a
much larger reserve of quiescent units from which it may
recruit. The increase in the number of phrenic motoneurons
that remain inactive during inspiration is correlated to a decreased input resistance and increased rheobase of these
cells between 2 and 5 weeks after birth. Without an increase in total membrane surface area in these neurons, the
change must be occurring at the level of specific membrane
resistance. The appearance of phrenic motoneurons with
the decreased input resistance (lower specific membrane resistance) coincides with the disappearance of polyneuronal
innervation of the kitten diaphragm (Sieck and Fournier,
personal communication). It is possible that events in the
muscle (i.e., the elimination of supernumerary synapses on
the muscle fibers) may trigger events in the motoneurons
that, in turn, shape the discharge properties of these respiratory neurons.

This chapter provides a brief review of the changes that
occur during development in the sensory and motor limbs
of the respiratory reflexes. In general, maturation of respiratory reflexes can be characterized by several processes:
first, the quickening of conduction due to myelination of
peripheral axons; second, the alteration of the central reflex
gain due to synaptic remodeling; third, a change in the nature of the central pattern generator; and finally, a conversion of the respiratory motor nuclei and muscles from one
where most units were activated for each breath in the

newborn to one where the majority of units were not recruited during normal inspiration by the first postnatal month.

REFERENCES

1. Anderson, J.W., F.B. Sant'Ambrogio, O.P. Mathew, and G. Sant'Ambrogio. Water-responsive laryngeal receptors in the dog are not specialized endings. *Resp. Physiol.* 79:33-44, 1990.

2. Blanco, C.E., G.S. Dawes, M.A. Hanson, and H.B. McCooke. The response to hypoxia of arterial chemoreceptors in fetal sheep and new-born lambs. *J. Physiol.* (London) 351:25-37, 1984.

3. Bodegard, G., G.H. Schwieler, S. Skoglund, and R. Zetterstrom. Control of respiration in newborn babies. I. The development of the Hering-Breuer inflation reflex. *Acta Paediat. Scand.* 58:567-571, 1969.

4. Bodegard, G., and G.H. Schwieler. Control of respiration in newborn babies. II. The development of the thoracic reflex response to an added respiratory load. *Acta Paediat. Scand.* 60:181-186, 1971.

5. Boggs, D.F., and D. Bartlett. Chemical specificity of a laryngeal apneic reflex in puppies. *J. Appl. Physiol.* 53:455-462, 1982.

6. Brown, J.W. Prenatal development of the human nucleus ambiguus during the embryonic and early fetal periods. *Am. J. Anat.* 189:267-282, 1990.

7. Bruce, E.N. Significance of high-frequency oscillations as a functional index of respiratory control. In *Neurobiology of the control of breathing,* ed. C. von Euler and H. Lagercrantz, 75-80. New York: Raven Press, 1987.

8. Cameron, W.E., F. He, B.S. Brozanski, and R.D. Guthrie. The postnatal growth of motoneurons at three levels of the cat neuraxis. *Neurosci. Lett.* 104:274-280, 1989.

9. Cameron, W.E., F. He, P. Kalipatnapu, and R.D. Guthrie. Three-dimensional analysis of dendrite development in phrenic motoneurons. *Soc. Neurosci. Abstr.* 16:730, 1990.

10. Cameron, W.E., B.S. Brozanski, and R.D. Guthrie. Postnatal development of phrenic motoneurons in the cat. *Dev. Brain Res.* 51:142-145, 1990.

11. Cameron, W.E., J.S. Jodkowski, F. He, and R.D. Guthrie. Electrophysiological properties of developing phrenic motoneurons in the cat. *J. Neurophysiol.* 65:671-679, 1991.

12. Cooke, I.R.C., and P.J. Berger. Precursor of respiratory pattern in the early gestation mammalian fetus. *Brain Res.* 522:333-336, 1990.

13. de Neef, K.J., J.R.C. Jansen, and A. Versprille. Developmental morphometry and physiology of the rabbit vagus nerve. *Dev. Brain Res.* 4:265-274, 1982.

14. Downing, S.E., and J.C. Lee. Laryngeal chemosensitivity: a possible mechanism for sudden infant death. *Pediatrics* 55:640-649, 1975.

15. Duron, B., and D. Marlot. Postnatal evolution of inspiratory activity in the kitten. In *Central nervous control mechanisms in breathing,* ed. C. von Euler and H. Lagercrantz, 327-336. New York: Pergamon Press, 1979.

16. England, S.J., G. Kent, and H.A.F. Stogryn. Laryngeal muscle and diaphragmatic activities in conscious dog pups. *Resp. Physiol.* 60:95-108, 1985.

17. Farber, J. Medullary inspiratory activity during opossum development. *Am. J. Physiol.* 254:R578-R584, 1988.

18. Farber, J. Medullary expiratory activity during opossum development. *J. Appl. Physiol.* 66:1606-1612, 1989.

19. Farber, J., J.T. Fisher, and G. Sant'Ambrogio. Airway receptor activity in the developing opossum. *Am. J. Physiol.* 246:R752-R758, 1984.

20. Fillenz, M., and J.G. Widdicombe. Receptors of the lungs and airways. In *Handbook of Sensory Physiology,* ed. E. Neil, vo. 3, 81-112. Heidelberg: Springer-Verlag, 1971.

21. Fisher, J.T., and G. Sant'Ambrogio. Location and discharge properties of respiratory vagal afferents in the newborn dog. *Resp. Physiol.* 50:209-220, 1982.

22. Fisher, J.T., and G. Sant'Ambrogio. Airway and lung receptors and their reflex effects in the newborn. *Pediatr. Pulmonol.* 1:112-126, 1985.

23. Fisher, J.T., O.P. Mathew, F.B. Sant'Ambrogio, and G. Sant'Ambrogio. Reflex effects and receptor responses to upper airway pressure and flow stimuli in developing puppies. *J. Appl. Physiol.* 58:258-264, 1985.

24. Hanson, M.A. Maturation of the peripheral chemoreceptor and CNS components of respiratory control in perinatal life. In *Neurobiology of the control of breathing.* ed. C. von Euler and H. Lagercrantz, 59-65. New York: Raven Press, 1987.

25. Krous, H.F., J. Jordan, J. Wen, and J.P. Farber. Developmental morphometry of the vagus nerve in the opossum. *Dev. Brain Res.* 20:155-159, 1985.

26. Lawson, E.E., D.W. Richter, and A. Bischoff. Intracellular recordings of respiratory neurons in the lateral medulla of piglets. *J. Appl. Physiol.* 66:983-988, 1989.

27. Lee, J.C., B.J. Stoll, and S.E. Downing. Properties of the laryngeal chemoreflex in neonatal piglets. *Am. J. Physiol.* 233:R30-R36, 1977.

28. Lucier, G.E., A.T. Storey, and B.J. Sessle. Effects of upper respiratory tract stimuli on neonatal respiration: Reflex and single neuron analyses in the kitten. *Biol. Neonate* 35:82-89, 1979.

29. Marlot, D., and B. Duron. Postnatal maturation of phrenic, vagus and intercostal nerves in kittens. *Biol. Neonate* 36:264-272, 1979.

30. Marlot, D., and B. Duron. Postnatal development of vagal control of breathing in the kitten. *J. Physiol.* (Paris) 75:891-900, 1979.

31. Miller, A.J., and C.R. Dunmire. Characterization of the postnatal development of superior laryngeal nerve fibers in the postnatal kitten. *J. Neurobiol.* 7:483-494, 1976.

32. Miller, L.S., and M. Kalia. Early development of nucleus ambiguus neurons: Implications in the control of airway smooth muscle in the neonate. *FASEB J.* 4(7):A406, 1990.

33. Purves, M.J. Onset of respiration at birth. *Arch. Dis. Child.* 49:333-343, 1974.

34. Rigatto, H. Control of ventilation in the newborn. *Ann. Rev. Physiol.* 46:661-674, 1984.

35. Rigatto, H., J.P. Brady, and R. dela Torre Verduzco. Chemoreceptor reflexes in preterm infants. I. The effect of gestational and postnatal age on the ventilatory response to inhalation of 100% and 15% oxygen. *Pediatrics* 55:604-613, 1975.

36. Schwieler, G.H. Respiratory regulation during postnatal development in cats and rabbits and some of its morphological substrate. *Acta Physiol. Scand.* 304 (suppl.):1-123, 1968.

37. Sica, A.L., and M.R. Gandhi. Efferent phrenic nerve and respiratory neuron activity in the developing kitten: Spontaneous discharges and hypoxic responses. *Brain Res.* 524:254-262, 1990.

38. Smejkal, V., F. Palecek, and M. Frydrychova. Développement postnatal du reflexe de Breuer-Hering chez le rat. *J. Physiol.* (Paris) 80:173-176, 1985.

39. Smith, J.C., G. Liu, and J.L. Feldman. Intracellular recording from phrenic motoneurons receiving respiratory drive *in vitro. Neurosci. Lett.* 88:27-32, 1988.

40. Suthers, G.K., D.J. Henderson-Smart, and D.J.C. Read. Postnatal changes in rate of high frequency bursts of inspiratory activity in cats and dogs. *Brain Res.* 132:537-540, 1977.

41. Suzue, T. Respiratory rhythm generation in the *in vitro* brainstem–spinal cord preparation of the neonatal rat. *J. Physiol.* (London) 354:173-183, 1984.

42. Trippenbach, T., and G. Kelly. Respiratory effects of cigarette smoke, dust, and histamine in newborn rabbits. *J. Appl. Physiol.* 64:837-845, 1988.

33

Central Effect of Hypoxia in the Neonate

Sandra J. England

In both adult (9, 29) and newborn (4, 6, 14) animals, the ventilatory response to hypoxia is characterized by a biphasic pattern. Ventilation initially increases due to stimulation of peripheral chemoreceptors but this hyperventilation is not sustained. The secondary decline in ventilation is most prominent in newborn animals in which ventilation can fall below normoxic levels within minutes after the initiation of the hypoxic exposure. Several mechanisms for the secondary ventilatory depression have been proposed and investigated (14, 19).

PERIPHERAL MECHANISMS OF HYPOXIC DEPRESSION OF VENTILATION

Adaptation of the afferent output of peripheral chemoreceptors during hypoxia has been demonstrated in some (4, 24) but not all investigations (1, 2, 28). Hypoxia-induced alterations in respiratory system mechanics (increased resistance, decreased compliance) which limit the transduction of respiratory drive to effective ventilation do occur but are of insufficient magnitude to explain the reduction in ventilation (18). Furthermore, it is clear that central respiratory drive is decreased since both phrenic nerve and diaphragmatic activities are reduced during the secondary decline in ventilation (2, 19). Metabolic rate has been shown to decline during hypoxia in unanesthetized animals (13, 23), a response which undoubtedly contributes to the secondary ventilatory decline. However, decreases in metabolism cannot be invoked as the sole mechanism since phrenic nerve activity follows a biphasic pattern even when metabolism is unchanged or increased during hypoxia (19). Thus mechanisms for central inhibition of respiration during hypoxia have been invoked to account for the secondary decline in ventilation during hypoxia in newborns.

CENTRAL MECHANISMS OF HYPOXIC DEPRESSION OF VENTILATION

Three mechanisms for central hypoxic depression have been previously elucidated based on the responses observed in both anesthetized and unanesthetized adult animals (26). Brain blood flow increases in response to hypoxia resulting in a washout of CO_2 from the brainstem. In addition, a decrease in arterial PCO_2 is induced by the initial hyperventilation in response to peripheral chemoreceptor

stimulation by hypoxia. Both of these factors will lead to reduced excitation of central chemoreceptors, which could result in a decreased respiratory drive. In adult animals, the reduction in ventilation due to increased brain blood flow has been shown to be a transitory phenomenon insufficient to account for the reduced ventilation observed during hypoxia under the majority of conditions (25, 26). In addition, the secondary depression is present even when isocapnia is maintained during hypoxia (9). Recent investigations in newborn animals have shown that there is an increase in brainstem blood flow during acute hypoxia (7, 11) leading to decreased extracellular fluid PCO_2 and $[H^+]$ which will negatively modulate the increase in respiratory drive during hypoxia. However, Brown and Lawson (3) have demonstrated that a secondary decline in phrenic nerve activity occurs during hypoxia in newborn animals under conditions in which brainstem extracellular pH is acidotic and arterial PCO_2 is maintained at eucapnic levels. Thus decreased central chemoreceptor activity during hypoxia is not the sole mechanism for central respiratory depression during hypoxia.

The second central mechanism for hypoxic depression that has been shown is a graded inhibition of brainstem respiratory neurons (26). In peripherally chemodenervated adult animals exposed to progressive central hypoxia induced with carbon monoxide (CO), this graded inhibition is characterized by the presence of normal extracellular potassium levels (22) and an intact phrenic nerve response to excitatory stimuli such as elevated arterial CO_2 (20) and electrical stimulation of the carotid sinus nerve (26). Central respiratory inhibition under these conditions is presumably mediated by release of inhibitory neurotransmitters such as GABA induced by brainstem acidosis during hypoxia (17, 21, 26). Adenosine and endorphins have also been implicated as inhibitory neuromodulators (6, 12, 19).

The final mechanism for central hypoxic depression is failure of cellular integrity in the brainstem respiratory neurons due to hypoxic cellular damage. Such failure occurs during severe hypoxia and, in contrast to the graded inhibition discussed above, is accompanied by gasping, increases in extracellular potassium levels, and lack of response to respiratory stimuli (26). The latter two mechanisms discussed have not been comprehensively evaluated in the newborn animal and were the focus of the study presented here.

HYPOXIC CENTRAL RESPIRATORY DEPRESSION IN THE NEONATAL PIGLET

The model used to investigate central depression during hypoxia in neonatal piglets was based on that previously used in adult cats (20). Eleven piglets (6 ± 3 [SD] days old, 2.4 ± 0.5 kg) were anesthetized with acepromazine (1 mg/kg im) and ketamine (10 mg/kg im). Brachial venous and arterial catheters were inserted and a cervical tracheostomy was performed. Anesthesia was maintained with alpha-chloralose (30–40 mg/kg iv). The vagi and carotid sinus nerves were sectioned bilaterally to eliminate peripheral chemoreceptor influences. The animals were paralyzed and mechanically ventilated (40% O_2) with central respiratory output monitored from the central cut end of one C5 root of the phrenic nerve. Phrenic nerve activity was quantitated from the moving time average as the peak inspiratory amplitude and as minute activity (peak χ frequency of inspirations). A cannula was placed in the abdominal aorta and attached to a reservoir containing blood obtained from another piglet for maintenance of arterial blood pressure. Body temperature was maintained at 38 ± 1°C with a heating blanket.

The animal was exposed to progressive hypercapnia by rebreathing to determine the relationship between arterial PCO_2 and the magnitude of phrenic nerve activity and to obtain a maximum value of phrenic nerve activity for standardization of activities subsequently observed during hypoxia. Rebreathing was performed before each of two hypoxic exposures induced by adding 0.5 to 1% CO to the breathing mixture. The two exposures were performed at different levels ("low" and "normal") of underlying respiratory drive achieved by adjusting arterial PCO_2 (table 33.1). Between hypoxic exposures, reoxygenation was achieved by ventilating the animal with 40% O_2 until oxygen content returned to the prehypoxic level.

Table 33.1. Conditions Immediately Preceding Exposure to Progressive Hypoxemia

| | Respiratory Drive[1] | |
	"Low"	"Normal"
Phrenic Nerve Activity		
Peak (% value at 9% CO_2)	26 (8)[2]	57 (11)
Minute (% value at 9% CO_2)	35 (12)	84 (17)
Frequency (min⁻¹)	20 (3)	22 (5)
Arterial P_{CO_2} (mm Hg)	27 (2)	31 (3)
Arterial Oxygen Content	12.2 (0.9)	11.8 (0.8)

[1] The only significant change made between "low" and "normal" drive was to increase arterial CO_2 slightly by adjusting the ventilator.

[2] Each value is mean (± SD).

At normal or eupneic levels of respiratory drive, no evidence of progressive central respiratory depression was observed during the initial stages of hypoxia (fig. 33.1). Both the amplitude and frequency of phrenic nerve activity

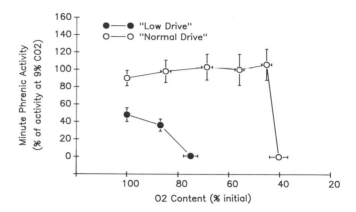

FIG. 33.1 Minute activity of the phrenic nerve (amplitude × frequency) as a function of arterial oxygenation during progressive hypoxemia during "low" and "normal" drive conditions. The circles represent the mean values for eleven piglets obtained in paired experiments. Bars represent SEM and if not shown lie within the symbols for the mean value.

were essentially unaltered until oxygen content was reduced to approximately 40% of control. At that point, expiratory time lengthened dramatically over several breaths culminating in central apnea. At this point, addition of CO_2 to the breathing mixture did not restore phrenic nerve activity.

When underlying respiratory drive was reduced by a small decrease in arterial PCO_2, progressive hypoxemia was accompanied by a progressive decline in the amplitude of phrenic nerve activity (fig. 33.1). Apnea was observed at a mean oxygen content of 75% of control. Addition of CO_2 to the breathing mixture during apnea resulted in an immediate and brisk return of phasic phrenic nerve activity. Saetta and Mortola (27) have demonstrated that the respiratory control system is also capable of responding to increased CO_2 during the secondary decline in respiration in the acutely hypoxic rat.

These data suggest that central hypoxic depression originating from two potential mechanisms is present in the newborn. At low to moderate levels of hypoxemia, a reversible inhibition of respiratory output can be observed if underlying respiratory drive is low. The source of this inhibition may be hyperpolarization of neurons in response to increased levels of inhibitory neurotransmitters as proposed in adult animals (26). Hyperpolarization of neurons in hippocampal slices has been demonstrated during hypoxia (10, 16) but only depolarization has been reported in hypoxic hypoglossal tissue slices from adult animals (15). Hypoglossal neurons from neonatal animals showed neither hyperpolarization nor depolarization when exposed to hypoxia (15). The response of medullary neurons of the respiratory control center have not been studied to date. Hyperpolarization and active inhibition are likely to be present in individual neurons whenever hypoxemia occurs but reduction of integrated and summated neuronal activities such as the phrenic will be evident only when excitatory inputs are insufficient to bring respiratory neurons from their hyperpolarized membrane potential to threshold during inspiration. Inspiratory premotor neuronal activity during hypoxia represents a balance between excitatory and inhibitory inputs with the predominant effect of central hypoxemia being inhibitory. Thus at low levels of CO_2 in the anesthetized, peripherally chemodenervated animal a reversible depression of respiratory center activity occurs.

A similar reduction in ventilation might be expected to occur in the unanesthetized animal during acute hypoxia when hyperventilation results in a decreased arterial PCO_2, brain blood flow is increased further reducing brainstem tissue PCO_2 and metabolism is reduced. All of the aforementioned factors will reduce excitatory inputs to respiratory neurons and the inhibition induced by central hypoxia may be unmasked. It is of interest that in piglets the magnitude and even the existence of a biphasic hypoxic response have been controversial. Darnall et al. (6) demonstrated a substantial reduction in ventilation in anesthetized piglets during hypoxia while Davis et al. (8) showed a sustained hyperventilation in unanesthetized piglets. Davis et al. (8) measured ventilation in unanesthetized animals using a face mask that would increase dead space and thus PCO_2, stimulate trigeminal afferents, and provide a small resistive load to breathing. All of these factors would be expected to enhance the excitation of respiratory neurons.

The sudden decline of phrenic nerve activity to apnea observed at low levels of oxygenation under "normal" drive, which was not reversed by inhalation of CO_2, is likely to result from neuronal insufficiency rather than from the graded inhibition just discussed. This response occurs near the same level of hypoxemia at which adult animals begin gasping (26). Bureau et al. (5), in a study of unanesthetized lambs subjected to progressive CO-induced hypoxia, observed responses similar to those reported here. Ventilation was maintained during hypoxemia until levels of arterial oxygen saturation declined to 35 to 40%, at which point ventilatory depression was observed in all animals with two exhibiting ventilatory arrest. This mechanism is unlikely to be apparent at the levels of hypoxemia normally observed in spontaneously breathing neonates.

SUMMARY

Central hypoxic depression arising from several mechanisms dependent on the level and duration of hypoxemia has been observed in the newborn piglet. The degree to which ventilation decreases during any given hypoxic exposure will depend on the balance between excitatory and inhibitory influences at the level of the brainstem respiratory controller.

ACKNOWLEDGMENTS

My thanks to Norman H. Edelman for agreeing to present this work at the symposium in my absence. This work was supported by National Heart, Lung and Blood Institute Grant HL-16022.

REFERENCES

1. Biscoe, T.J., and M.J. Purves. Carotid body chemoreceptor activity in the newborn lamb. *J. Physiol.* (London) 190:443-454, 1967.

2. Blanco, C.E., M.A. Hanson, P. Johnson, and H. Rigatto. Breathing pattern of kittens during hypoxia. *J. Appl. Physiol.* 56:12-17, 1984.

3. Brown, D.L., and E.E. Lawson. Brain stem extracellular fluid pH and respiratory drive during hypoxia in newborn pigs. *J. Appl. Physiol.* 64:1055-1059, 1988.

4. Bureau, M.A., A. Cote, P.W. Blanchard, S. Hobbs, P. Foulon, and D. Dalle. Exponential and diphasic ventilatory response to hypoxia in conscious lambs. *J. Appl. Physiol.* 61:836-842, 1986.

5. Bureau, M.A., J.L. Carroll, and E. Canet. Response of newborn lambs to CO-induced hypoxia. *J. Appl. Physiol.* 64:1870-1877, 1988.

6. Darnall, R.A., and R.D. Bruce. Aminophylline reduces hypoxic ventilatory depression: Possible role of adenosine. *Pediatric Res.* 19:706-710, 1985.

7. Darnall, R.A., G. Green, L. Pinto, and N. Hart. Effect of acute hypoxia on respiration and brain stem blood flow in the piglet. *J. Appl. Physiol.* 70:251-259, 1991.

8. Davis, G.M., M.A. Bureau, and C. Gaultier. The sustained ventilatory response to hypoxic challenge in the awake newborn piglet with an intact upper airway. *Resp. Physiol.* 71:307-318, 1988.

9. Easton, P.A., L.J. Slyderman, and N.R. Anthonisen. Ventilatory response to sustained hypoxia in normal adults. *J. Appl. Physiol.* 61:906-911, 1986.

10. Fujiwara, N., H. Higashi, K. Shimoji, and M. Yoshimura. Effects of hypoxia on rat hippocampal neurones *in vitro*. *J. Physiol.* (London) 384:131-151, 1987.

11. Goplerud, J.M., L.C. Wagerle, and M. Delivoria-Papadopoulos. Regional cerebral blood flow response during and after acute asphyxia in newborn piglets. *J. Appl. Physiol.* 66:2827-2832, 1989.

12. Grunstein, M.M., T.A. Hazinski, and M.A. Schlueter. Respiratory control during hypoxia in newborn rabbits: Implied action of endorphins. *J. Appl. Physiol.* 51:122-130, 1981.

13. Haddad, G.G., M.R. Gandhi, and R.B. Mellins. Maturation of ventilatory response to hypoxia in puppies during sleep. *J. Appl. Physiol.* 52:309-314, 1982.

14. Haddad, G.G., and R.B. Mellins. Hypoxia and respiratory control in early life. *Ann. Rev. Physiol.* 46:629-643, 1984.

15. Haddad, G.G., and D.F. Donnelly. O_2 deprivation induces a major depolarization in brain stem neurons in the adult but not in the neonatal rat. *J. Physiol.* (London) 429:411-428, 1990.

16. Hansen, A.J., J. Hounsgaard, and H. Jahnsen. Anoxia increases potassium conductance in hippocampal nerve cells. *Acta Physiol. Scand.* 115:301-310, 1982.

17. Hedner, J., T. Hedner, P. Wessberg, and J. Jonason. An analysis of the mechanism by which gamma-aminobutyric acid depresses ventilation in the rat. *J. Appl. Physiol.* 56:849-856, 1984.

18. Laframboise, W.A., R.D. Guthrie, T.A. Standaert, and D.E. Woodrum. Pulmonary mechanics during the ventilatory response to hypoxemia in the newborn monkey. *J. Appl. Physiol.* 55:1008-1014, 1983.

19. Lawson, E.E., and W.A. Long. Central origin of biphasic breathing pattern during hypoxia in newborns. *J. Appl. Physiol.* 55:483-488, 1983.

20. Melton, J.E., J.A. Neubauer, and N.H. Edelman. CO_2 sensitivity of cat phrenic neurogram during hypoxic respiratory depression. *J. Appl. Physiol.* 65:736-743, 1988.

21. Melton, J.E., J.A. Neubauer, and N.H. Edelman. GABA antagonism reverses hypoxic respiratory depression in the cat. *J. Appl. Physiol.* 69:1296-1301, 1990.

22. Melton, J.E., L.O. Chae, J.A. Neubauer, and N.H. Edelman. Extracellular potassium homeostasis in the cat medulla during progressive brain hypoxia. *J. Appl. Physiol.* 70:1477-1482, 1991.

23. Mortola, J.P., and R. Rezzonico. Metabolic and ventilatory rates in newborn kittens during acute hypoxia. *Resp. Physiol.* 73:55-68, 1988.

24. Mulligan, E., and S. Bhide. Non-sustained responses to hypoxia of carotid body chemoreceptor afferents in the piglet. *FASEB J.* 3:A399, 1989.

25. Neubauer, J.A., T.V. Santiago, M.A. Posner, and N.H. Edelman. Ventral medullary pH and ventilatory responses to hyperperfusion and hypoxia. *J. Appl. Physiol.* 58:1659-1668, 1985.

26. Neubauer, J.A., J.E. Melton, and N.H. Edelman. Modulation of respiration during brain hypoxia (review). *J. Appl. Physiol.* 68:441-451, 1990.

27. Saetta, M., and J. P. Mortola. Interaction of hypoxic and hypercapnic stimuli on breathing pattern in the newborn rat. *J. Appl. Physiol.* 62:506-512, 1987.

28. Schweiler, G.H. Respiratory regulation during postnatal development in cats and rabbits and some of its morphological substrate. *Acta Physiol. Scand. Suppl.* 304:49-63, 1968.

29. Vizek, M., C.K. Pickett, and J.V. Weil. Biphasic ventilatory response of adult cats to sustained hypoxia has central origin. *J. Appl. Physiol.* 63:1658-1664, 1987.

34

Mechanisms of Apnea in the Newborn

Edward E. Lawson, Maria F. Czyzyk-Krzeska, and Roger C. Rudesill

In various animal species the respiratory central pattern generator of adults as well as newborns consists of three phases identified as inspiration and two distinctly different periods of expiration (15, 22, 31). The two phases of expiration are termed postinspiration (passive expiration) and stage II (active) expiration. The postinspiratory phase appears to mediate cessation of inspiration and to provide a transition to active stage II expiration (24) and, therefore, postinspiration might be the phase most sensitively affecting the respiratory rhythm.

Introduction of smoke or water into the larynx activates medullary post-inspiratory mechanisms resulting in slowing of the respiratory rhythm or apnea, a phenomenon which may be simulated by superior laryngeal nerve (SLN) stimulation (21, 25). Similar activation of upper airway reflexes in newborns of various species results in strong, protracted apnea which appears more powerful than that of adults (6, 16, 18, 28, 30). We have previously shown that SLN stimulation of piglets results in a protracted apnea which persists even following cessation of the stimulus (12, 13). Further, stimulation of upper airway receptors is recognized as a major cause of clinically important apnea, particularly in newborns (8, 19, 20), but the central neuronal mechanism of this reflex in infants has not been thoroughly identified. The purpose of these studies was to demonstrate neurophysiologic mechanisms by which respiration is perturbed by laryngeal receptor activation.

METHODS

The studies were performed in neonatal piglets (1–17 days of age; 1.1–4.0 Kg) because their size allowed intubation, controlled ventilation, maintenance of adequate acid-base balance, and surgical exposure of the peripheral and central neural structures needed to facilitate identification of afferent inputs and the specific elements of the central respiratory network. The piglets were anesthetized with pentobarbital (30 mg/kg ip with supplementary iv doses of 2–6 mg/kg as needed). For approximately one-half of the piglets the trachea was cannulated just below the larynx by a dual lumen cannula. One caudally directed lumen was used for mechanical ventilation and a rostrally directed second lumen was used for insufflation of aromatic ammonia spirits or water into the larynx. In the remaining piglets, a single lumen tracheal cannula was used for mechanical ventilation only. All pigs were paralyzed and mechanically ventilated. Polyethylene catheters were inserted into a femoral artery and a femoral vein for monitoring arterial pressure, controlling acid-base balance, and continuous administration of 5% dextrose in water, gallamine, and other drugs. Rectal temperature was continuously measured and maintained between 38–39°C with radiant heat lamps and ventral heating blankets.

The vagal nerves were sectioned bilaterally, the nerve ipsilateral to the recording site was placed on a bipolar stimulating electrode. The cervical phrenic nerve contralateral to the neuronal recording site was prepared for recording of the respiratory rhythm. The medulla oblongata was exposed by occipital craniotomy for recording of respiratory neurons of the ventral respiratory group. Intracellular recording of respiratory neurons was accomplished using a standard protocol described previously (15, 21, 25).

Two stimuli were administered via the rostrally directed tracheal lumen in order to activate laryngeal receptors. One stimulus was water instilled into the larynx and the other was air saturated with ammonia "smelling salts" insufflated into the larynx. During electrical stimulation of the SLN poststimulus membrane potential averaging (ASYST Software Technologies, Inc.) of intracellularly recorded neurons was used to determine synaptic events occurring during laryngeal induced apnea.

RESULTS

Ammonia or water stimuli usually resulted in obliteration of neural activity in the phrenic nerve (fig. 34.1), but on occasion, the initial poststimulus phrenic activity response resembled the "aspiration reflex" described by Tomori and Widdicombe (29) and Batsel and Lines (3). A rapid respiratory pattern (data not shown) was observed in approximately one-third of the piglets, but an apnea, similar to that induced in the remaining piglets, could be evoked in the same piglets by using a stimulus of greater volume. In most instances the protracted period of phrenic silence following the laryngeal stimulus ended with a ramplike phrenic burst having characteristics very similar to those of the control breaths except for a reduction in amplitude and duration (12).

The effect of laryngeal mucosal stimulation on membrane potential trajectory was dependent upon the type of neuron. Prior to laryngeal stimulation all respiratory neurons displayed the expected three distinct levels of membrane potential, including depolarization during the respective respiratory phase for which the cell was named

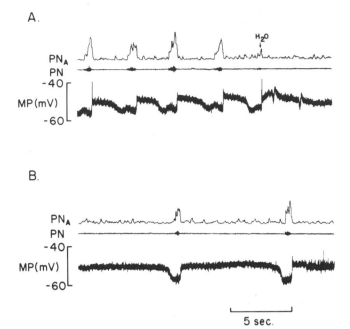

FIG. 34.1 Effect of laryngeal water upon phrenic activity and membrane potential of a non-antidromically activated postinspiratory neuron. A and B are continuous records. In this example the postinspiratory period is relatively prolonged, even in the control breaths. Nevertheless, water instillation (A) results in dramatic phrenic apnea associated with protracted depolarization of the membrane potential. Just prior to onset of the first recovery phrenic breath (B) the membrane potential hyperpolarizes for the stage II expiratory phase, which, in turn, is followed by a slight change in membrane potential associated with the onset of inspiration. This pattern of hyperpolarization is similar to that seen in the control breaths. PN, phrenic nerve; PN_A, averaged phrenic nerve; MP, membrane potential.

(e.g., inspiratory neurons depolarized during inspiration) followed by two levels of hyperpolarization corresponding to the other two phases of the respiratory cycle. Laryngeal insufflation of ammonia or water could prematurely terminate inspiratory and expiratory depolarization. During the apneic period following laryngeal stimulation, the neurons displayed a prolonged stable membrane potential at levels which were similar to that of the postinspiratory level regardless of the cell type. Before onset of the subsequent phrenic inspiratory activity the membrane potential transiently shifted to a level consistent with that of the stage II expiratory level. During recovery, when the initial inspiratory phrenic activity was diminished compared with control breaths, the magnitude of inspiratory neuron depolarization was also diminished.

Figure 34.1 demonstrates the response of a postinspiratory neuron following water instillation into the larynx, which caused a rather protracted apnea. This neuron was not antidromically activated by spinal or vagal stimulation and was therefore considered to be a propriobulbar postinspiratory neuron (22, 25). Under control conditions postinspiratory neurons hyperpolarized abruptly during

inspiration, depolarized sharply immediately at the end of inspiration, and repolarized at the onset of stage II expiration. During the early phase of laryngeal-induced central apnea these postinspiratory neurons were strongly depolarized (fig. 34.1) and they remained relatively depolarized until transition to stage II expiration, which invariably preceded onset of the first recovery ramplike inspiration. During the phrenic apnea, inspiratory and expiratory neurons also displayed stable membrane potentials at levels approximating those of the control postinspiration. Before onset of the first recovery ramp-like inspiration, the membrane potential of all cells shifted from the postinspiratory level in the direction consistent with a shift to the expiratory level. An example of this membrane potential shift is shown for a postinspiratory neuron (fig. 34.1) as an abrupt decline in membrane potential preceding onset of phrenic activity.

To further investigate the nature of the membrane potential changes observed during laryngeal-induced apnea we used trains of electrical stimuli delivered to the SLN (3–9 V, 7–10 Hz). Similar to the respiratory response to chemical laryngeal stimulation, onset of SLN stimulation was associated with cessation of phrenic nerve activity and cessation of the triphasic pattern of membrane potential changes in simultaneously recorded respiratory neurons. Stimulus-triggered averaging of the respiratory neuron membrane potential was used to determine the synaptic events occurring during apnea.

Among all inspiratory neurons recorded during the course of electrically induced apnea lasting for longer than several seconds, the membrane potential initially hyperpolarized to the control postinspiratory level and thereafter it gradually became more hyperpolarized during the remainder of the apnea. Stimulus-triggered averaging was successful in 7 of 10 recorded inspiratory neurons. Four of these, all bulbospinal, demonstrated biphasic post-stimulus membrane potential changes. The first component of these changes was a brief wave of depolarization (mean latency to onset 3.3 msec) followed by the second component which was a protracted hyperpolarizing wave (fig. 34.2A). In the remaining three inspiratory neurons (one was antidromically activated by spinal stimulation) only the late hyperpolarizing wave was observed. Based upon differential reversal of the membrane voltage trajectory (fig. 34.2B) by chloride injection or passage of negative current, the late membrane hyperpolarization seemed to consist of two distinctly different phases of inhibition. The first of these readily reversed while the neuron displayed a nonreversing late component. Similarly, the gradual hyperpolarizing trajectory of the membrane throughout the period of SLN stimulation also did not change despite reversal of the earlier component.

Of twenty recorded expiratory neurons, ten were antidromically activated by spinal cord stimulation. SLN stimulation during intracellular recording of these neu-

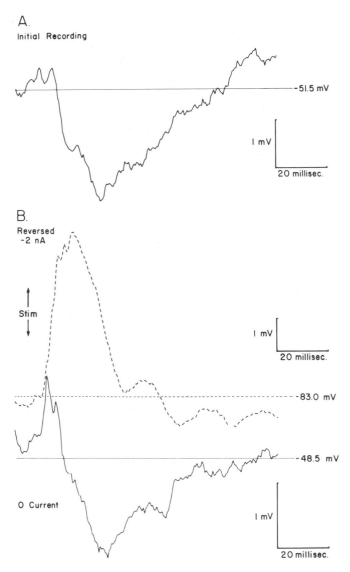

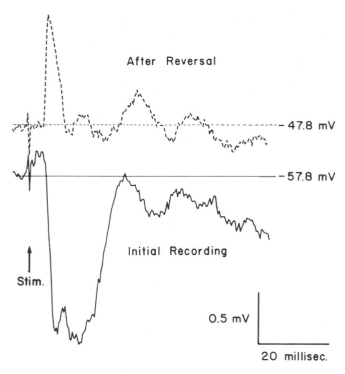

FIG. 34.2 Effect of superior laryngeal nerve stimulation on membrane potential of an inspiratory neuron. (A) Stimulus-triggered averaging of the membrane potential immediately following cell impalement. Note the short depolarization prior to the protracted hyperpolarizing component. (B) The effects of negative current passage on the poststimulus wave pattern. The pattern with the continuous line indicates control activity before current passage, and the dashed line indicates the pattern during negative current passage throught the recording electrode while stimulating the superior laryngeal nerve. The recording electrode was not exactly balanced.

FIG. 34.3 Effect of superior laryngeal nerve stimulation on membrane potential of an expiratory neuron. A pattern having two peaks of hyperpolarization occurs during the first 30 msec following the stimulus. Chloride iontophoresis resulted in dramatic reversal of the early component, but lesser change in the latter component.

rons resulted in a stable membrane potential at a level similar to that which occurred immediately following the cessation of inspiration in control breaths. Stimulus-triggered averaging of the expiratory cell membrane potential during apnea evoked a dual-phased wave again having two separable components. Among the bulbospinal expiratory neurons 88% displayed a short latency hyperpolarization followed by a long lasting depolarization. In contrast, both components of the averaged membrane

potential were hyperpolarizing in six of seven non-antidromically activated expiratory neurons. In either case, the latency to the onset of the first hyperpolarizing component in the expiratory cells correlated temporally with the onset of the early depolarizing component of the inspiratory neurons. Both hyperpolarizing components of the expiratory neurons reversed following chloride injection or passage of negative current (fig. 34.3), but the early component reversed earlier and more extensively than the later component.

During apnea induced by SLN stimulation, postinspiratory neurons were depolarized to the membrane potential associated with the control postinspiratory level. Repetitive firing of action potentials following a single stimulus often accompanied this depolarization. Stimulus triggered averaging of the membrane potential during apnea revealed excitatory postsynaptic potentials having two distinct components. The latency of the early component (mean: 3.6 msec) was similar to that of the early components of inspiratory and expiratory neurons. However, the late depolarizing wave peaked earlier than the second components of the inspiratory and expiratory neurons.

DISCUSSION

Despite earlier work (17), the mechanisms of central apnea in newborns induced by stimulation of the larynx have not been elucidated. The work reported in this paper demonstrates that, in the newborn pig, laryngeal stimulation very sensitively perturbs the respiratory cycle by activating neuronal mechanisms within the brainstem which are associated with the postinspiratory phase of breathing. Activation of these postinspiratory mechanisms was demonstrated using both chemical stimuli delivered to the laryngeal mucosa and electrical stimulation of the principal sensory nerve of the larynx, the SLN. In general, apnea-producing stimuli resulted in excitation of the postinspiratory neurons and inhibition of the inspiratory and expiratory neurons. These findings are similar to those described by Remmers et al. (21) and Richter et al. (25), who demonstrated that brief electric stimulation of the SLN and laryngeal receptor activation by chemical stimuli such as water, dilute hydrochloric acid solution, and smoke, activated postinspiratory mechanisms in the adult cat. Further, they demonstrated that the postinspiratory inhibition was associated with activation of chloride-mediated postsynaptic potentials in inspiratory and expiratory neurons (1, 2, 25). However, the synaptic activity was not specifically characterized and the relevance of these findings to the mechanisms of apnea remained unclear for newborns.

The stimulus-triggered averaging experiments demonstrated that the synaptic events resulting in apnea characteristically consisted of an early and a late component. For each cell recorded, the direction of the late component determined the overall membrane potential level throughout apnea. This is particularly illustrated by the inspiratory neurons which had an early excitatory component that was strongly inhibited by the protracted late component. The direct effect of the laryngeal afferents has been assumed to be mediated through oligosynaptic connections with the dorsal group of respiratory neurons in the nucleus of the solitary tract (5) where SLN afferents project (4, 26). In the current experiments, the short latency to the early component of the compound postsynaptic potential supports the concept of direct mono- or oligosynaptic contacts by laryngeal afferents with ventral respiratory group neurons. In piglets, Goding et al. (10) demonstrated that sensory SLN fibers also terminate in the nucleus ambiguus, suggesting a more direct influence of the laryngeal sensory receptors on these ventral respiratory neurons. This may be a species difference or, alternatively, increased numbers of synaptic connections may be present among newborns. If the latter possibility is found to be correct then this increased synaptic interconnectivity, involving both ventral respiratory group as well as dorsal respiratory group neurons, may explain the apparent increased inhibitory effect of laryngeal stimuli in newborns.

The ionic mechanisms associated with the compound postsynaptic pattern seen after an SLN stimulus are likely to represent both chloride and non-chloride channels. Those portions of waves readily reversing with negative current or iontophoresis of chloride are likely to be mediated by chloride. In contrast, the late phase of the second component of the pattern seen in inspiratory neurons seems not to be mediated by chloride as it neither reversed nor even lessened its degree of polarization despite reversal of the earlier phase.

Onset of recovery ramp inspiratory breaths only occurred following evidence of stage II expiration. This suggests that stage II expiration may be essential for initiation of breaths characterized by ramp inspiration. Phrenic inspiratory activity occurs when bulbospinal inspiratory neurons are released from stage II inhibition and the ramp pattern is shaped by decrementing inhibition of the early-inspiratory neurons (23). The current models of respiratory control (7, 23) support early-inspiratory cell inhibition by postinspiratory neurons, but no significant inhibition of early-inspiratory neurons by stage II expiratory neurons is postulated. Our observation suggests that stage II expiratory activity must somehow condition the early-inspiratory neurons so they do not provide the usual decrementing inhibition in certain circumstances. Presumably, in addition to postinspiratory inhibition, the stage II expiratory activity inhibits early inspiratory neurons which, upon release, activates membrane ion currents resulting in a lower membrane potential threshold for action potential generation than would exist otherwise. The ionic mechanism responsible for this relative excitation could involve membrane post-inhibitory rebound in order to activate the early-inspiratory neurons and to restart the normal three-phase cycle (23). In the absence of stage II expiration a two-phased respiratory cycle, characterized as an oscillation between postinspiration and inspiration, occurs. In this latter pattern the phrenic activity does not show the ramp inspiratory pattern, the inspiratory time is short, and the cycle time is short. Such respiratory patterns as the "aspiration reflex," sniffing, swallowing, sneezing, and coughing (3, 9, 29) often coexist with laryngeal stimulation, and they may represent a two-phase respiratory pattern.

In summary, we have shown in newborns that apnea produced by laryngeal stimuli is associated with activation of postinspiratory neurons and inhibition of the other two principal respiratory classes of neurons represented in the ventral respiratory group. The clinical relevance of these findings are, at present, speculative. Gastroesophageal reflux is increasingly recognized as an important aspect of significant respiratory control disorders in the newborn. Upper airway stimuli have been shown to stimulate respiratory abnormalities similar to those elicited during gastroesophageal reflux (8, 11, 17, 19, 20, 27). This suggests that laryngeal, postinspiratory mechanisms are activated during many episodes clinically recognized as apnea. Apnea induced by SLN stimulation overcomes even markedly increased peripheral chemosensitive afferent activity (14). Hence, disappearance of significant apnea events with advancing postnatal age may indicate reduction in the inhibition of the respiratory network induced after respiration, rather than an increase in peripheral or central chemosensitivity. Further investigation along this line may reveal specific neuromodulators or other unique aspects of the postinspiratory neuronal network allowing development of specific strategies for directed therapy of symptomatic infants. A means to clinically investigate the role of postinspiration in newborns would be recording of laryngeal muscles which have strong postinspiratory activity.

ACKNOWLEDGMENTS

This work was supported in part by grants received from the U.S. Public Health Service (HD00475 and HL34919), the Deutsche Forschungsgemeinschaft (Ri279/7–10), the American Lung Association of North Carolina, the Alexander von Humboldt Stiftung (Bonn, FRG), and the Burroughs-Wellcome Trust Fund.

REFERENCES

1. Ballantyne, D., and D.W. Richter. Post-synaptic inhibition of bulbar inspiratory neurones in the cat. *J. Physiol.* (London) 348:67-87, 1984.

2. Ballantyne, D., and D.W. Richter. The non-uniform character of expiratory synaptic activity in expiratory bulbospinal neurones of the cat. *J. Physiol.* (London) 370:433-456, 1986.

3. Batsel, H.L., and A.J. Lines. Bulbar respiratory neurons participating in the sniff reflex in the cat. *Exp. Neurol.* 39:469-481, 1973.

4. Bellingham, M., and J. Lipski. Morphology of superior laryngeal nerve afferents and first order interneurones involved in reflex inhibition of respiration. *Neurosci. Lett.* Suppl. 30:S48, 1988.

5. Berger, A.J. Dorsal respiratory group neurons in the medulla of cat: Spinal projections, responses to lung inflation and superior laryngeal nerve stimulation. *Brain Res.* 135:231-254, 1977.

6. Boushey, H.A., P.S. Richardson, and J.G. Widdicombe. Reflex effects of laryngeal irritation on the pattern of breathing and total lung resistance. *J. Physiol.* 224:501-513, 1972.

7. Connor, K.M., D.G. Ferrington, and M.J. Rowe. Tactile sensory coding during development: Signaling capacities of neurons in kitten dorsal column nuclei. *J. Neurophysiol.* 52:86, 1984.

8. Davies, A.M., J.S. Koenig, and B.T. Thach. Upper airway chemoreflex responses to saline and water in preterm infants. *J. Appl. Physiol.* 64:1412-1420, 1988.

9. duPont, J.S. Firing patterns of bulbar respiratory neurones during sniffing in the conscious, non-paralyzed rabbit. *Brain Res.* 414:163-168, 1987.

10. Goding, G.S., M.A. Richardson, and R.E. Trachy. Laryngeal chemoreflex: Anatomic and physiologic study by use of the superior laryngeal nerve in the piglet. *Otolaryngol. Head Neck Surg.* 97:28-38, 1987.

11. Johnson, P., D.M. Salisbury, and A.T. Storey. Apnoea induced by stimulation of sensory receptors in the larynx. In *Development of upper respiratory anatomy and function: Implications for sudden infant death syndrome*, ed. J.F. Bosma and J. Showacre, 160-178. Washington, D.C.: DHEW, 1975.

12. Lawson, E.E. Prolonged central respiratory inhibition following reflex-induced apnea. *J. Appl. Physiol.* 50:874-879, 1981.

13. Lawson, E.E. Recovery from central apnea: Effect of stimulus duration and end-tidal CO_2 partial pressure. *J. Appl. Physiol.* 53:105-109, 1982.

14. Lawson, E.E., and W.A. Long. Interaction of excitatory and inhibitory respiratory afterdischarge mechanisms in piglets. *J. Appl. Physiol.* 55:1299-1304, 1983.

15. Lawson, E.E., D.W. Richter, and A.M. Bischoff. Intracellular recordings of respiratory neurons in the lateral medulla of piglets. *J. Appl. Physiol.* 66:983-988, 1989.

16. Lee, J.C., and S.E. Downing. Laryngeal reflex inhibition of breathing in piglets: Influences of anemia and catecholamine depletion. *Am. J. Physiol.* 239:R25-R30, 1980.

17. Lucier, G.E., A.T. Storey, and B.J. Sessle. Effects of upper respiratory tract stimuli on neonatal respiration: Reflex and single neuron analyses in the kitten. *Biol. Neonate* 35:82-89, 1979.

18. Marchal, F., B.C. Corke, and H. Sundell. Reflex apnea from laryngeal chemo-stimulation in the sleeping premature newborn lamb. *Pediatric Res.* 16:621-627, 1982.

19. Perkett, E.A., and R.L. Vaughan. Evidence for a laryngeal chemoreflex in some human preterm infants. *Acta Paediat. Scand.* 71:969-972, 1982.

20. Pickens, D.L., G. Schefft, and B.T. Thach. Prolonged apnea associated with upper airway protective reflexes in apnea of prematurity. *Am. Rev. Resp. Dis.* 137:113-118, 1988.

21. Remmers, J.E., D.W. Richter, D. Ballantyne, C.R. Bainton, and J.P. Klein. Reflex prolongation of stage I of expiration. *Pflügers Arch.* 407:190-198, 1986.

22. Richter, D.W. Generation and maintenance of the respiratory rhythm. *J. Exp. Biol.* 100:93-107, 1982.

23. Richter, D.W., D. Ballantyne, and J.E. Remmers. How is the respiratory rhythm generated? A model. *NIPS* 1:109-112, 1986.

24. Richter, D.W., and D. Ballantyne. On the significance of postinspiration. In: *Funktionanalyse biologischer Systeme* 18, ed. J. Grote, 149-156. Stuttgart: Gustav Fischer Verlag, 1988.

25. Richter, D.W., D. Ballantyne, and J.E. Remmers. The differential organization of medullary postinspiratory activities. *Pflügers Arch.* 410:420-427, 1987.

26. Schwarzacher, S.W., K. Anders, and D.W. Richter. Terminale projektion laryngealer afferenzen im hirnstamm der katze. *Pflügers Arch.* 415: in press, 1990.

27. Sessle, B.J., L.F. Greenwood, J.P. Lund, and G.E. Lucier. Effects of upper respiratory tract stimuli on respiration and single respiratory neurons in the adult cat. *Exp. Neurol.* 61:245-259, 1978.

28. Storey, A.T., and P. Johnson. Laryngeal water receptors initiating apnea in the lamb. *Exp. Neurol.* 47:42-55, 1975.

29. Tomori, Z., and J.G. Widdicombe. Muscular, bronchomotor and cardiovascular reflexes elicited by mechanical stimulation of the respiratory tract. *J. Physiol.* (London) 200:25-49, 1969.

30. Trippenbach, T., and G. Kelly. Respiratory effects of cigarette smoke, dust, and histamine in newborn rabbits. *J. Appl. Physiol.* 64:837-845, 1988.

31. Wilhelm, Z., S.W. Schwarzacher, K. Anders, and D.W. Richter. Medullary respiratory neurones in rat. *Pflügers Arch.* 415 (supplement): R94, 1990.

35

Developmental Influences on Breathing Pattern by the Vagus Nerve: Some Correlations with Activities of Medullary Respiratory Neurons and Lung Mechanoreceptors

Jay P. Farber

The role of vagally mediated pulmonary afferents in the generation and maintenance of breathing rhythm has been studied extensively. Of interest has been not only the breath by breath regulation of inspiration and expiration, but also maintenance of an adequate minute ventilation through vagal input. Thus, Sullivan et al. (23) noted that vagal blockade greatly decreased breathing rate in sleeping dogs. With respect to development, it has been shown that some anesthetized and/or unanesthetized neonatal mammals (e.g., the rat [14], the cat [6, 22], and the monkey [20]) have difficulty maintaining an adequate level of ventilation after bilateral vagotomy, due to slowing of breathing. The latter observations have been interpreted to suggest that vagal input to the central nervous system in early life is particularly important for the maintenance of effective pulmonary ventilation. One possible explanation is that immaturity of peripheral chemoreceptor function in the newborn (1) could, in part, account for the greater reliance on vagal input since removal of arterial chemoreceptor and vagal information in the sleeping adult dog resulted in near cessation of breathing efforts (23).

In contrast with the preceding, loss of vagal input in newborn pigs and rabbits produces only moderate decreases in breathing rate (4, 21). Moreover, in anesthetized opossum sucklings tested at 3 to 4 weeks of age, vagal section had little effect on breathing pattern (fig. 35.1; top two sets of raw diaphragm electromyograms [EMGs]). On the other hand, vagotomy exerted more prominent effects as the animals matured (fig. 35.1; lower two sets of diaphragm EMGs). In opossums approaching weaning age (3 postnatal months), prolongation of the inspired breath (Ti) and an increase in the peak diaphragm EMG was the typical result of bilateral vagotomy. Increases in expiratory duration (Te) also occurred.

In addition to the preceding, vagally mediated effects during the inspired breath can be examined. Withdrawal of lung volume-dependent information from the vagi using end-expiratory airway occlusion causes prolongation of Ti in adult cats (3) and opossums (13). However, in opossums tested during the third to fourth postnatal week using end-expiratory occlusion applied through a tracheal cannula, no consistent effects on duration of diaphragm EMG discharge were obtained (fig. 35.2). With respect to end-expiratory occlusions in other species, human neonates, for example,

show prolongation of inspiration. In premature infants the response may be complicated by reflexes from the chest wall which apparently act to shorten the breath (17, 18, 19, 24).

The opossum, a marsupial mammal, is particularly immature at birth; it requires about 8 postnatal weeks to achieve the gross motor activity, appearance, and vagal myelination of a newborn placental mammal such as the cat or the rabbit (see 10, 12). It might be suspected that the particular immaturity of this preparation during the first few weeks of life accounts for the lack of response to elimination of vagal input. I have examined this issue using single unit recordings from respiratory neurons in the medulla as well as from vagal afferent fibers whose discharge is modulated by lung inflation.

In opossums 3–4 weeks of age, Ti values of only 100 msec are common (7). Increased age and surgical manipulation during anesthesia in open-chested animals tend to increase Ti (10). Very few action potentials per breath are generated in inspiration-related neurons in the young opossums (10). For animals between the fourth and ninth postnatal week of age, only about two spikes per breath occurred on average; this included inspiratory neurons with bulbospinal connections. While the few spikes per breath in these young animals must be in part related to the brevity of Ti, we also found that peak rates of firing were low (17 Hz on average). Other potential mechanisms to explain the paucity of discharge among inspiration-related neurons in the young opossum are high thresholds for synaptic activation and/or limited release of neurotransmitters. For any of the preceding reasons, it may take a relatively large afferent input to alter discharge of the medullary neurons. Nevertheless, there are clearly functional connections between peripheral afferents and central mechanisms because lung inflation results in apnea and other responses (see below) in suckling opossums of similar age (8, 9).

Combined with reduced responsiveness of medullary neurons, the amount of afferent traffic originating from slowly adapting airway receptors (SARs) could help account for the lack of effective vagal regulation of Ti. It is thought that slowly adapting airway receptors, which have afferent fibers in the vagus, are largely responsible for lung volume–related reductions in Ti (2, 3, 5), but if receptor activity does not reach a threshold level then the inspired

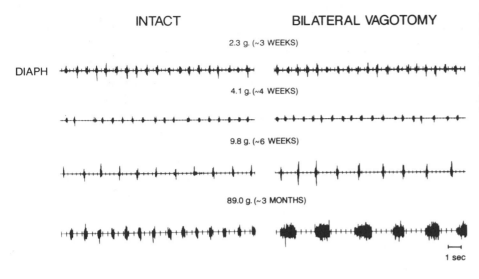

INTACT   BILATERAL VAGOTOMY

FIG. 35.1 Effects of bilateral vagotomy on breath-by-breath diaphragm EMG activity in opossums of different postnatal ages. Records of raw diaphragm EMG activity are from intact animals (*left*); and during the first minute after bilateral vagotomy (*right*). Animals were anesthetized with the thiobarbiturate derivative Inactin.

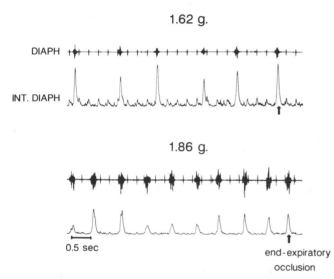

FIG. 35.2 Effects of end-expiratory airway occlusion on diaphragm EMG activity in two animals during the third postnatal week. Raw (*upper traces*) and moving average (*lower traces*) of diaphragm EMG activity are shown in each case. Animals were anesthetized as in figure 35.1 and were breathing through a tracheal cannula. During the expiratory interval before the arrow associated with each record, a piece of soft clay was pushed over the tracheal cannula. This manipulation was timed to occur after the animal had exhaled and was verified by lack of prolongation of the expired breath.

breath is unaffected (3). In the youngest opossums tested (about 3 weeks of age) rates of receptor firing for a given transpulmonary pressure were always low in comparison with older animals (12). In older sucklings, rates of SAR firing were mainly lower at high transpulmonary pressures. The transpulmonary pressure range required for normal inspiration in sucklings is unlikely to exceed 5 cm H_2O (Fisher, Farber, and Sant'Ambrogio, unpublished results). In 30-day-old animals, for example, peak firing rates of SARs might dynamically reach 40 Hz, based on 25–30%

overshoot from static values at 5 cm H_2O (12). Despite this, little phasic information from SARs reaches the medulla within the time that medullary inspiratory circuitry is active during a brief inspired breath. This phenomenon is described in figure 35.3.

In the model of figure 35.3, the top panel shows activation of the medullary inspiratory neuronal network for a 100 msec inspired breath. With this brief Ti, latencies for activating inspiratory muscles and latencies for SAR action potentials to reach the medulla become important. For a 5 g animal (30–35 days of age), path lengths from lung receptor to medulla (afferent path) and from medulla to diaphragm (efferent path) total approximately 20 mm; conduction velocity for a typical fiber in the largely unmyelinated nervous system was chosen as 0.5 m/sec based on values obtained from bulbospinal neurons in opossums of similar age (10). About two-thirds of the conduction delay to the motor endplate is caused by the 13 mm path length on the efferent side, so that there would be a delay of about 26 msec before central events (top panel) could influence contraction of the diaphragm (second panel down). Because of the delay in diaphragm contraction, lung inflation (third panel down) is also delayed relative to central inspiratory events (top panel). In the two examples (*A* and *B*) illustrated in the fourth panel down, airway receptor excitability is assumed to increase as a ramp function so that a discharge at the rate of 40 Hz occurs by the end of lung inflation. In example *A* (solid line) there is a 10 Hz discharge rate at end-expiration while in example *B* (dashed line) there is no end-expiratory firing.

Most receptor stimulation caused by inflation of the lungs will arrive and be processed by the brainstem relatively late in inspiration, and the largest effects occur when off-switching mechanisms for inspiration are already committed. The arrival in the medulla of action potentials from pulmonary afferents are illustrated in the lowest panel of figure 35.3. Note that an extra 14 msec latency needs to be added for getting afferent information from the receptor to

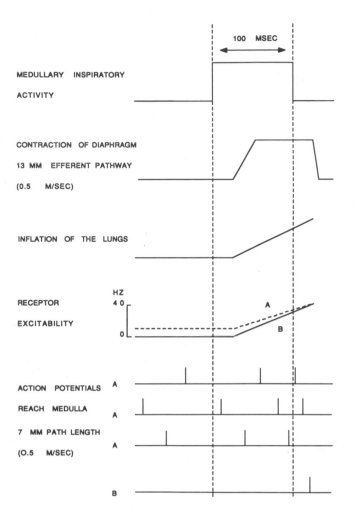

FIG. 35.3 Model showing paucity of lung volume–related airway receptor discharge during neural inspiration in a suckling opossum. Values are based on a 5-g animal with a Ti of 100 msec. In the lowest panel, intervals between action ptentials in the four traces were obtained using an integrative technique. It was assumed that a given total amount of excitation was required to fire an action potential, and that amount of excitation was reached sooner as receptor excitability (fourth panel down) was increased. (For further explanation see text.)

the medulla as the result of a 7 mm path length. Because the increase in receptor excitability is slow relative to the inspiratory event, very few action potentials can actually be produced. In example A, the end-expiratory discharge at 10 Hz would cause one spike to occur during a 100 msec inspiration without any phasic influence. Based on when the spontaneous spike occurs, the increased excitability during the inflation process may or may not produce a single extra spike within the time of neural inspiration marked by the two vertical dashed lines (note the three illustrated examples labeled A in the bottom panel). When there is no end-expiratory receptor activity, as shown in example B of the bottom panel, the increase in receptor excitability is insufficient to produce an action potential within the time of neural inspiration. A third category of response was not in-

cluded on the figure, namely, the response from a receptor with a dynamic threshold. That is, the receptor is not excited until a certain transpulmonary pressure value occurs. Even if the firing rate at the dynamic threshold is relatively high, it is clear that many cells will not fire within the time frame of central inspiratory events. It has been noted previously that dynamic thresholds can be unstable for SARs in young animals (12).

In contrast with a clear inability to influence the inspired breath, under some circumstances feedback from the lungs in young opossums can strongly influence the character of the expired breath. By the third to fourth postnatal week lung inflation causes prolongation of the expired breath and tonic activation of laryngeal dilator muscles. By the fourth to fifth postnatal week, animals also recruit expiratory muscles of the abdominal wall during lung inflation or positive pressure breathing (PPB) as well as during ventilatory chemostimulation (8, 9). These effects depend on an intact vagal innervation (8, 9). Despite the preceding, bilateral vagotomy of the very young opossum has a trivial effect on the expired breath as was shown during inspiration (fig. 35.1).

Considering the above effects with respect to events in the medulla, medullary expiratory neurons in anesthetized young opossums often had no rhythmic discharge, except during PPB (11). This contrasts with adults where rhythmic discharge was most often obtained on and off load. Most expiratory neurons obtained from young opossums were expected to be from the caudal medulla, and the lack of discharge of such cells during unloaded breathing is consistent with the lack of effects on expiratory timing accompanying vagotomy. However, other studies suggest that caudal medullary expiratory neurons do not help set respiratory timing (11); instead, they may regulate motor (e.g., abdominal muscle) output. Discharge rates of expiratory neurons were remarkably low, even during PPB in the youngest animals tested (e.g., <5 Hz at about 4 weeks of age), and rose as a function of age toward values obtained in adults (on average, 42 Hz in the caudal medulla and 33 Hz in the rostral medulla). These findings probably do not simply result from an age-related effect of anesthesia on opossums; even an unanesthetized opossum younger than about 3–4 weeks of age fails to recruit expiratory muscles with PPB (8), and the very low discharge rates of many medullary expiratory neurons could be responsible. In turn, the low rate of discharge of medullary expiratory neurons could, in part, reflect the relative paucity of input from airway receptors.

Whatever the cause of the deterioration of breathing in other neonates after bilateral vagotomy, the present studies suggest that immaturity of central and/or peripheral pathways are not sufficient to produce the effect. The clear difference between the present marsupial preparation and placental mammals is the transition from uterine to extrauterine life. How this factor could influence the response to loss of vagal input is unclear, especially considering that lung volume related vagal afferent activity may be very low in the newborn (15,16). For those species strongly affected by vagotomy, it would also be of considerable interest to know whether effects of vagotomy are similar in newborns delivered prematurely and then allowed to develop further in the *extra-utero* environment to normal term. From such data we might learn whether (1) the less-developed animal has a reduced dependence on vagal input and (2) it is the transition to extrauterine life that results in the greatest susceptibility to vagotomy.

REFERENCES

1. Blanco, C.E., G.S. Dawes, M.A. Hanson, and H.B. Mc-Cooke. The response to hypoxia of arterial chemoreceptors in fetal sheep and new-born lambs. *J. Physiol.* (London) 351:25-37, 1985.

2. Citterio, G., S. Piccoli, and E. Agostoni. Breathing pattern and diaphragm EMG after SO$_2$ in rabbit intra- or extrathoracic airways. *Resp. Physiol.* 59:169-183, 1985.

3. Clark, F.J., and C. von Euler. On the regulation of rate and depth of breathing. *J. Physiol.* (London) 222:267-295, 1972.

4. Clement, M.G., J.P. Mortola, M. Albertini, and G. Aguggini. Effects of vagotomy on respiratory mechanics in newborn and adult pigs. *J. Appl. Physiol.* 60:1992-1999, 1986.

5. Davies, A., M. Dixon, A. Callanan, A. Huszczuk, J.G. Widdicombe, and J.C.M. Wise. Lung reflexes in rabbits during pulmonary stretch receptor block by sulphur dioxide. *Resp. Physiol.* 34:83-101, 1978.

6. Duron, B., and D. Marlot. Nervous control of breathing during postnatal development in the kitten. *Sleep* 3:323-330, 1980.

7. Farber, J.P. Laryngeal effects and respiration in the suckling opossum. *Resp. Physiol.* 35:189-201, 1978.

8. Farber, J.P. Expiratory motor responses in the suckling opossum. *J. Appl. Physiol.* 54:919-925, 1983.

9. Farber, J.P. Motor responses to positive-pressure breathing in the developing opossum. *J. Appl. Physiol.* 58:1489-1495, 1985.

10. Farber, J.P. Medullary inspiratory activity during opossum development. *Am. J. Physiol.* 254:R578-R584, 1988.

11. Farber, J.P. Medullary expiratory activity during opossum development. *J. Appl. Physiol.* 66:1606-1612, 1989.

12. Farber, J.P., J.T. Fisher, and G. Sant'Ambrogio. Airway receptor activity in the developing opossum. *Am. J. Physiol.* 246:R753-R758, 1984.

13. Farber, J.P., and T.A. Marlow. Pulmonary reflexes and breathing pattern during sleep in the opossum. *Resp. Physiol.* 27:73-86, 1976.

14. Fedorko, L., E.N. Kelly, and S.J. England. Importance of vagal afferents in determining ventilation in newborn rats. *J. Appl. Physiol.* 65:1033-1039, 1988.

15. Fisher, J.T., and G. Sant'Ambrogio. Location and discharge properties of respiratory vagal afferents in the newborn dog. *Resp. Physiol.* 50:209-220, 1982.

16. Fisher, J.T., and G. Sant'Ambrogio. Airway and lung receptors and their reflex effects in the newborn. *Pediatr. Pulmonol.* 1:112-126, 1985.

17. Gerhardt, T., and E. Bancalari. Maturational changes of reflexes influencing inspiratory timing in newborns. *J. Appl. Physiol.* 50:1282-1285, 1981.

18. Gerhardt, T., and E. Bancalari. Apnea of prematurity. II. Respiratory reflexes. *Pediatrics* 74:63-66, 1984.

19. Knill, R., and A.C. Bryan. An intercostal-phrenic inhibitory reflex. *J. Appl. Physiol.* 40:352-356, 1976.

20. LaFramboise, W.A., D.E. Woodrum, and R.D. Guthrie. Influence of vagal activity on the neonatal response to hypoxemia. *Pediatric Res.* 19:903-907, 1985.

21. Mortola, J.P., J.T. Fisher, and G. Sant'Ambrogio. Vagal control of breathing pattern and respiratory mechanics in the adult and newborn rabbit. *Euro. J. Physiol.* 401:281-286, 1984.

22. Schwieler, G.H. Respiratory regulation during postnatal development in cats and rabbits, and some of its morphological substrate. *Acta Physiol. Scand.* Suppl. 304:1-123, 1968.

23. Sullivan, C.E., L.F. Kozar, E. Murphy, and E.A. Philipson. Primary role of respiratory afferents in sustaining breathing. *J. Appl. Physiol.* 45:11-17, 1978.

24. Thach, B.T., I.D. Frantz III, S.M. Adler, and H.W. Taeusch, Jr. Maturation of reflexes influencing inspiratory duration in human infants. *J. Appl. Physiol.* 45:203-211, 1978.

36

Adaptation and Acclimatization in the Hypoxic Newborn Mammal

Jacopo P. Mortola, Robin D. Gleed, and Chikako Saiki

For any given inspired O_2 concentration, the alveolar and arterial O_2 pressures are mainly determined by the ratio between oxygen consumption ($\dot{V}O_2$) and alveolar ventilation ($\dot{V}_A$). This suggests that the general mechanisms for protection of arterial PO_2 against hypoxia could consist of a reduction in $\dot{V}O_2$ (metabolic adaptation), an increase in $\dot{V}_A$ (respiratory acclimatization), or a combination of the two. This paper is a brief analysis of how the newborn mammal combines metabolic adaptation and ventilatory acclimatization to cope with acute and chronic hypoxia. It also discusses some of the short- and long-term effects of these strategies.

METABOLIC ADAPTATION TO ACUTE HYPOXIA

In adult mammals, including humans, ventilatory acclimatization is a primary response to acute hypoxia, although several species, especially small rodents, combine it with metabolic adaptation. On the other hand, most newborn mammals including the human infant, respond to acute hypoxia with a brisk drop in metabolic rate (1, 3, 6, 7). The absolute level of ventilation ($\dot{V}_E$) in hypoxia is often not much higher, and is sometimes even lower, than the normoxic value (7). Although these latter results are often interpreted as indicating an absence of the ventilatory response, in reality, because of the significant fall in metabolic rate, $\dot{V}_E/\dot{V}O_2$ is consistently increased (6, 7) and PCO_2 decreased (6). Thus, the hyperventilatory response is also occurring in the newborn.

It is not clear why in the acutely hypoxic newborn the ventilatory response is relatively less important than metabolic adaptation. The observations that $\dot{V}_E$ eventually increases after several hours of hypoxia (12) and that high levels of $\dot{V}_E$ can be sustained for many days during chronic hypercapnia (13) suggest that the respiratory pump and muscles are not a limiting factor. Neural afferent recordings have excluded the possibility of adaptation of the chemoreceptors to the hypoxic stimulus (2, 14); in addition, the common observation that the newborn's breathing rate during hypoxia is immediately increased and maintained at a steady high value seems to eliminate the possibility of a central adaptation to the peripheral inputs.

The metabolic adaptation may itself have some influence on the level of $\dot{V}_E$ during hypoxia. The decrease in metabolic rate leads to reduced CO_2 production ($\dot{V}CO_2$), which, in turn, affects $\dot{V}_E$. Since CO_2 production seems to be a key element in maintaining $\dot{V}_E$ (11), and hypercapnia mostly stimulates the depth of breathing, the hypothesis could be made that a drop in $\dot{V}CO_2$ during the hypoxia-induced hypometabolism decreases the drive to tidal volume, yielding the characteristic rapid and shallow pattern. In an attempt to test this hypothesis, kittens were exposed to 10% inspired O_2 with and without an inspiratory CO_2 load. When the inspired gas was not enriched with CO_2, the level of $\dot{V}_E$ during hypoxia was little different from the normoxic value, and the breathing pattern was rapid and shallow (fig. 36.1, open circles). However, if the animals were CO_2 loaded (by breathing 5% CO_2), exposure to hypoxia produced a sustained increase in tidal volume and $\dot{V}_E$ (fig. 36.1, filled circles). Similar levels of $\dot{V}_E$ were reached by adding the CO_2 load after the onset of hypoxia. These and similar experiments are compatible with the hypothesis that the level of CO_2, via the control of tidal volume, represents the link between the newborn's metabolic and ventilatory responses to acute hypoxia.

If the above interpretation was correct, it should follow that the hypoxia-induced hypometabolism, by reducing the drive to breathe, may allow arterial PO_2 to be lower than it would be otherwise in some cases of mild or moderate hypoxia. This possibility is presented graphically in figure 36.2. Values are average data of $\dot{V}_E$ and $\dot{V}O_2$ (both in STPD) in newborn and 50-day-old (i.e., postpuberty) rats. In normoxia, the $\dot{V}_E/\dot{V}O_2$ ratio is approximately the same at both ages. Alveolar ventilation was computed assuming a dead space equal to one-third of the normoxic tidal volume; this, according to the alveolar gas equation, would yield an alveolar PO_2 (P_AO_2) of approximately 105 mmHg. During 10% O_2 breathing, if no changes in metabolism and breathing pattern were taking place, P_AO_2 should fall to about 36 mmHg. The 50-day-old rats, by combining hyperventilation and hypometabolism, increase the $\dot{V}_E/\dot{V}O_2$ ratio to about 300% of the normoxic value, which would maintain P_AO_2 at about 60 mmHg. The newborns have a more important hypometabolic response, but little hyperventilation; the effect of the smaller increase in $\dot{V}_E/\dot{V}O_2$ is a lower P_AO_2 than in the 50-day-old, to only about 50 mmHg. In conclusion, it seems probable, on the basis of the data available, that for a similar acute hypoxic challenge of moderate level the adult should protect arterial PO_2 better than the newborn.

On the other hand, in the case of severe hypoxia or anoxia, the adult's pronounced ventilatory response should

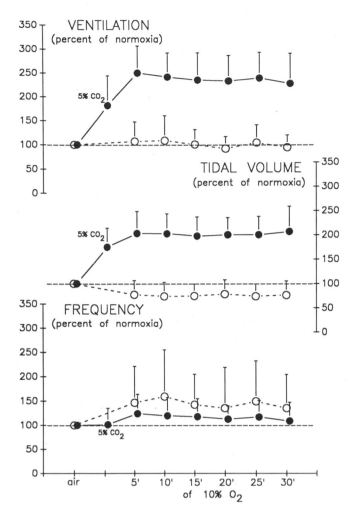

FIG. 36.1 Ventilation ($\dot{V}_E$) during normoxia and acute hypoxia in kittens a few days old. Hypoxia in normocapnic conditions (open circles, N = 14) had little effect on the absolute value of $\dot{V}_E$ and decreased tidal volume. However, hypoxia in the presence of hypercapnia (5% CO_2, filled circles, N = 20) caused a significant rise in $\dot{V}_E$, because of a rise in tidal volume. Symbols represent group averages, bars are 1 standard deviation. Fourteen kittens were subjected to both procedures.

FIG. 36.2 Average values of ventilation and oxygen consumption in newborn rats (triangles) and 50-day-old rats (squares) during normoxia (open symbols) and acute hypoxia (filled symbols). (For explanations see text.)

offer little benefit; in fact, it may be so energetically expensive as to be inefficient and hindering, rather than assisting the response to hypoxia. In these severe cases, the hypometabolic response would seem to be the only viable option. The newborn is renowned for its ability to resist extreme levels of hypoxia. In anoxia, the newborn rat drops $\dot{V}O_2$ within a few minutes to a value which is a very small fraction of the normoxic value, continuing a low frequency breathing pattern for half an hour, while the adult ceases breathing within 3–5 min.

HYPOMETABOLISM AND CHRONIC HYPOXIA

The newborn's strategy of hypoxia-induced hypometabolism has serious drawbacks when the hypoxic condition becomes chronic. The drop in energy production has profound effects not only on body growth (fig. 36.3, top) but also, because of differences in O_2 requirements and blood flow distribution, on the relative development of individual organs. In the 1-week-old newborn rat in chronic hypoxia of moderate level ($F_IO_2 = 15\%$) body weight is slightly decreased (−10%), the weight and cellular content of the lungs are little affected, and the heart is hyperplastic. In severe hypoxia ($F_IO_2 = 10\%$), body growth is drastically blunted (−50%), with hypoplasia of both lungs and heart (fig. 36.3, bottom). Whether organs with such noticeable deviations from the normal developmental pattern may still be functional and suitable for life depends not only, as one may expect, on the duration and magnitude of hypoxia, but also on the developmental period during which the hypoxic stimulus occurred. In the developing rat a critical period seems to occur during the first few days after birth. For example, most newborn rats survive well if exposed after the fourth day of age to a simulated altitude of 4500 m (PO_2 about 90 mmHg), but they die within 2–3 weeks if the exposure to hypoxia starts in the first 1–3 days after birth (fig. 36.4). Similarly, most rats born after gestation in hypoxia and raised in hypoxia die before weaning age, unless

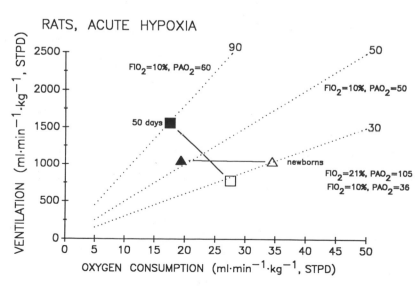

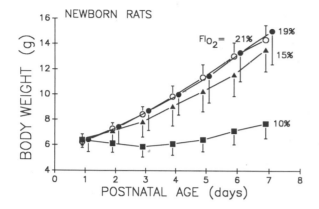

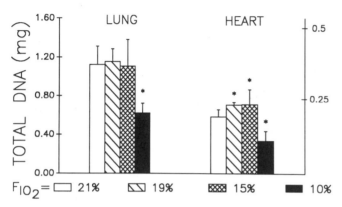

FIG. 36.3 *Top:* Body weight during the first days after birth in newborn rats exposed to various O_2 concentrations. Symbols are means of six litters of ten pups each, bars are 1 standard deviation. *Bottom:* Total DNA content in lung and heart of 7-day-old rats exposed since day 1 to various O_2 concentrations. Columns are group means, bars are standard deviations. Asterisk indicates significant difference from $F_IO_2 = 21\%$. (From 5.)

normoxia is reestablished for the first 4 days after birth. On the other hand, adult rats show no obvious problems at these degrees of hypoxia. Hence, the hypoxia-induced hypometabolism seems to more severely penalize organisms in rapid growth (which have higher O_2 requirements) and produces alterations which may be incompatible with survival.

LONG-TERM EFFECTS OF NEONATAL HYPOXIA

A question of obvious practical interest is to what extent the structural and functional changes of neonatal hypoxia can be reversed upon reestablishment of the normoxic condition. Experiments on rats maintained in 10% O_2 for 6 days after birth and returned to normoxia thereafter indicate that many alterations are still present at day 50, which in the rat corresponds to the early postpubertal period. These alterations include hypertrophy of the right heart, increased resistance of the pulmonary vasculature, and relatively larger lungs with high compliance and low resistance of the respiratory system (4, 9, 10). In normoxia, these 50-day-old rats moderately hyperventilate, with higher tidal volume and $\dot{V}_E$ (Fig. 36.5, top panel), normal $\dot{V}O_2$, and a mild noncompensated respiratory alkalosis (8, 10). In acute hypoxia, the ventilatory response is about half normal (Fig. 36.5, bottom panel). Because these differences are not seen in rats made chronically hypoxic at weaning age (i.e., at a later stage of postnatal development), it seems that the early postnatal period is very sensitive to hypoxia and that chronic hypoxia during this developmental phase is more likely to leave long-lasting alterations.

It is also of interest that some of the structural and functional changes observed in adult rats exposed to hypoxia in the neonatal period resemble characteristics of high altitude inhabitants (10). This gives support to the hypothesis that the highlander's attributes are the result of prolonged postnatal hypoxia during early development, and are not solely genetic characteristics.

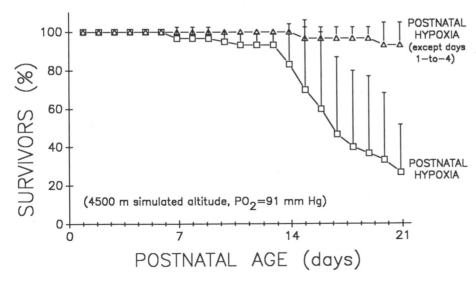

FIG. 36.4 Percent of newborn rats surviving at a simulated altitude of 4500 m. In one group of rats (squares) the hypoxic exposure started at day 1, in the other (triangles), at day 5. Symbols are averages from three litters, each litter limited to ten pups at day 1.

FIG. 36.5 *Top:* ventilation (ml/min/kg), breathing rate (breaths/min), and tidal volume (ml/kg) in 50-day-old control rats (open columns) or same-age rats exposed to 10% O_2 for 6 days after birth (filled columns) or at puberty (crosshatch columns). *Bottom:* Ventilatory response to acute hypoxia (10 min, 10% O_2) in the three groups represented at top. Columns and symbols are mean values, bars are 1 standard deviation. Asterisk indicates significant difference from the other two groups (P<0.05) (From 10.)

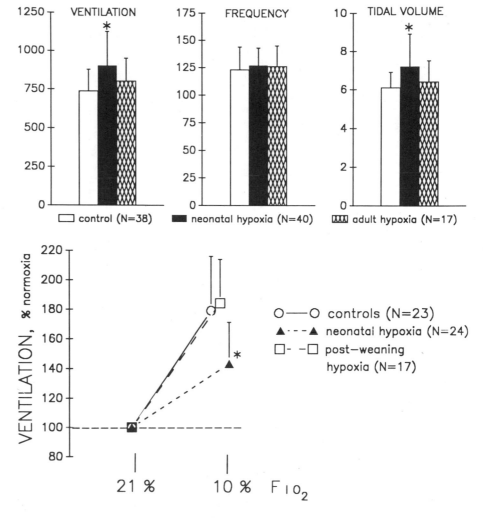

CONCLUSION

The hypometabolic response is a fundamental part of the newborn's strategy for survival against hypoxia. The much smaller ventilatory response may be the result of the drop in CO_2 production or a parallel and independently controlled phenomenon. The combination of metabolic adaptation with small ventilatory acclimatization probably does not protect arterial PO_2 as well as in the adult in the case of mild hypoxia, but it is a formidable defense against severe hypoxia or periods of anoxia. When the hypoxia persists, the hypometabolism poses a serious threat to homogeneous organ development and may have long-term functional effects or may even be incompatible with survival.

REFERENCES

1. Adolph, E.F., and P.A. Hoy. Ventilation of lungs in infants and adult rats and its responses to hypoxia. *J. Appl. Physiol.* 15:1075-1086, 1960.

2. Blanco, C.E., M.A. Hanson, P. Johnson, and H. Rigatto. Breathing pattern in kittens during hypoxia. *J. Appl. Physiol.* 56:12-17, 1984.

3. Cross, K.W., J.P.M. Tizard, and D.A.H. Trythall. The gaseous metabolism of the newborn infant breathing 15% oxygen. *Acta Paediatr.* 47:217-237, 1958.

4. Hakim, T., and J.P. Mortola. Pulmonary vascular resistance in adult rats exposed to hypoxia in the neonatal period. *Can. J. Physiol. Pharmacol.* 68:419-424, 1990.

5. Mortola, J.P., L. Xu, and A.-M. Lauzon. Body growth, lung and heart weight and DNA content in newborn rats exposed to different levels of chronic hypoxia. *Can. J. Physiol. Pharmacol.* 68:1590-1594, 1990.

6. Mortola, J.P., and R. Rezzonico. Metabolic and ventilatory rates in newborn kittens during acute hypoxia. *Resp. Physiol.* 73:55-68, 1988.

7. Mortola, J.P., R. Rezzonico, and C. Lanthier. Ventilation and oxygen consumption during acute hypoxia in newborn mammals: a comparative analysis. *Resp. Physiol.* 78:31-43, 1989.

8. Okubo, S., and J.P. Mortola. Long-term respiratory effects of neonatal hypoxia in the rat. *J. Appl. Physiol.* 64:952-958, 1988.

9. Okubo, S., and J.P. Mortola. Respiratory mechanics in adult rats hypoxic in the neonatal period. *J. Appl. Physiol.* 66:1772-1778, 1989.

10. Okubo, S., and J.P. Mortola. Control of ventilation in adult rats hypoxic in the neonatal period. *Am. J. Physiol.* 259:R836-R841, 1990.

11. Phillipson, E.A., J. Duffin, and J.D. Cooper. Critical dependence of respiratory rhythmicity on metabolic CO_2 load. *J. Appl. Physiol.* 50:45-54. 1981.

12. Piazza, T., A.-M. Lauzon, and J.P. Mortola. Time course of adaptation to hypoxia in newborn rats. *Can. J. Physiol. Pharmacol.* 66:152-158, 1988.

13. Rezzonico, R., and J.P. Mortola. Respiratory adaptation to chronic hypercapnia in newborn rats. *J. Appl. Physiol.* 67:311-315, 1989.

14. Schwieler, G.H. Respiratory regulation during postnatal development in cats and rabbits and some of its morphological substrate. *Acta Physiol. Scand.* (Suppl.) 304:1-123, 1968.

37

Birth-Related Activation of the "Substance P Gene" in Central Respiratory Neurons and Dopaminergic Disinhibition of Carotid Bodies at Birth

Hugo Lagercrantz, Torbjörn Hertzberg, Håkan Persson, Meera Srinivasan, and Yuji Yamamoto

Breathing movements are episodic and partially inhibited before birth (3). The peripheral chemoreceptors are active, but their sensitivity is set at the low-PO_2 level of the fetus, and they do not seem to contribute to the ventilatory drive before birth (2). The prenatal inhibition of breathing can be assumed to be due to the possibility that excitatory neurotransmitters stimulating breathing are not sufficiently expressed before birth and/or inhibitory neuroactive agents dominate in the fetus (9). To save oxygen consumption it might be appropriate to decrease breathing movements as well as general motor activity, particularly during asphyxia when the fetus reacts with apnea. The existence of a tonic neurochemical suppression of fetal breathing is corroborated by the finding that specific blockers of endogenous inhibitors can induce continuous breathing. For example, the cyclooxygenase inhibitor indomethacin can induce continuous breathing in the fetal sheep (10) indicating that prostaglandins are involved in the inhibition of fetal breathing. The adenosine antagonist theophylline can also stimulate fetal breathing (8), suggesting an endogenous inhibition of breathing mediated by adenosine. Increased tissue concentrations of adenosine can be expected to occur in the fetus in view of the low fetal PO_2 level (7).

We have been interested in studying the neurochemical events behind the transition of breathing control at birth. In this brief review we report the changes of substance P expression in the brainstem and dopamine turn-over in the carotid bodies that occur around birth. These two neurotransmitters are of particular interest in view of their involvement in the mediation of the hypoxic ventilatory drive.

SUBSTANCE P EXPRESSION

Substance P (SP) is probably the main neurotransmitter mediating the hypoxic ventilatory drive both at a peripheral and central level. This is based on classical criteria of a neurotransmitter such as synaptic mimicry, anatomical localization in the peripheral chemoreceptor arch, and blocking the hypoxic drive stimulation with a specific SP-antagonist (11, 12, 16). Furthermore, moderate hypoxia has been found to stimulate release of SP in the nucleus tractus solitarius (NTS), as detected with a microdialysis technique. This release was abolished by bilateral sinus nerve denervation (14).

Since SP does not seem to be involved in the control of fetal breathing movements (1), we wondered whether it could be expressed at birth and be involved in the changes in respiratory control occurring at that time. SP immunoreactivity had been analyzed both in the brainstem of the rabbit pup and in the peripheral chemoreceptors of the kitten. It was found to peak at day 7 in NTS of rabbit pups (4). The appearance of SP in the glomus cells coincided with the development of the hypoxic response (13).

We determined the ontogenesis of SP neurons in the NTS by analyzing the expression of mRNA for preprotachykinin A (PPT-A), which also encodes the SP precursor (15). The dorsal respiratory group containing the NTS, the ventral medullary surface and the striatum were dissected from rabbit fetuses one day before birth and from rabbit pups. Tissue from 4–6 pups were pooled for each age and the RNA was isolated by conventional CsCl density gradient centrifugation. mRNA for PPT-A was identified by the Northern blot technique (15).

We found that the mRNA coding for the SP precursor increased 380% in NTS from the 1-day-old rabbit pups as compared with fetuses taken out one day before expected delivery. The level decreased 25% from day 1 to 2 and even more to day 3, but it was higher than in adult controls. In the ventral surface structures of the medulla, the prenatal expression was higher than on the day of birth, but a gradual increase occurred after a few days of birth until adulthood. To study more specifically whether this increased expression of the "SP gene" was related to breathing, we compared half the litter of pups delivered by caesarean section, which were allowed to breathe for two hours, with the other half which were immediately sacrificed. We then found that the SP mRNA in the breathers was 370% of that of the nonbreathers. No difference in mRNA expression was seen in the striatum, which was used as the hybridization control. This finding suggests that SP is involved in the changes in respiratory control.

DOPAMINE TURNOVER

Physiological studies have demonstrated that there is essentially no peripheral chemoreceptor drive during normoxia in the newborn lamb, human, or rat the first day after birth (2, 5, 6). This is assumed to be due to the fact that the chemoreceptors still retain their low threshold for hypoxia (about 4 kiloPascals) from fetal life, and they adapt to the higher extrauterine PO_2 slowly.

We have investigated the neurochemical events behind this resetting. Although the occurrence of SP in the carotid bodies is very sparse in the fetus and the newborn and increases rapidly during infanthood (13), we believe that the removal of some kind of inhibition is more important for the resetting. Since dopamine has been ascribed such a modulatory role (e.g., during acclimatization), we decided to analyze dopamine turn-over in relation to chemoreceptor sensitivity in the newborn period (5).

To test the peripheral chemoreflex, non-anaesthetized rat pups (days -1 to $+7$), were exposed to hyperoxia and their ventilation was monitored with a body plethysmograph. No response was seen in the preterm rat pups, which were delivered by caesarean section, and in the <1-day-old ones. From 1 day of age onwards the peripheral chemoreflex increased significantly, up to 30% of the ventilatory drive after 3 days.

In a parallel study, dopamine turnover was assessed in the carotid bodies, by blocking the synthesis with α-methyl-p-tyrosine. The turnover rate of dopamine was found to be high during the first 6 hours after birth but then dropped markedly and was low throughout the first postnatal week. The decrease in dopamine turnover was found to precede the increased ventilatory reflex response.

To further corroborate the role of dopamine for the resetting of the peripheral chemoreceptors, another series of rat pups were allowed to be born and reared in a hypoxic environment. These animals were found to have attenuated chemoreflexes, which coincided with maintained increased turnover of carotid body dopamine. After termination of hypoxia the turnover rate decreased and the chemoreceptor reflex increased.

The interpretation of these findings is that the relatively low PO_2 in the fetus maintains a high dopamine release to suppress the sensitivity of the peripheral chemoreceptors. When PO_2 increases after birth, the relatively high dopamine release is turned off, initially leading to accumulation of dopamine before a new steady state is reached. Infants with sustained low PO_2 can retain their high dopamine turnover and low set-point for their carotid body sensitivity.

CONCLUSIONS

These studies demonstrate that the transition from the intrauterine to extrauterine environment is associated with striking changes in the expression of the "SP-gene" in the central respiration-related structures and in dopamine turnover in the carotid body. The increased expression of mRNA for SP at birth was found to be related to air breathing. The triggering mechanism of the enhanced SP expres-

sion has not yet been elucidated. Alternatively, it could be due to removal of some kind of prenatal inhibition. The decrease of dopamine turnover in the carotid bodies was related to the increase of the PO_2 level. Since the sensory neurons involved in the chemoreceptor arch are bipolar, we can speculate about the possibility that a relatively high dopamine turnover inhibits the SP expression in the brainstem before birth.

ACKNOWLEDGMENTS

Supported by the Swedish MRC 5234, Bergvall Foundation and the Heart and Lung Foundation.

REFERENCES

1. Bennet, L. Neuropeptides and respiratory control in the fetal sheep. Master's thesis, University of Auckland, Auckland, 1989.

2. Blanco, C.E., M.A. Hanson, P. Johnson, and H. Rigatto. Breathing pattern of kittens during hypoxia. *J. Appl. Physiol.* 56:12-17, 1984.

3. Bryan, A.C., G. Bowes, and J.E. Maloney. Control of breathing in the fetus and the newborn. In *Handbook of Physiology,* Section 3, vol. 2, ed. N.S. Cherniack and J.G. Widdicombe, 621-647. Baltimore, Md.: American Physiological Society, 1989.

4. Gingras, J.L., S.L. Brunner, and M.C. McNamara. Developmental characteristics of substance P immunoreactivity within specific rabbit brainstem nuclei. *Regulatory Peptides* 23:183-192, 1988.

5. Hertzberg, T., S. Hellstrom, H. Lagercrantz, J.M. Pequignot. Resetting of arterial chemoreceptors and carotid body catecholamines in the newborn rat. *J. Physiol.* 425:211-225, 1990.

6. Hertzberg, T., and H. Lagercrantz. Postnatal sensitivity of the peripheral chemoreceptors in newborn infants. *Arch Dis. Child.* 62:1238-1241, 1987.

7. Irestedt, L., I. Dahlin, T. Hertzberg, A. Sollevi, and H. Lagercrantz. Adenosine concentration in umbilical cord blood of newborn infants after vaginal delivery and cesarean section. *Pediatric Res.* 26:106-108, 1989.

8. Koos, B.J., and K. Matsuda. Fetal breathing, sleep state and cardiovascular responses to adenosine in sheep. *J. Appl. Physiol.* 68:489-495, 1990.

9. Lagercrantz, H. and M. Srinivasan. Development and function of neurotransmitter/modulator systems in the brainstem. In *Fetal and Neonatal Brainstem,* ed. M. Hanson, 1-19. Cambridge, U.K.: Cambridge University Press, 1991.

10. Murai, D.T., C.C. Lee, L.D. Wallen, and J.A. Kitterman. Denervation of peripheral chemoreceptors decreases breathing movements in fetal sheep. *J. Appl. Physiol.* 59:575-579, 1985.

11. Prabhakar, N.R., S.C. Landis, G.K. Kumar, D. Mullikan-Kilpatrick, N.S. Cherniack, and S. Leeman. Substance P and neurokinin A in the cat carotid body: Localization, exogenous effects and changes in content in response to arterial PO_2. *Brain Res.* 481:205-214, 1989.

12. Prabhakar, N.R., M. Runold, Y. Yamamoto, and H. Lagercrantz. Effect of substance P antagonist on the hypoxia-induced carotid chemoreceptor activity. *Acta Physiol. Scand.* 121:301-303, 1984.

13. Scheibner, T., D.J.C. Read, and C.E. Sullivan. Distribution of substance P-immunoreactive structures in the developing cat carotid body. *Brain Res.* 453:72-78, 1988.

14. Srinivasan, M., M. Goiny, T. Pantaleo, E. Brodin, and Y. Yamamoto. Enhanced *in vivo* release of substance P in the nucleus tractus solitarius during hypoxia in the rabbit: Role of peripheral input. *Brain Res.* 546:211-216, 1991.

15. Srinivasan, M., Y. Yamamoto, H. Persson, and H. Lagercrantz. Birth-related activation of preprotachykinin-A mRNA in the respiratory neural structures of the rabbit *Pediatric Res.* 29:369-371, 1991.

16. Yamamoto, Y., and H. Lagercrantz. Some effects of substance P on central respiratory control in rabbit pups. *Acta Physiol. Scand.* 124:449-455, 1985.

Part VIII

Behavioral Control of Breathing

38

An Overview

John Orem

Behavioral control of breathing may be reflexive, as in sneezing, coughing, vomiting, and eructation, or voluntary (or learned), as during speaking, breathholding, and playing a wind instrument. These behavioral acts involve integration of large amounts of information in the brainstem and spinal circuits that produce automatic breathing. This information is nonrespiratory in form. It is not known for any of the acts of behavioral control listed above exactly how the control occurs.

SOURCES AND SITES OF BEHAVIORAL CONTROL

The list of structures that can control brainstem and spinal respiratory neurons is long and includes structures from all levels of the neuraxis. For example, hypothalamic control occurs in relation to temperature regulation and to locomotion (8) and telencephalic structures can control breathing— a control exerted presumably in relation to emotional and volitional acts (30, 32). The central nucleus of the amygdala, the anterior cingulate gyrus, the orbital frontal cortex, and the central gray contain cells that have state-dependent respiratory relations (9, 10, 16, 35). Stimulation or inactivation of these limbic structures (15, 16, 20, 32, 36) and other telencephalic (3, 18), subcortical (4, 5), and cerebellar (19, 34) structures can influence the respiratory system.

Thus, many areas of the brain when stimulated or lesioned affect respiration. These areas project either to pontomedullary respiratory areas or to respiratory motoneurons (or their internuncial neurons) or to both. Current knowledge indicates that different behavioral respiratory acts involve different pathways. For each act (e.g., sneezing, coughing, breathholding) the level within the respiratory system (brainstem or spinal) at which non-respiratory control occurs is the first issue to resolve, and no simple generalization can be made about this. Expiratory control in sneezing, vomiting, coughing, and straining occurs, at least in part, within the brainstem (7, 11–14, 22, 31), but an expiratory effort elicited by superior laryngeal nerve stimulation does not involve brainstem expiratory neurons (17). Similarly, inspiratory control during behavioral apneas and the sniff reflex occurs through control of brainstem inspiratory neurons (6, 26, 28), but diaphragmatic activation during straining and crural diaphragmatic inhibition during swallowing does not occur by control of medullary inspiratory neurons (1, 11–14). Thus, the picture emerges that behavioral control *in toto* involves many levels of the respiratory neural network. Earlier experimental results had indicated that nonrespiratory control of respiratory muscles could be unexpectedly complex. Aminoff and Sears (2) showed that excitation of internal intercostal nerves by cortical stimulation was mediated by direct (corticospinal) connections, whereas the attendant inhibition of external intercostal nerves was mediated by indirect connections, possibly to medullary respiratory areas.

LEARNED AND VOLUNTARY CONTROL OF BREATHING

In humans, destruction of corticofugal fibers can cause loss of voluntary control of breathing (29, 30); however, corticofugal fibers comprise both corticobulbar and corticospinal fibers, and it is uncertain whether one or both mediate voluntary control. Patients without automatic breathing because of lesions of the brainstem ponto-medullary respiratory areas can breathe rhythmically and adequately while awake (presumably via functional corticospinal pathways) but have reduced maximal voluntary efforts (30). If voluntary control occurs via corticospinal connections, then selective destruction of the latter should produce a syndrome of automatic breathing without voluntary control. The patient of Meyer and Herndon (21) is cited by some authors (23) as evidence of this. This patient, however, who had a bilateral infarction of the pyramids and adjoining ventromedial medulla, had pharyngeal and hypoglossal motor paralysis as well as a loss of voluntary control. This deficit indicates that corticobulbar as well as corticospinal pathways were interrupted by the infarction.

In contrast to this uncertainty over the mechanism of voluntary control in humans, there is evidence that a learned respiratory response in cats occurs through behavioral control of medullary respiratory neurons (26, 28). The learned response is a rapid termination of inspiration when a conditioning stimulus is presented (figure 38.1). Orem and his colleagues showed that medullary inspiratory neurons are inactivated when inspiration is inhibited in this task (figure 38.2), or, precisely, that high η^2-valued inspiratory cells are inactivated, because some low η^2-valued inspiratory cells are, paradoxically, activated during the response (24, 26, see note 1). Thus behavioral control for this task occurs apparently within the brainstem (which does not mean that it cannot occur also at spinal levels).

DIAPHRAGM

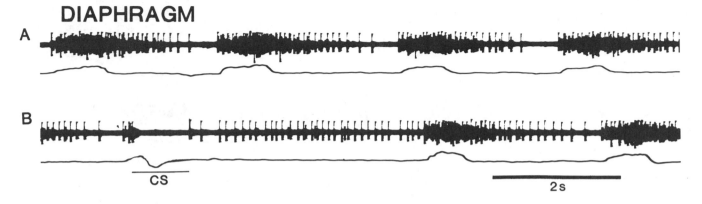

FIG. 38.1 Diaphragmatic activity during behavioral inhibition of inspiration. (*A*) Activity of the diaphragm (top trace) and intratracheal pressure (bottom trace) during eupnea. (*B*) Activity during the behavioral response. CS, conditioning response. (From 26)

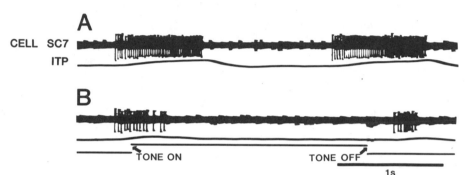

FIG. 38.2 Inactivation of a high η^2-valued ventral group inspiratory neuron when inspiration is stopped behaviorally. (*A*) Control record showing two inspirations: action potentials of the neuron (*top trace*), and intratracheal pressure (ITP) with negative pressures (inspiration) signaled by upward deflections (*bottom trace*). (*B*) Inactivation of the cell in response to the conditioning stimulus (tone). (Adapted from 27)

The inhibition of inspiration in Orem's experiments was obtained with a paradigm involving both escape or avoidance and operant characteristics. A conditioning stimulus was presented at the onset of an inspiration and failure to stop that inspiration within 0.5 sec was "punished" by presentation of an aerosol of ammonium hydroxide (smelling salts). This is an easy and atraumatic task for the cat, and the evidence already presented indicates that in this case, control of the respiratory system occurs within the respiratory centers of the medulla. The source and mechanism of this control are, however, unknown. The respiratory centers of the medulla contain various cell types presumed to be interrelated to produce rhythmogenesis (33). The termination and suppression of inspiration is a complex event produced, it is believed, by the inhibitory action of at least three cell types: late-onset inspiratory cells, decrementing (or postinspiratory) and augmenting expiratory cells. Interestingly, late-onset inspiratory cells and augmenting expiratory cells do not mediate the behavioral inhibition because they too are inhibited during the response (25, 27); there has been no report on the behavior of postinspiratory cells during this response. Orem (24, 26) has demonstrated that some respiratory cells are activated intensely during the behavioral apnea and therefore may cause the inactivation of the high η^2-valued inspiratory cells (figure 38.3). These cells are of all types (inspiratory, expiratory, phase-

spanning) but they share the common feature of having low η^2-valued activity.

Thus, inspiratory cells with high η^2-valued activity are inhibited when inspiration is stopped behaviorally, and the respiratory cells that are activated during the behavioral inhibition have low η^2-valued activity. These results have been interpreted (24, 26) as follows: the high η^2-valued cells are parts of the oscillator or are rigidly controlled by it, and their inactivation during the behavioral task reflects inactivation of the oscillator. The low η^2-valued cells that are activated when inspiration is stopped behaviorally act as an interface between behavioral influences and the respiratory oscillator (figure 38.4).

CONCLUSION

Behavioral control of breathing comprises many subjects related by the common feature that they all involve control of the respiratory system for functions other than gas exchange. Essentially all parts of the brain outside the primary respiratory areas in the pons and medulla are involved potentially in some kind of behavioral control of breathing; therefore, the need is to understand which parts are related to what kind of behavioral control and how this control occurs. The relevance of this issue of nonrespiratory control extends beyond the mechanisms of the various kinds of control: indeed, it may be that understanding of differences

CELL C10

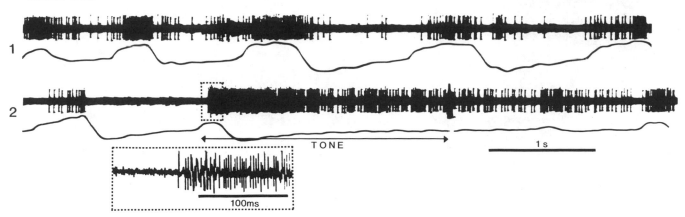

FIG. 38.3 Activity of an inspiratory cell that was activated when inspiration was inhibited behaviorally. The upper traces (1) show spontaneous activity of this cell. Note the breath-to-breath variability in the activity, giving it a low η^2-value (0.30). In the lower traces (2), the conditioning stimulus (tone) is presented and inspiration is stopped behaviorally. The cell is activated intensely during the behavioral inhibition. The insert below shows a high-speed trace of the onset of the activation and corresponds to the boxed area shown in 2. (From 24)

FIG. 38.4 A schema showing hypothesized relationships among nonrespiratory inputs and respiratory pre-motor and motor neurons.

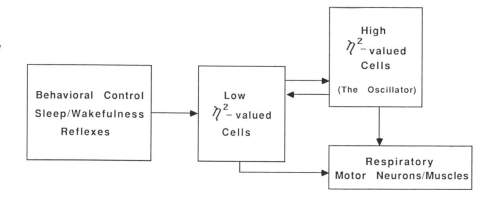

in breathing during sleep and wakefulness lies in understanding the influences of behavioral control in wakefulness (and perhaps in REM sleep) and the absence of these influences in sleep.

ACKNOWLEDGMENT

Experiments of J. Orem were supported by NHLBI grant HL21257.

NOTE

1. η^2 is an estimate of the magnitude of an experimental effect. Its value can vary from 1.0 to 0.0, indicating, respectively, that all or none of the variability in a set of data is accounted for by the treatment variable.

η^2 is the proportion of the total variance (σ_t^2) of the neuronal activity over a series of breaths that is made up by the variance across fractions of the respiratory cycle (σ_m^2)

$$\eta^2 = \sigma_m^2/\sigma_t^2 = \sigma_m^2/(\sigma_m^2 + \sigma^2) \qquad \text{(Equation 1)}$$

where σ^2 is the variance within fractions of the respiratory cycle and σ_m^2 is the variance of means across fractions.

The two terms in equation 1, σ_m^2 and σ^2, have the following meanings when applied to an analysis of the degree of respiratory activity. The term σ_m^2 represents the variance of activity across fractions of the respiratory cycle. This term depends on the range of means across fractions of the cycle and also on how the means are dispersed over this range, σ_m^2 increases both as the range increases and as the values of the individual means tend to be distributed at the end points of the range (one-half at one end of the range; the other half at the other end). For example, σ_m^2 would be large in the case of a respiratory neuron that discharged at a uniformly high rate for half of the respiratory cycle and then was silent for the other half of the cycle. In contrast, σ_m^2 decreases as the degree and duration of modulation of activity within the respiratory cycle decreases.

The other term in equation 1, σ^2, is the variance within treatment groups. In the case of respiratory activity, it is the variance across breaths within the individual fractions of the respiratory cycle. If the activity of a cell varies greatly from breath to breath, σ^2 will be large. Conversely, as the consistency of the discharge pattern across breaths increases, σ^2 will decrease and η^2 will increase. Therefore, $1/\sigma^2$ is an index of the consistency of the respiratory activity of a cell.

REFERENCES

1. Altschuler, S., R.O. Davies, J.T. Boyle, and A.I. Pack. Control of the crural diaphragm during gastroesophageal reflexes. In: *Respiratory muscles and their neuromotor control*, ed. G.C. Sieck, S.C. Gandevia, and W.E. Cameron, 449-453. New York: Alan R. Liss, 1987.

2. Aminoff, M.J., and T.A. Sears. Spinal integration of segmental, cortical and breathing inputs to thoracic respiratory motoneurons. *J. Physiol.* (London) 215:557-575, 1971.

3. Bassal, M., and A.L. Bianchi. Effects de la stimulation des structures nerveuses centrales sur les activities respiratoires efferentes chez le chat. I. Responses a la stimulation corticale. *J. Physiol.* (Paris) 77:741-757, 1981.

4. Bassal, M., and A.L. Bianchi. Effects de la stimulation des structures nerveuses centrales sur les activities respiratoires efferentes chez le chat. II. Responses a la stimulation sous corticale. *J. Physiol.* (Paris) 77:759-777, 1981.

5. Bassal, M., A.L. Bianchi, and M. Dussardier. Effects de la stimulation des structures nerveuses centrales sur l'activite des neurones respiratoires chez le chat. *J. Physiol.* (Paris) 77:779-795, 1981.

6. Batsel, H.L., and A.J. Lines, Jr. Bulbar respiratory neurons participating in the sniff reflex in the cat. *Exp. Neurol.* 39:467-481, 1973.

7. Batsel, H.L., and A.J. Lines, Jr. Neural mechanisms of sneeze. *Am. J. Physiol.* 229:770-776, 1975.

8. Eldridge, F.L., D.E. Millhorn, and T.G. Waldrop. Exercise hyperpnea and locomotion: Parallel activation from the hypothalmus. *Science* 211:844-846, 1981.

9. Frysinger, R.C., and R.M. Harper. Cardiac and respiratory relationships with neural discharge in the anterior cingulate cortex during sleep-waking states. *Exp. Neurol.* 94:247-263, 1986.

10. Frysinger, R.C., J. Zhang, and R.M. Harper. Cardiovascular and respiratory relationships with neuronal discharge in the central nucleus of the amygdala during sleep-waking states. *Sleep* 11:317-322, 1988.

11. Fukuda, H., and K. Fukai. Postural change and straining induced by distension of the rectum, vagina and urinary bladder of decerebrate dogs. *Brain Res.* 380:276-286, 1986.

12. Fukuda, H., and K. Fukai. Location of the reflex centre for straining elicited by activation of pelvic afferent fibers of decerebrate dogs. *Brain Res.* 380:287-296, 1986.

13. Fukuda, H., and K. Fukai. Ascending and descending pathways of reflex straining in the dog. *Jpn. J. Physiol.* 36:905-920, 1986.

14. Fukuda, H., and K. Fukai. Discharges of bulbar respiratory neurons during rhythmic straining evoked by activation of pelvic afferent fibers in dogs. *Brain Res.* 449:157-166, 1988.

15. Harper, R.M., and R.C. Frysinger. Suprapontine mechanisms underlying cardiorespiratory regulation: Implications for the Sudden Infant Death Syndrome. In *Sudden Infant Death Syndrome: Risk factors and basic mechanisms,* ed. R.M. Harper and H.J. Hoffman, 399-414. New York: PMA Publishing, 1988.

16. Harper, R.M., R.C. Frysinger, R.R. Terreberry, J.D. Marks, J.X. Zhang, and H.F. Ni. Suprapontine control of respiratory activity. In *Respiratory Muscles and Their Neuromotor Control,* ed. G.C. Sieck, S.C. Gandevia, and W.E. Cameron, 93-101. New York: Alan R. Liss, 1987.

17. Jodkowski, J.S. and A.J. Berger. Influences from laryngeal afferents on expiratory bulbospinal neurons and motoneurons. *J. Appl. Physiol.* 64:1337-1345, 1988.

18. Lipski, J., A. Bektas, and R. Porter. Short latency input to phrenic motoneurons from sensorimotor cortex in the cat. *Exp. Brain Res.* 61:280-290, 1986.

19. Lutherer, L.O., and J.L. Williams. Stimulating fastigial nucleus pressor region elicits patterned respiratory responses. *Am. J. Physiol.* 250:R418-R426, 1986.

20. Marks, J.D., R.C. Frysinger, and R.M. Harper. State-dependent respiratory depression elicited by stimulation of the orbital frontal cortex. *Exp. Neurol.* 95:714-729, 1987.

21. Meyer, J.S., and R.M. Herndon. Bilateral infarction of the pyramidal tract in man. *Neurology* 12:637-642, 1962.

22. Miller, A.D., L.K. Tan, and I. Suzuki. Control of abdominal and expiratory intercostal muscle activity during vomiting: Role of ventral respiratory group expiratory neurons. *J. Neurophysiol.* 57:1854-1866, 1987.

23. Mitchell, R.A., and A.J. Berger. Neural regulation of respiration. *Am. Rev. Resp. Dis.* 111:206-224, 1975.

24. Orem, J. Inspiratory neurons that are activated when inspiration is inhibited behaviorally. *Neurosci. Lett.* 83:282-286, 1987.

25. Orem, J. The activity of late inspiratory cells during the behavioral inhibition of inspiration. *Brain Res.* 458:224-230, 1988.

26. Orem, J. Behavioral inspiratory inhibition: Inactivated and activated respiratory cells. *J. Neurophysiol.* 62:1069-1078, 1989.

27. Orem, J., and E.G. Brooks. The activity of retrofacial expiratory cells during behavioral respiratory responses and active expiration. *Brain Res.* 374:409-412, 1986.

28. Orem, J., and A. Netick. Behavioral control of breathing in the cat. *Brain Res.* 366:238-253, 1986.

29. Plum, F. Neurological integration of behavioral and metabolic control of breathing. In *Breathing: Hering-Breuer Centenary Symposium,* ed. R. Porter, 159-175. London: Churchill, 1970.

30. Plum, F. and R.J. Leigh. Abnormalities of central mechanisms. In *Regulation of Breathing,* Part 2, ed. T.F. Hornbein, 989-1067. New York: Marcel Dekker, 1981.

31. Price, W.H., and H.L. Batsel. Respiratory neurons participating in sneeze and in response to resistance to expiration. *Exp. Neurol.* 29:554-570, 1970.

32. Reis, D.J., and P.R. McHugh. Hypoxia as a cause of bradycardia during amygdala stimulation in monkey. *J. Appl. Physiol.* 214:601-610, 1968.

33. Richter, D.W., D. Ballantyne, and J.E. Remmers. How is the respiratory rhythm generated? A model. *NIPS* 1:109-112, 1986.

34. Williams, J.L., P.J. Robinson, and L.O. Lutherer. Inhibitory effects of cerebellar lesions on respiration in the spontaneously breathing, anesthetized cat. *Brain Res.* 399:224-231, 1986.

35. Zhang, J., R.M. Harper, and R.C. Frysinger. Respiratory modulation of neuronal discharge in the central nucleus of the amygdala during sleep and waking states. *Exp. Neurol.* 91:193-207, 1986.

36. Zhang, J.-X., R.M. Harper, and H. Ni. Cryogenic blockade of the central nucleus of the amygdala attenuates aversively conditioned blood pressure and respiratory responses. *Brain Res.* 386:136-145, 1986.

39

Respiratory Responses to Prolonged Central or Peripheral Hypoxia

G.E. Bisgard, M.J.A. Engwall, W.Z. Niu, L. Daristotle and J. Pizarro

Prolonged hypoxic exposure results in a time-dependent ventilatory increase that is termed ventilatory acclimatization to hypoxia (VAH). This process requires up to one week to complete in humans and a much shorter period in animals (7). The process is completed sufficiently in four hours in the goat to make the goat a convenient animal model to investigate mechanisms of ventilatory control in hypoxic states including VAH (2, 4, 11, 18).

We have examined the separate roles of carotid body (CB) and central nervous system (CNS) hypoxia on ventilatory control in the awake goat using isolated perfusion of the CB (1, 2, 4). Our previous work has primarily been aimed at defining the role of the CB in VAH and has shown that VAH can be produced by isolating the hypoxic stimulation to the CB while maintaining systemic arterial (and CNS) normoxia. These studies have tended to downplay an important role for CNS mechanisms in VAH. Nevertheless, CNS effects are known to occur during hypoxia, including changes in neurotransmitter metabolism (17), brain blood flow (13) and acid-base balance (9). Thus, it would seem likely that there would be numerous possible influences on ventilatory control during hypoxic exposure. Therefore, we sought to determine the changes in ventilation during a 4-hour period of CNS hypoxia. In addition, we wished to examine the influence of prolonged CNS hypoxia on ventilatory stimuli confined primarily to the CNS or to the CB. To achieve these goals we measured the time course of ventilatory variables over a 4-hour hour period of systemic (CNS) hypoxia while maintaining CB normoxia. Before and after the hypoxic exposure we assessed the central chemoreceptor sensitivity by carrying out CO_2 response curves. We also assessed the CNS response to acute CB stimulation before and after prolonged hypoxia to determine if the central respiratory controller would respond differently to a peripheral chemoreceptor stimulation after prolonged hypoxia. These studies differ from CB denervation experiments in that the CB is intact and functioning and providing some tonic ventilatory drive. In addition, because these animals were not subjected to chronic chemoreceptor denervation, no compensatory mechanisms for the chronic hypoventilation that follows CB denervation were present.

METHODS

Five adult goats were trained to accept a respiratory mask and stand quietly in a stanchion. Prior to experiments the animals were surgically prepared for perfusion of the CB by an extracorporeal circuit. The procedures used to prepare the animals have been described and validated previously (2, 4). Briefly, under general anesthesia (Halothane, nitrous oxide, and oxygen) sterile surgery was carried out to remove one CB and ligate the occipital artery on one side. This became the brain perfusion side. On the opposite side arteries above the CB were ligated and cannulas were inserted in the common carotid artery and jugular vein for later access to venous blood for perfusion (jugular vein) and to the CB circulation (carotid artery). Animals were given 40,000 units of heparin daily to maintain patency of the cannulas. At least 1 week was allowed to pass before a CB perfusion study was undertaken.

In preparation for a perfusion, an airtight muzzle mask was placed on the animal and attached to a low-resistance, one-way breathing valve (Hans Rudolf). Inspired gases were mixed with a bank of rotameters for room air, O_2, N_2 and CO_2 and delivered to the goat via large-bore flexible tubing. A pneumotachograph (Fleisch, T-2) was used to measure inspiratory flows, which were integrated to give inspired tidal volumes. A CO_2 analyzer was used to measure inspired and expired CO_2 levels from a port in the face mask. A polygraph was used to record respiratory variables and the analog signal output was digitized and analyzed using a computer to calculate breathing frequency and inspired minute ventilation ($\dot{V}_I$). Variables were stored on disk for later analysis.

The perfusion circuit drew blood from the right atrium via the jugular vein and circulated it through an oxygenator/ heat exchanger and filter and then into the carotid artery for perfusion of the CB. Blood gases perfusing the CB were controlled by the gas mixtures used to ventilate the oxygenator. This blood perfused the CB and surrounding local tissue and venous outflow from the area returned via the normal venous drainage. Systemic arterial blood and CB perfusion blood were analyzed for PO_2, PCO_2, and pH on a Radiometer system (BMS3-MK2) with blood values tonometer and temperature corrected.

Before instituting a study of systemic hypoxia, evidence for extracarotid body peripheral chemoreceptor sensitivity (aortic bodies) was tested by injecting 50 μg/kg NaCN iv while perfusing the CB from a blood reservoir containing no NaCN. Five goats that were selected for study exhibited an average increase in $\dot{V}_I$ following NaCN injection of less than 1 l/min from a control mean of 7.5 l/min (not significantly changed, P>0.5). One goat was eliminated because of an increase in V_T of 30% following iv cyanide.

The protocol for the studies was to first carry out a CO_2 ventilatory response curve to assess central chemosensitivity. Inspired CO_2 was increased in steps during room air inhalation while the CB was maintained normoxic and normocapnic. Ventilatory variables were measured at each step. The response to CB hypoxia ($P_{cb}O_2$ 40 torr) was then measured during systemic arterial (CNS) normoxia and normocapnia. After return to CB and systemic normoxia a control measurement of ventilatory and blood variables was made and systemic hypoxia was instituted by reducing inspired O_2, with frequent measurement of arterial blood gases until reaching a P_aO_2 of near 40 torr. The CB was maintained normoxic and normocapnic during the entire 4-hour systemic hypoxic exposure. Ventilatory variables were measured frequently throughout the period of hypoxic exposure. Upon return to normoxic conditions, the ventilatory responses to CB hypoxia and systemic hypercapnia were again measured as done prior to the 4-hour hypoxic exposure.

RESULTS

Systemic arterial and CB blood values before and after 4 hours of systemic hypoxia are shown in table 39.1. There were no differences between these conditions. During systemic hypoxia arterial and CB blood values were maintained within the following limits respectively: $P_aO_2 = 40 \pm 5$ torr, $P_aCO_2 = 34 \pm 3$ torr, pH = 7.40 ± 0.05; $P_{cb}O_2 = 90$–120 torr, $P_{cb}CO_2 = 34 \pm 2$ torr, pH = 7.40 ± 0.05 torr. Decreases in systemic P_aCO_2 were prevented by adding CO_2 to the inspired air.

Ventilation was increased by systemic hypoxia, primarily due to an increase in respiratory frequency (fig. 39.1). The increase in $\dot{V}_I$ and f was slow to develop, reaching a peak after 30 min of systemic hypoxia. By 1 hour of hypoxia, $\dot{V}_I$ decreased somewhat and then remained stable for the remaining period of hypoxia.

The response to acute CB hypoxia during systemic normoxia was unchanged by 4 hours of systemic hypoxia (table 39.1). Similarly the central chemoreceptor response to hypercapnia during CB normoxia/normocapnia was not affected by exposure of the systemic circulation to 4 hours of hypoxia (table 39.2).

DISCUSSION

Ventilatory stimulation by hypoxia in the presence of only the tonic level of peripheral chemoreceptor input typical of

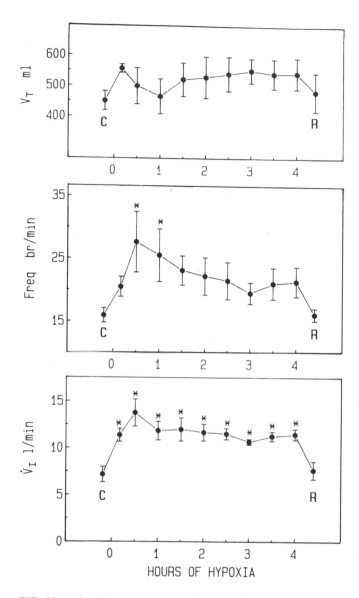

FIG. 39.1 Ventilatory response to 4 hours of systemic isocapnic arterial hypoxia during maintenance of carotid body normoxia and normocapnia. C, control value with systemic normoxia; R, return to systemic arterial normoxia. Asterisk indicates significant difference from the control value, C (P<0.05).

normoxic-normocapnic conditions may be unexpected. However, the findings of the present studies are consistent with previous experiments demonstrating hypoxic tachypnea in awake CB denervated animals (12), in CB perfused goats subjected to acute systemic hypoxia (6), and in goats exposed to CO (5). What we have documented for the first time are the time-dependent characteristics of the response. No one has systematically evaluated this response over a 4-hour period. Previous studies of CB denervated animals found mild hyperventilation in ponies and goats during hypoxic exposure that was very much attenuated compared to animals with intact CBs (10, 11, 18). Ventilatory pattern was not determined in those studies.

Table 39.1. Blood Gases and pH, Ventilation, and Ventilatory Response to Carotid Body (CB) Hypoxia

| | Before Systemic Hypoxia | | After Systemic Hypoxia[1] | |
	Control	CB Hypoxia	Control	CB Hypoxia
Systemic Arterial				
pH	7.42±0.01[2]	7.41±0.02	7.41±0.02	7.40±0.01
PCO_2[3]	34.3 ±1.1	34.0 ±0.4	33.1 ±1.7	34.0 ±1.0
PO_2	96.2 ±2.4	120.0 ±2.0	89.3 ±3.3	119.8 ±4.1
Carotid Body				
pH	7.43±0.01	7.44±0.01	7.43±0.01	7.42±0.01
PCO_2	34.2 ±0.5	32.9 ±0.2	32.5 ±1.0	34.3 ±0.9
PO_2	100.8 ±5.6	37.4 ±1.0	100.5 ±4.8	37.7 ±0.4
V_I (l/min)	7.04±0.76	21.97±1.68	7.24±1.68	23.32±3.09

[1] After 4 hours of systemic (CNS) hypoxia.
[2] Values are means ± SEM.
[3] Values of PCO_2 and PO_2 are given in torr.

Table 39.2. Ventilatory Response to Change in Systemic Arterial PCO_2[1]

| | Systemic Hypoxia | |
	Before	After
Slope[2]	1.87±0.26[3]	1.68±0.18
$PaCO_2$ Intercept[4]	29.2 ±0.45	29.1 ±1.8
R^2	0.84±0.02	0.92±0.03

[1] During carotid body normoxia/normocapnia.
[2] In l • min^{-1} • torr^{-1}.
[3] Values are means ± SEM.
[4] In torr.

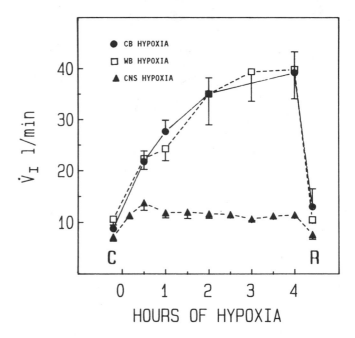

FIG. 39.2 Ventilatory response to isocapnic hypoxia (PO_2 near 40 torr) applied to the whole intact animal (WB) or to the carotid body (CB) while systemic (and CNS) normoxia is maintained, and to the systemic circulation (CNS) while the CB is maintained normoxic and normocapnic. (Data for CB from 2, for WB from 8.)

Previous studies of VAH in goats specifically examining the first 4 hours of either whole-animal hypoxia or isolated CB hypoxia with systemic normoxia have shown further time-dependent increasing $\dot{V}_I$ due to an increase in V_T and f (2, 8). The time course and magnitude of increasing $\dot{V}_I$ are strikingly different from the present findings, in which no further time-dependent increase in $\dot{V}_I$ was present after 30 min of hypoxia (fig. 39.2).

The present data do not indicate the persistent hyperventilation on return to normoxic conditions that is well documented following VAH in intact animals (7, 8, 10, 11, 18). Recent studies suggest that persistent hyperventilation following acclimatization requires the presence of hypocapnic alkalosis, that is, it does not occur in goats if systemic isocapnia is maintained during exposure to hypoxia (2, 8). The present studies are consistent with this: there was no hypocapnic alkalosis and no persistent hyperventilation.

Ventilatory responses to peripheral chemoreceptor stimulation were unchanged in the goats after 4 hours of CNS hypoxia. This is in marked contrast to findings in animals with whole-body or isolated CB hypoxia where the ventilatory response to acute hypoxia was significantly increased after 4 hours of hypoxic exposure (2, 8). This has been a controversial topic in human studies, although a recent experiment found increasing hypoxic ventilatory gain during VAH in human subjects (20). Increased hypoxic gain of the CB appears to be an important component of acclimatization in cats and goats (3, 16, 19).

The ventilatory response to CO_2 (CBs remaining normoxic and normocapnic) was not changed by exposure to 4 hours of systemic (CNS) hypoxia. A shift to the left of the CO_2 ventilatory response curve is a consistent finding following VAH in humans and animals, including the goat (7, 8, 14, 15). Increased CO_2 sensitivity or slope of the curve is also frequently reported (7). Since neither occurred in the present studies, we suggest that isocapnic brain hypoxia alone does not produce a change in the central chemoreceptor sensitivity.

We conclude that sustained CNS hypoxia produces a mild hyperventilation in the goat. However, in animals where carotid bodies are made hypoxic, either with or without CNS hypoxia, the increase is very different with respect to magnitude and time-dependency of increased ventilation. This suggests little role for CNS mechanisms in acclimatization to hypoxia in the goat.

ACKNOWLEDGMENTS

The authors thank Gordon Johnson and Margaret Rankin for their excellent technical assistance. This work was supported by NIH grants HL 15473 and HL 07654.

REFERENCES

1. Bisgard, G.E., M.A. Busch, L. Daristotle, A.D. Berssenbrugge, and H.V. Forster. Carotid body hypercapnia does not elicit ventilatory acclimatization in goats. *Resp. Physiol.* 65:113-125, 1986.

2. Bisgard, G.E., M.A. Busch, and H.V. Forster. Ventilatory acclimatization to hypoxia is not dependent on cerebral hypocapnic alkalosis. *J. Appl. Physiol.* 60:1011-1015, 1986.

3. Bisgard, G.E., W. Niu, and M.J.A. Engwall. Increased gain of carotid chemoreceptors in the goat during prolonged hypoxia. *FASEB J.* 4:A716, 1990.

4. Busch, M., G. E. Bisgard, and H. V. Forster. Ventilatory acclimatization to hypoxia is not dependent on arterial hypoxemia. *J. Appl. Physiol.* 58:1874-1880, 1985.

5. Chapman, R.W., T.V. Santiago, and N.H. Edelman. Brain hypoxia and control of breathing: Neuromechanical control. *J. Appl. Physiol.* 49:496-507, 1980.

6. Daristotle, L., M. Engwall, N. Weizhen, and G. Bisgard. Ventilatory responses to acute changes in systemic O_2 in awake goats. *FASEB J.* 3:A401, 1989

7. Dempsey J.A., and H.V. Forster. Mediation of ventilatory adaptations. *Physiol. Rev.* 62:262-346, 1982.

8. Engwall, M.J.A., and G.E. Bisgard. Ventilatory responses to chemoreceptor stimulation after hypoxic acclimatization in awake goats. *J. Appl. Physiol.* 69:1236-1243, 1990.

9. Fencl, V., R.A. Gabel, and D. Wolfe. Composition of cerebral fluids in goats adapted to high altitude. *J. Appl. Physiol.* 47:508-513, 1979.

10. Forster, H.V., G.E. Bisgard, B. Rassmussen, J.A. Orr, D.D. Buss, and M. Manohar. Ventilatory control in peripheral chemoreceptor denervated ponies during chronic hypoxemia. *J. Appl. Physiol.* 41:878-885, 1976.

11. Forster, H.V., G.E. Bisgard, and J.P. Klein. Effect of peripheral chemoreceptor denervation on acclimatization of goats during hypoxia. *J. Appl. Physiol.* 50:392-398, 1981.

12. Gautier, H., and M. Bonora. Possible alterations in brain monoamine metabolism during hypoxia-induced tachypnea in cats. *J. Appl. Physiol.* 49:769-777, 1980.

13. Krasney, J.A., K. Miki, K. McAndrews, G. Hajduczok, and D. Curran-Everett. Peripheral circulatory responses to 96 h of hypoxia in conscious sinoaortic-denervated sheep. *Am. J. Physiol.* 250:R868-R874, 1986.

14. Lahiri, S., N.S. Cherniack, N.H. Edelman, and P. Fishman. Regulation of respiration in goat and its adaptation to chronic and life-long hypoxia. *Resp. Physiol.* 12:388-403, 1971.

15. Mines, A.H., and S.C. Sorensen. Ventilatory responses of awake normal goats during acute and chronic hypoxia. *J. Appl. Physiol.* 28:826-831, 1970.

16. Nielsen, A.M., G.E. Bisgard, and E.H. Vidruk. Carotid chemoreceptor activity during acute and sustained hypoxia in goats. *J. Appl. Physiol.* 65:1796-1802, 1988.

17. Olson, E.B., Jr., E.H. Vidruk, D.R. McCrimmon, and J.A. Dempsey. Monoamine neurotransmitter metabolism during acclimatization to hypoxia in rats. *Resp. Physiol.* 54:79-96, 1983.

18. Smith, C.A., G.E. Bisgard, A.M. Nielsen, L. Daristotle, N.A. Kressin, H.V. Forster, and J.A. Dempsey. Carotid bodies are required for ventilatory acclimatization to moderate and severe chronic hypoxemia. *J. Appl. Physiol.* 60:2403-2410, 1986.

19. Vizek, M., C.K. Pickett, and J.V. Weil. Increased carotid body hypoxic sensitivity during acclimatization to hypobaric hypoxia. *J. Appl. Physiol.* 63:2403-2410, 1987.

20. White, D.P., K. Gleeson, C.K. Pickett, A.M. Rannels, A. Cymerman, and J.V. Weil. Altitude acclimatization: Influence on periodic breathing and chemoresponsiveness during sleep. *J. Appl. Physiol.* 63:401-412, 1987.

40

Forebrain-Brainstem Interactions Modulating Respiratory Patterning

Ronald M. Harper, C.A. Richard, H. Ni, J.X. Zhang, and R.K. Harper

Although it is essential to consider the microenvironment of the local brainstem and spinal cord circuitry which allows for cyclic activation of respiratory musculature, the reality of moment-by-moment respiratory control in behaving animals is that a large number of external forces modify respiratory patterning. The "external influences" include mechanisms which can affect breathing on a breath-by-breath or an overall basis, and are brought into play when the organism encounters particular needs. These needs include such actions as dissipation of excess heat through air exchange, or enhancing oxygen capacity in anticipation of exercise.

On occasion, organisms need to recruit respiratory musculature in a transient and massive manner. Apneusis associated with sudden fright is one such occasion; this action recruits the respiratory musculature to greatly enhance thoracic pressure. The resulting increased pressure, together with enhanced tension on abdominal and upper airway musculature, provides the potential for an extreme locomotor escape response without collapse of the thoracic cage. Vocalization represents a "transient" use of the respiratory musculature which can be intermittently recruited and, on occasion, massively so with sounds of distress. The complexities of vocalization suggest extremely complex integration of a sophisticated motor control system which incorporates respiratory musculature.

Respiratory pattern changes observed during different sleep states far exceed the variation expected from metabolic demands necessitated by physiological alterations within each sleep condition. A portion of the state-related patterning changes requires the integrity of forebrain structures, since quiet sleep, a condition characterized by prolonged inspiratory times and extreme cycle regularity, depends on the presence of rostral structures for its maintenance, and possibly its initiation (20). Sleep states can, under some conditions, paralyze large regions of the respiratory musculature, such as the thoracic wall and abdominal muscles in rapid eye movement (REM) sleep. A portion of the respiratory variability during REM sleep, and the upper airway and skeletal respiratory muscle atonia during that state, can be maintained with caudal brain regions (11). However, some of the respiratory patterning influences during REM sleep may be mediated by rostral brain/midbrain interactions. This potential derives from the demonstration of pronounced, and reciprocal, projections from rostral sites to midbrain areas that appear to be "pre-motor" to respiratory musculature; these rostral and midbrain sites have the potential to modify particular influences on respiration, including temperature and affect. The median preoptic region, for example, an area which plays a critical role in temperature regulation and sleep maintenance, projects heavily to the midbrain periaqueductal gray (PAG), regions of which are pre-motor to laryngeal and abdominal wall expiratory muscles (18). The central nucleus of the amygdala (ACE), a rostral brain region mediating components of conditioned negative affect, and a region with a demonstrated potential to modify respiratory patterns, has projections to the PAG as well (10).

The need for understanding that rostral brain mechanisms exert profound influences on respiratory patterning becomes critical when assessing effects of particular pharmacologic agents, such as cocaine. Cocaine has a particular affinity for regions of mesolimbic structures; local administration to the medial frontal cortex or the nucleus accumbens elicits extensive locomotor activity, and the rewarding aspects of this drug appear to be at least partially dependent on dopaminergic neurons projecting from the ventral tegmental area to this region. Intravenous or cerebral intraventricular cocaine delivery results in an extreme tachypnea, accompanied by apneustic efforts (6).

The nucleus accumbens and the medial frontal cortex contain cells with a number of common features, including common neurotransmitters, functional relationships, and common developmental origins (8). The group of structures including the ACE, bed nucleus of the stria terminalis (BNST), the nucleus accumbens (NA), and the medial frontal cortex (MFC), have been termed the "extended amygdala" by Heimer (8) to designate a commonality of structure and function for that region.

A number of these rostral structures including the ACE (22) and BNST (21) contain neurons which discharge on a breath-by-breath basis with the respiratory cycle. In all these structures, neuronal discharge relationships of both tonic and breath-by-breath dependencies are state-specific; i.e., discharge dependencies occur strongly in some states, and disappear or are greatly reduced in others. Local cocaine administration into particular regions of the ACE profoundly modifies neural discharge patterns; both overall rate and breath-by-breath dependencies are greatly modified (15,24).

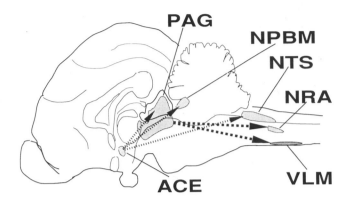

FIG. 40.1 Several rostral structures can impinge on brainstem respiratory regions, including the amygdala central nucleus (ACE), which projects to the periaqueductal gray (PAG), parabrachial pons (NPBM), and the nucleus of the solitary tract (NTS); the PAG, in turn, projects to the nucleus retroambiguus (NRA), a pre-motor nucleus to the upper airway musculature, and to the ventrolateral medulla (VLM).

The means by which these far-rostral structures can modify respiratory patterning can be readily understood from the destiny of their descending projections to the brainstem "respiratory" regions, and reciprocal projections from these structures. Both the ACE and NA project heavily to the parabrachial pons. The nucleus parabrachialis medialis and Kölliker-Fuse nuclei of the parabrachial pons have long been implicated in respiratory phase switching (1) and contain neurons which discharge on a breath-by-breath basis in a state-related manner (19). The portion of the "extended amygdala" represented by the ACE, BNST, and medial frontal cortex may provide some of the excitation to the parabrachial pons and contribute to phase switching.

These regions exact an additional and perhaps more profound influence on upper airway musculature through a pathway which is not commonly recognized in the neurophysiologic literature. Structures within the "extended amygdala", particularly the ACE, project heavily to medial lateral regions of the PAG (10; fig. 40.1). Regions within the PAG, in turn, project to the nucleus retroambiguus, which supplies laryngeal motor neurons and motor neurons of the abdominal musculature (9).

We examined discharge properties of neurons in PAG and rostral brain sites during different sleep-waking states to determine respiratory dependencies. Bundles of microwires were stereotaxically placed into the ACE, anterior cingulate cortex, and PAG of cats, together with electrodes to assess electrophysiological indices of state. After surgery, the drug-free animals were allowed to sleep unrestrained, and cross-correlation histograms were calculated between inspiratory onset and neuronal discharge; linear regressions were also calculated between respiratory rate and cell discharge rates.

The NA-ACE-PAG-retroambiguus pathway has the potential to greatly modify upper airway and abdominal res-

piratory action. The abdominal musculature tends to be active during the expiratory phase of the respiratory cycle. Thus, instances of forced expiration, respiratory braking, and increasing upper airway resistance are contenders for particular control by this pathway. We examined neural discharge in a portion of the PAG in freely moving animals and related this discharge to respiratory patterns during different sleep states. A substantial percentage (20%) of PAG neurons discharged on an overall tonic or phasic relationship to the respiratory cycle (14; fig 40.2). The percentage of cells phasically related to the respiratory cycle is similar to that found for the ACE and larger than that for the anterior cingulate cortex (2, 22).

The finding of respiratory neurons in the PAG may be related to the description of "vocalization" neurons in the PAG (12,13). In the monkey, Larson (13) found a set of neurons which became active, particularly during the inspiratory phase of the vocalization effort. The cells were slightly more lateral than the region surveyed in the cat, but that region also receives major projections from the "extended amygdala."

Respiratory rates are extremely dependent on temperature (16). Intravenous or cerebral ventricular cocaine delivery results in extreme tachypnea and a rise in core and brain temperature (fig. 40.3); this may result partially from a direct cocaine action on hypothalamic sites in the forebrain, or by indirect effects, such as vasoconstriction, which may alter heat dissipation. Localized microinjection of cocaine into the ACE, however, causes a decline in temperature (4) while tachypnea remains, suggesting a direct, but perhaps temperature independent, action of cocaine on the ACE.

Regions within the extended amygdala have been associated with mechanisms of reward (17) and with mechanisms of negative affect. Thus, cold blockade of the ACE can abolish a negative conditioned respiratory response (23). Apparently both positive and negative affect may be partially mediated by regions of this extended amygdala. These structures also exhibit influences on respiratory patterning: trains of electrical stimulation to the ACE elicit sustained inspiration (3, 5) and single pulse stimulation can entrain inspiratory onset (7). Finally, the evidence that neurons in both the ACE and BNST exhibit discharge dependency on a breath-by-breath basis to the respiratory cycle is substantial (21, 22).

The collection of stimulation, lesion, recording, and pharmacologic evidence suggests a role for the extended amygdala in exerting respiratory patterning influences, partially through projections to the PAG and to the parabrachial pons, and partially through projections to the nucleus of the solitary tract. The role of rostral amygdala regions in respiratory patterning may be largely one of providing excitatory or inhibitory tone to phase switching, since the region is heavily involved in aspects of affect and defensive reactions, behaviors which strongly recruit respiratory muscles.

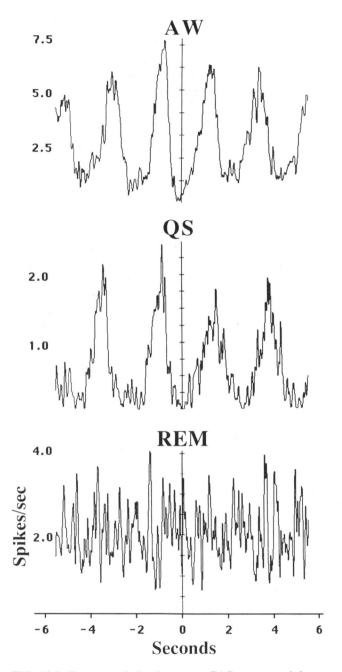

FIG. 40.2 Cross-correlation between a PAG neuron and the respiratory cycle. A subset of PAG neurons discharges phasically with the respiratory cycle, but that relationship is state dependent; here the relationship disintegrates during rapid eye movement (REM) sleep. AW, awake; QS, quiet sleep. (Reproduced from *Brain Research*, ref. 14).

The need for recruitment of respiratory musculature for defensive reactions stems from incorporation of breathing muscles in escape behavior. We speculate that the respiratory-related involvement of structures associated with reward behavior relates to the generalized somatomotor tone increase which accompanies excitement of reinforcement. The respiratory musculature constitutes one

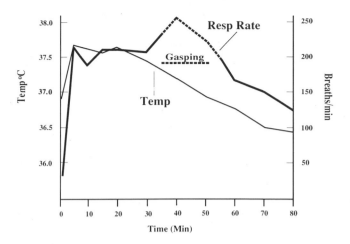

FIG. 40.3 Response to intravenous or cerebral ventricular cocaine administration. A 2.5-mg ventricular dose raises brain and core temperature and induces an extreme tachypnea; a portion of the respiratory response may result from the elevated temperature. (From 6).

component of the somatomotor system and is closely integrated with generalized motor functions. Thus, actions which recruit overall locomotor responses also recruit respiratory muscles.

ACKNOWLEDGMENTS

This work was supported by DAO4913; the basic sleep studies were supported by NIH HL22418.

REFERENCES

1. Cohen, M.I. Switching of the respiratory phases and evoked phrenic responses produced by rostral pontine electrical stimulation. *J. Physiol.* (London) 136:444-446, 1982.
2. Frysinger, R.C., and R.M. Harper. Cardiac and respiratory relationships with neural discharge in the anterior cingulate cortex during sleep-waking states. *Exp. Neurol.* 94:247-263, 1986.
3. Frysinger, R.C., R.M. Harper, and R.J. Hackel. State-dependent cardiac and respiratory changes associated with complex partial epilepsy. In *Fundamental mechanisms of human brain function.* ed. J. Engel, Jr., G.A. Ojemann, H.O. Lüders, and P.D. Williamson, 219-226. New York: Raven Press, 1987.
4. Harper, R.K., R.R. Terreberry, R.C. Frysinger, C.A. Richard, and R.M. Harper. Respiratory patterning following cocaine administration to the central nucleus of the amygdala. *Soc. Neurosci. Abstr.* 16:1063, 1990.
5. Harper, R.M., R.C. Frysinger, J.D. Marks, J.X. Zhang, and R.D. Frostig. Forebrain control of the respiratory rhythm. In *Neurogenesis of central respiratory rhythm.* ed. A.L. Bianchi, and M. Denavit-Saubie, 91-98. Boston: MTP Press, 1985.
6. Harper, R.M., R.R. Terreberry, C.A. Richard, and R.K. Harper. Upper airway and diaphragmatic muscle activity following acute cocaine administration. *Pharmacol. Biochem. Behav.* In press, 1991.

7. Harper, R.M., R.C. Frysinger, R.B. Trelease, and J.D. Marks. State-dependent alteration of respiratory cycle timing by stimulation of the central nucleus of the amygdala. *Brain Res.* 306:1-8, 1984.

8. Heimer, L., J. de Olmos, G.F. Alheid, and L. Zaborszky. "Perestroika" in the basal forebrain: Opening the border between neurology and psychiatry. *Prog. Brain Res.* In press, 1991.

9. Holstege, G. Anatomical study of the final common pathway for vocalization in the cat. *J. Comp. Neurol.* 284:242-252, 1989.

10. Hopkins, D.A., and G. Holstege. Amygdaloid projections to the mesencephalon, pons and medulla oblongata in the cat. *Exp. Brain Res.* 32:529-547, 1978.

11. Jouvet, M. Paradoxical sleep: A study of its nature and mechanisms. In *Progress in brain research,* vol. 18, ed. K. Alert, C. Bally, and J.P. Schade, 20-62. Amsterdam: Elsevier, 1965.

12. Jurgens, U., and R. Pratt. Role of the periaqueductal grey in vocal expression of emotion. *Brain Res.* 167:367-378, 1979.

13. Larson, C.R. On the relation of PAG neurons to laryngeal and respiratory muscles during vocalization in the monkey. *Brain Res.* In press, 1991.

14. Ni, H., J. Zhang, and R.M. Harper. Respiratory-related discharge of periaqueductal gray neurons during sleep-waking states. *Brain Res.* 511:319-325, 1990.

15. Ni, H., J.X. Zhang, R.K. Harper, and R.M. Harper. Amygdala central nucleus neuronal discharge following localized microinjection of cocaine. *Soc. Neurosci. Abstr.* 16:582, 1990.

16. Parmeggiani, P.L., A. Azzaroni, D. Cevolani, and G. Ferrari. Responses of anterior hypothalamic-preoptic neurons to direct thermal stimulation during wakefulness and sleep. *Brain Res.* 269:382-385, 1983.

17. Roberts, D.C.S., G.F. Koob, P. Klonoff, and H.C. Fibiger. Extinction and recovery of cocaine self-administration following 6-hydroxydopamine lesions of the nucleus accumbens. *Pharmacol. Biochem. Behav.* 12:781-787, 1980.

18. Shipley, M.T., M. Ennis, T.A. Rizvi, and M.M. Behbehani. Forebrain inputs to the midbrain periaqueductal grey: Evidence for discrete longitudinally organized input columns. In *The midbrain periaqueductal grey matter: Functional, anatomical and immunohistochemical organization,* ed. A. Depaulis and R. Bandler. New York: Plenum Publishing Corp. (NATO ASI Series). In press, 1991.

19. Sieck, G.C., and R.M. Harper. Discharge of neurons in the parabrachial pons related to the cardiac cycle: Changes during different sleep-waking states. *Brain Res.* 199:385-399, 1980.

20. Sterman, M.B., and C.D. Clemente. Forebrain mechanisms for the onset of sleep. In *Basic sleep mechanisms,* ed. O. Petre-Quadens and J.D. Schlag, 83-97. New York: Academic Press, 1974.

21. Terreberry, R.R., R.C. Frysinger, H. Ni, M. Oguri, and R.M. Harper. Respiratory-related neuronal discharge in the BNST during sleep-waking states in the drug-free cat. *Soc. Neurosci. Abstr.* 13:1638, 1987.

22. Zhang, J.X., R.M. Harper, and R.C. Frysinger. Respiratory modulation of neuronal discharge in the central nucleus of the amygdala during sleep and waking states. *Exp. Neurol.* 91:193-207, 1986.

23. Zhang, J.X., R.M. Harper, and H. Ni. Cryogenic blockade of the central nucleus of the amygdala attenuates aversively conditioned blood pressure and respiratory responses. *Brain Res.* 386:136-145, 1986.

24. Zhang, J.X., H. Ni, and R.M. Harper. Discharge dependencies of amygdala central nucleus neurons to the cardiac and respiratory cycle following local cocaine administration. *Soc. Neurosci. Abstr.* 16:559, 1990.

41

State-Dependent Variations in Medullary Respiratory-Related Discharge Patterns

Fat-Chun T. Chang

Modifications of brainstem respiratory neuronal activities by physiological and behavioral changes have been investigated in unanesthetized preparations by several laboratories. These studies showed that brainstem respiratory neuronal activities can undergo marked variations not only with sleep/wakefulness cycles (22, 28, 30, 31, 35, 38, 40), but also with changes in cardiovascular activities (14, 36), and during the execution of a conditioned inspiratory inhibition response (23–25, 29). More recently, a freely behaving guinea pig model system has been developed in my laboratory (8, 9). This model system permits hours of stable recording from single medullary respiratory neurons in freely behaving animals and is therefore ideally suited for a variety of investigations into the extent of state and behavior-dependent variations in medullary respiratory neuronal discharge patterns.

When instrumented, the model system allows concurrent recordings of electrocorticogram (ECoG), medullary respiratory-related unit activity (RRU; see 9 for details), and diaphragmatic electromyogram (see 8 for details). RRU activities are recorded from either the Bötzinger Complex (BOT) or nucleus para-ambiguus (NpA). A miniature, skull-mounted microdrive is used to isolate units. Once isolated, the unit can frequently be recorded for several hours with only occasional movement-induced signal amplitude diminution. Prior to each recording session, the animal is acclimated in a noise-attenuated Faraday recording chamber (W×L×H = 30×30×40 cm). Aside from the minor restriction imposed by the signal transmission tether, the animal is free to move about within the perimeter of the recording cage.

As a technical note, there are two major differences between the present model system and that used by Orem and Dement (26). First, the unanesthetized preparations used in this study are allowed to freely behave. Orem and Dement's technique requires the use of a head restraint, thereby limiting the animal's movement during single unit recording. Second, the fine-wire recording electrode used in this study is implanted stereotaxically at the time of surgery under pentobarbital anesthesia. Once the respiratory neuron of interest is identified, the tip of the fine wire is raised by approximately 100 µm to avoid unnecessary damage to the target area during the postoperative recovery period. The chronically implanted microdrive provides high-resolution forward-reverse mobility so the electrode can be maneu-

vered to reach the target neuron at the time of unit isolation and recording. It has long been known that barbiturate causes a dose-dependent depression and inactivation of selected populations of ponto-medullary respiratory neurons (1, 3, 4, 15, 34). Thus, the present approach has the distinct disadvantage of not sampling bulbar RRUs that are inactivated by pentobarbital during surgery. In Orem and Dement's procedure, electrode placement and unit isolation are performed while the animals are awake, therefore significantly increasing the probability of encountering medullary RRUs that may be overlooked in the present study. The impact of this sampling problem on some of the experimental outcomes in this and Orem's (e.g., 24) studies will be discussed later.

Modification of medullary respiratory unit activities by sleep and wakefulness influences has been studied by Orem and co-workers (22, 28, 30, 31). This chapter focuses on the modulation of discharge patterns of BOT and NpA neurons by sleep, wakefulness, volitional behavior, phonation, barbiturate anesthesia, and a variety of reflex-mediated respiratory behaviors.

PATTERN VARIATIONS DURING BEHAVING STATES

In awake, behaving states, the temporal attributes (cycle duration, burst duration, and spike frequency) of BOT and NpA unit activities rarely adhere to a fixed, immutable pattern for any extended period of time. They frequently exhibit marked variations with discrete changes during ongoing behaviors such as postural modification, phonation, deglutition, sniffing, alerting/startle reflexes, and so on. RRU patterns of reasonably stationary periodicity and invariant temporal attributes can be observed only during sleep, and on occasions when the animal assumes a motionless, resting posture.

One of the most intriguing phenomenon is the varying degrees of fluctuation in the within-burst frequency modulation. Examples of this phenomena are illustrated in figure 41.1. In the left panel, a BOT (expiratory) unit is seen to undergo a "reversal" of its normally incrementing pattern, and to discharge, for a burst or two, in what appears to be a decrementing pattern. More perplexing is the degree of fluctuation of an NpA inspiratory unit (fig. 41.1; right panel). This unit normally discharges in a decrementing fashion. Here, within the span of a few seconds, the unit

FIG. 41.1 "Spontaneous" fluctuations in the within-burst frequency modulation of an expiratory BOT unit (*left*) and an inspiratory NpA unit (*right*). Single unit events delineated by the arrows are enlarged at the bottom of each figure panel. The emergence of these events are typically not accompanied by any recognizable behavioral correlates or changes in states of arousal. Signal trace description: ECoG, electrocorticogram; Unit, respiratory-related unit activity (left panel, BOT expiratory unit; right panel, NpA inspiratory unit); DEMG, diaphragmatic electromyogram; Int. DEMG, integrated diaphragmatic electromyogram ($\tau = 20$ msec). Time calibration: 2 sec. Voltage calibrations: ECoG, 295 μV; Unit, 135 μV; DEMG, 1.42 mV.

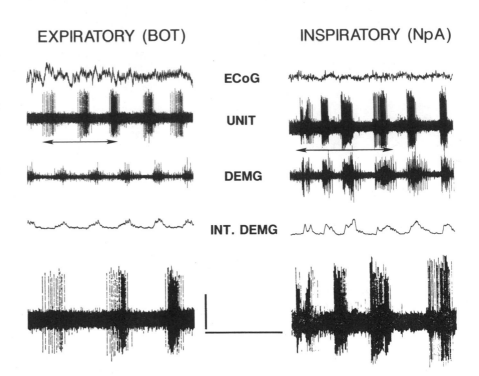

WITHIN-BURST SPIKE FREQUENCY MODULATION

EXPIRATORY (BOT) INSPIRATORY (NpA)

ECoG

UNIT

DEMG

INT. DEMG

repeatedly shows a transient decay in its within-burst spike frequency. Typically, these events are not accompanied by any recognizable behavioral correlates or changes in states of arousal.

When startled or aroused by a novel stimulus, guinea pigs often emit a rather high-pitch sound (which resembles purring or chirping) as well as engage in a series of sniffing/exploratory repertories. With the exception of Orem's (24) electrophysiographic depiction of changes in an inspiratory unit (dorsal respiratory group, DRG) during phonation (meowing), sniffing reflex, and purring in the cat, virtually nothing is known about the medullary RRU activity correlates during such behavioral repertories as phonation, sniffing, and others.

As electrophysiograms on the left side of figure 41.2 show, the generation of the chirping sound (15–30 Hz) in guinea pigs is associated with activation of only NpA inspiratory neurons, while BOT expiratory cells are completely quiescent. Whether the quiescence represents inhibition or removal of excitation is not known. However, since chirping is a volitional act, the source of entrainment of NpA oscillations, and that which causes the "inhibition" of BOT cells, are probably both derived from the forebrain and/or other suprasegmental areas.

In comparison to chirping, sniffing oscillations occur at a much lower frequency (5–8 Hz). As indicated in the electrophysiograms on the right side of figure 41.2, maintenance of the sniffing reflex is associated with activation of both BOT and NpA neurons. Holst and Kolb (16) were the first to suggest a correlation between sniffing activities and theta rhythm. To further examine the involvement of theta

rhythm in sniffing reflexes, segments of ECoG data temporally corresponding to periods of sniffing reflex were subjected to power spectral analysis (10). Noteworthy was the consistent emergence of a 6–10 Hz power spectral component (corresponding to theta rhythm) during sniffing. This finding suggests, therefore, that the maintenance of sniffing rhythm probably involves the entrainment of medullary RRUs by the theta rhythm.

A period of apnea occurs in most, if not all, cases subsequent to an augmented inspiration (sigh). This response pattern is depicted in the left panels of figure 41.3. The most interesting attributes of this response profile are a sustained BOT discharge throughout the apneic episode and a complete inhibition of NpA inspiratory activity. Note also that the diaphragmatic activity disappears entirely during the apneic episodes. An augmented breath (or sigh) increases the pulmonary compliance and functional residual capacity, opens up the partially collapsed alveolar units, and averts the development of atelectasis (39). Thus, the apnea seen in this case is probably due to an altered chemoreceptor input as the blood O_2 tension is transiently elevated shortly after a deep breath. The contributions of vagally mediated stretch and/or irritant receptor input to the development of apnea are probably minor in view of the latency (mean $\pm$ SEM = 3.8 $\pm$ 0.8 sec; n=47) of the apneic response.

BOT neurons have been shown to exert a powerful inhibitory influence over inspiratory neurons in the DRG, NpA, and phrenic motor nuclei (2, 12, 18–20), and an excitatory/facilitatory modulation of the expiratory neurons in nucleus retroambigualis (12). It is very likely, therefore,

PURRING
CHIRPING

SNIFFING REFLEX

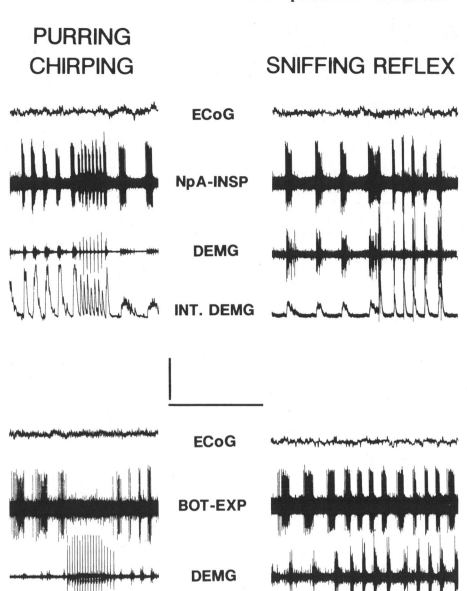

ECoG

NpA-INSP

DEMG

INT. DEMG

ECoG

BOT-EXP

DEMG

INT. DEMG

FIG. 41.2 Electrophysiological correlates of respiratory-related activities during emission of a high-pitch sound (purring, chirping; *left*) and sniffing (*right*). Inspiratory (NpA-INSP) activities are shown in the top two panels, and expiratory (BOT-EXP) activities are in the bottom two panels. Signal trace descriptions same as in figure 41.1. Time calibration: 1.5 sec. Voltage calibrations: ECoG, 295 μV; Unit 205 μV; DEMG, 5.65 mV (chirping; *left*) and 1.35 mV (sniffing; *right*).

that the inhibition of NpA activity during sigh-induced apnea is caused by the sustained BOT discharge. However, the nature of synaptic events that cause the BOT neuron to show a sustained discharge is unknown.

Postural modifications do not always modify respiration. Those that do exert an influence on the respiratory pattern all seem to have the quality of being able to interfere with ventilatory movements. Back scratching with a hindlimb, as illustrated in the right panels of figure 41.3, is a case in point. Changes in BOT and NpA activities during back scratching are very similar to the apneic response mentioned previously. Namely, there is inhibition of NpA and activation (albeit to a lesser extent than the sustained discharge seen in sigh-induced apnea) of BOT neurons. Parenthetically, the activity profile during the act of deglu-

tition is very similar to that of back scratching. A major difference is the relatively shorter periods of BOT activation and NpA inhibition.

Another intriguing feature can be seen upon closer examination of the NpA recording in the right upper panel of figure 41.3. There is a conspicuous elevation in the background activity level throughout the duration of NpA inhibition. This phenomenon is not only observed during back scratching but also during a variety of other behaviors such as radical turning behavior, deglutition, and defecation. The following can be inferred from this phenomenon. First, judging from the signal strength of the background activity, the unit(s) must be located in close proximity to the NpA unit under observation. These background cells may belong to the same category of inspiratory neurons reported by

APNEIC RESPONSES

FOLLOWING AUGMENTED INSPIRATION (SIGH)   DURING BEHAVIOR (BACK SCRATCHING)

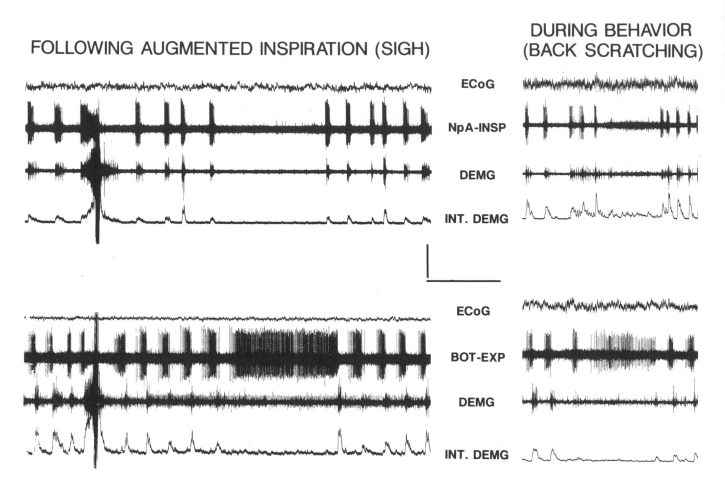

FIG. 41.3 Electrophysiographic depictions of respiratory-related unit activities during episodes of apneic responses after an augmented breath (sigh; left top and bottom panels) and during back scratching (right top and bottom panels). Signal trace descriptions same as in figure 41.1. Time calibration: 2 sec. Voltage calibrations: ECoG, 295 μV; Unit, 225 μV; DEMG, 3.42 mV.

Orem (23, 24) that are activated during conditioned inspiratory inhibition. The reason these units are not regularly encountered in this study may be attributed to the technical difference between the present model system and that of Orem mentioned above. Second, the phenomenon of background activity elevation can only be seen during inspiratory inhibition by volitional behaviors. Little, if any, change in the inspiratory background activity level can be detected during sigh-induced inspiratory inhibition (see fig. 41.3). These observations imply that the recruitment of background unit activities during inspiratory inhibition may involve synaptic input extrinsic to the network such as those of forebrain origin.

STATES OF AROUSAL

Generally speaking, transitions from behaving or resting states to slow-wave sleep (SWS) invariably cause an increase in RRU burst and cycle durations, and a decrease in

RRU spike frequencies. Referencing against the resting state (100%), the discharge rate can increase to as much as 200% in active behaving states and decrease to 30% during SWS. Incidentally, it should be pointed out that Orem and co-workers (31) have identified a small population of medullary RRUs that actually showed an increase in discharge rate during NREM sleep. Again, sampling problems mentioned above may very well account for this discrepancy.

BARBITURATE ANESTHESIA

Pentobarbital-induced changes in medullary RRU activity patterns (5), as demonstrated in figures 41.4–6, are even more striking. In this experiment, the effects of pentobarbital (35 mg/kg; ip) on medullary RRUs are evaluated before, throughout the course of, and during recovery from anesthesia in chronically instrumented guinea pigs. The most remarkable development following pentobarbital is a state of progressive bradypnea accompanied by a multitude

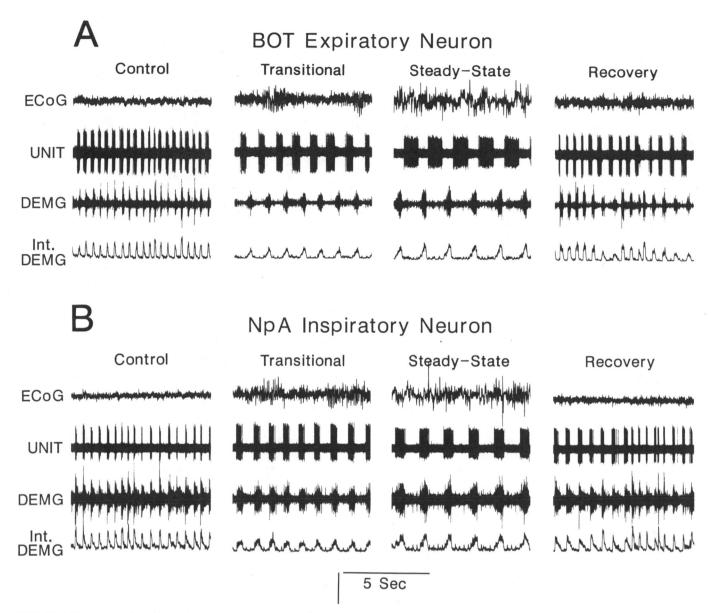

FIG. 41.4 Representative electrophysiograms of ECoG, RRU, and DEMG activities across control (wakefulness), transitional (2.32 min post-pentobarbital), steady-state (4.07 hr post-pentobarbital), and recovery (1.00 hr after the first attempt to right) periods. Response profile of a BOT expiratory unit (*top panel*). Response pattern of an NpA inspiratory neuron (*bottom panel*). Signal trace descriptions same as in figure 41.1. Experimental conditions: control (awake, resting) state; transitional period (period during which the animal loses consciousness; duration = 3.5 ± 1.6 min); steady-state period (anesthetized state; duration = 8.6 ± 2.1 hr), and recovery period (conscious, behaving states; a fixed duration of 2 hr). Voltage calibrations: ECoG, 290 μV; Unit, 235 μV; DEMG, 1.12 mV.

of profound changes in the amplitudes and temporal attributes of RRU (BOT and NpA units), DEMG and ECoG activities. As the anesthetic effect progresses, both BOT and NpA unit activities undergo remarkable transformations from a behavioral and state-dependent wakefulness pattern to a profile characterized by a significantly augmented RRU cycle duration (BOT, 340%; NpA 380%; fig. 41.5, upper left panel) and burst duration (BOT, 500%; NpA 350%; fig. 41.5, upper right panel). A somewhat paradoxical observation is a notable increase in the RRU spike frequencies (BOT, 170%; NpA 140%) during anesthesia. This "anomalous" phenomenon is currently being investi-

gated with the use of pentobarbital-anesthetized guinea pigs. Briefly, a segment of trachea between the larynx and the bronchial bifurcation point is replaced by a "T-shaped" shunt assembly so the path for air exchange can be switched to either the larynx or the shunt. Preliminary results suggest that the NpA discharge frequency is significantly reduced when the air flow is diverted from the larynx to the shunt. These findings suggest that the increased RRU spike frequency may be attributed, at least in part, to the hypercapnic burden (33, 37) which results from pentobarbital-induced inactivation of medullary neurons that normally control the airway muscles (27).

FIG. 41.5 Effects of pentobarbital on RRU cycle duration (top left panel), burst duration (top right panel), T_{Burst}/T_{Cycle} ratio (bottom left panel), and spike frequency (bottom right panel). Each epoch data point represents the average response magnitude of a specific activity category across all the BOT (n = 10; dash line) units or all the NpA (n = 9; solid line) cells. Abscissa labels: C, control (awake, resting) state; T1, S1, R1; T2, S2, R2; and T3, S3, R3 are the beginning, the midpoint, and the end of the transitional period, the steady-state period, and the recovery period, respectively. Each activity category is normalized and expressed as percent of control (quiet wakefulness). Error bars = SEM.

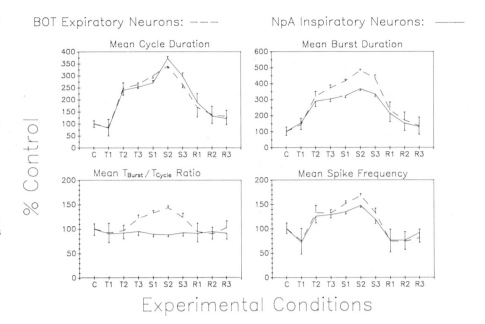

Figure 41.6 (*A* and *B*) is a summary of interspike-interval (ISI) analyses of pentobarbital-induced alterations of the within-burst spike frequency modulation patterns of a BOT (fig. 41.6*A*) and an NpA (fig. 41.6*B*) unit. For the BOT unit, the increase in spike frequency is represented in the ISI histograms as an increase in the number of spike events per bin. The profile of the ISI distribution remains essentially uni-modal, and the central tendency of the ISI distribution is unaltered throughout the course of anesthesia. Changes in the NpA unit are more complex. The most noticeable transformation in NpA histograms is the reorganization of a uni-modal ISI distribution to that of a dispersed, multimodal profile during the steady-state period of pentobarbital anesthesia. There is also a shift of the central tendency of the ISI distribution from the 14-msec bin to the 9-msec bin. These findings indicate that BOT and NpA units are differentially sensitive to pentobarbital anesthesia.

CONCLUSION

The notion that medullary respiratory-related rhythmogenic neurons are subject to modulation by states of consciousness, behaviors, and a multitude of supra-segmental and peripheral sensory influences is beyond dispute (see 11, 17, and 32 for reviews). Evidence abounds in the literature that ventilatory patterns can be modified by a variety of physiological and behavioral factors such as states of arousal, behaviors, emotions, temperature, blood O_2/CO_2 tensions, metabolism, vago-pulmonary and somatosensory afferent activities, forebrain and other suprasegmental activities, and hormonal activities (see 13). Step or ramp changes in respiratory patterns, be they volitional or automatic, are orchestrated to ensure adequate supply and prompt delivery of oxygen to tissues and organs in need and to maintain a chemostatic constancy of blood O_2/CO_2 tensions and pH. To effectively cope with fluctuating tissue oxygen demands across a wide range of behavioral and physiological condi-

tions, the rhythmogenic mechanism must be able to recognize the needs on a moment-to-moment basis and be amenable to modulation and entrainment by a multiplicity of intrinsic (network) and extrinsic (physiological and behavioral factors) synaptic events. Indeed, the remarkable differences in respiratory behaviors across different states of arousal and behaviors are clear indications of varying degrees of interaction and functional overlap between the brainstem rhythmogenic network and other CNS control and integrative mechanisms (14, 17, 21, 40).

Thus far, evidence derived from unanesthetized preparations in the laboratories of Harper and Orem, and more recently in my laboratory (5–7), have only begun to unfold the complex operational dynamics of brainstem rhythmogenic networks. Future investigations into the sites and mechanisms that underlie the state- and behavior-dependent aspects of respiratory control will be challenging. Investigators should always be mindful that in addition to the colossal puzzle of respiratory rhythmogenesis, there are also complexities of behavioral and physiological variables that are as yet incompletely understood. Progress toward understanding respiratory rhythmogenesis is most likely to take place as a result of multidisciplinary effort and the collective creativity of individuals involved in this area of research.

ACKNOWLEDGMENTS

The opinions and assertions contained in this report are the personal views of the author and are not to be construed as official or as reflecting the views of U.S. Army or the Department of Defense.

In conducting the research described in this report, the investigator adhered to the "Guide for the care and use of laboratory animals of the Institute of Laboratory Animal Resources, National Research Council."

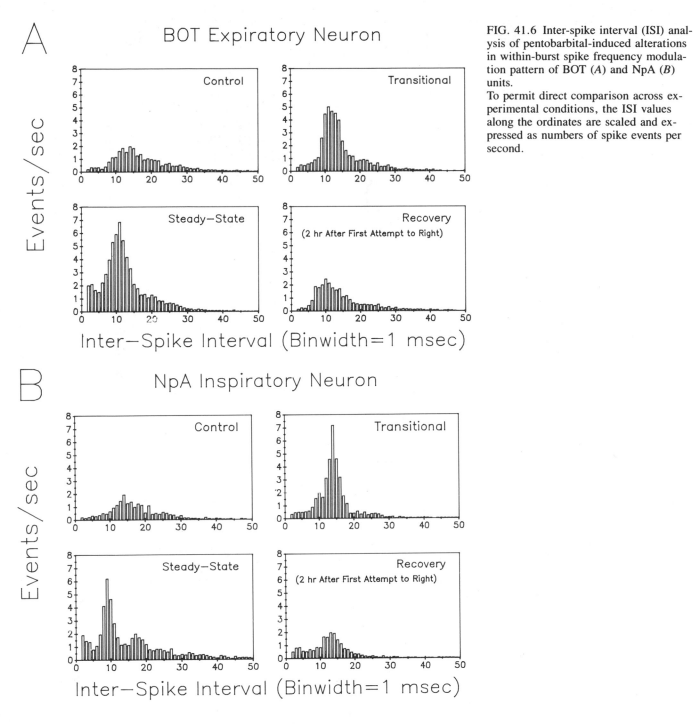

FIG. 41.6 Inter-spike interval (ISI) analysis of pentobarbital-induced alterations in within-burst spike frequency modulation pattern of BOT (*A*) and NpA (*B*) units.

To permit direct comparison across experimental conditions, the ISI values along the ordinates are scaled and expressed as numbers of spike events per second.

REFERENCES

1. Bianchi, A.L., and J.C. Barillot. Effects of anesthesia on activity patterns of respiratory neurones. *Adv. Exp. Med. Bio.* 99:17-22, 1978.

2. Bianchi, A.L., and J.C. Barillot. Respiratory neurons in the region of the retrofacial nucleus: Pontile, medullary, spinal and vagal projections. *Neurosci. Lett.* 31:277-282, 1982.

3. Brodie, D.A. The effect of thiopental and cyanide on the activity of inspiratory neurons. *J. Pharmacol. Exp. Therap.* 126:264-269, 1959.

4. Caille, D., J.-F. Vibert, F. Bertrand, H. Gromysz, and A. Hugelin. Pentobarbitone effects on respiration related units: selective depression of bulbopontine reticular neurones. *Resp. Physiol.* 36:201-216, 1979.

5. Chang, F.-C.T. Effects of pentobarbital on respiratory functional dynamics in chronically instrumented guinea pigs. *Brain Res. Bull.* 26(1):123-132, 1991.

6. Chang, F.-C.T., and R.E. Foster. Medullary inspiratory-related unit discharge patterns in awake, behaving guinea pigs. *Neurosci. Abstr.* 12:305, 1986.

7. Chang, F.-C.T., R.E. Foster, E.T. Beers, D.L. Rickett, and M.G. Filbert. Neurophysiological concomitants of soman-induced respiratory failure in awake, behaving guinea pigs. *Toxicol. Appl. Pharmacol.* 102:233-250, 1990.

8. Chang, F.-C.T., and R.M. Harper. A procedure for chronic recording of diaphragmatic electromyographic activity. *Brain Res. Bull.* 22:561-563, 1989.

9. Chang, F.-C.T., T.R. Scott, and R.M. Harper. Methods of single unit recording from medullary neural substrates in awake, behaving guinea pigs. *Brain Res. Bull.* 21:749-756, 1988.

10. Childers, D.G. *Modern spectrum analysis.* New York: IEEE Press, 1978.

11. von Euler, C. Brain stem mechanisms for generation and control of breathing pattern. In *Handbook of Physiology,* Section 3, vol. 2, ed. N.S. Cherniack and J.G. Widdicombe, 1-67. Bethesda, Md.: American Physiological Society, 1986.

12. Fedorko, L., and E.G. Merrill. Axonal projections from the rostral expiratory neurons of the Bötzinger Complex to medulla and spinal cord in the cat. *J. Physiol.* (London) 350:487-496, 1984.

13. Fishman, A.P., N.S. Cherniack, J.G. Widdicombe, and S.R. Geiger, eds. *Handbook of Physiology.* Section 3, vol. 2. Bethesda, Md.: American Physiological Society, 1986.

14. Frysinger, R.C., J.X. Zhang, and R.M. Harper. Cardiovascular and respiratory relationships with neuronal discharge in the central nucleus of the amygdala during sleep-waking states. *Sleep* 11:317-332, 1988.

15. Gautier, H. Pattern of breathing during hypoxia or hypercapnia of the awake or anesthetized cat. *Resp. Physiol.* 27:193-206, 1976.

16. Holst, D.V., and H. Kolb. Sniffing frequency of *tupaia belangeri:* Measurement of central nervous activity (arousal). *J. Comp. Physiol.* 105:243-258, 1976.

17. Hugelin, A. Forebrain and Midbrain influence on respiration. In *Handbook of Physiology,* Section 3, vol. 2, ed. N.S. Cherniack and J.G. Widdicombe, 69-91, Bethesda, Md.: American Physiological Society, 1986.

18. Lipski, J., and E.G. Merrill. Electrophysiological demonstration of the projection from expiratory neurones in the rostral medulla to contralateral dorsal respiratory group. *Brain Res.* 197:521-524, 1980.

19. Merrill, E.G., and L. Fedorko. Monosynaptic inhibition of phrenic motoneurons: A long descending projection from Bötzinger neurons. *J. Neurosci.* 4:2350-2353, 1984.

20. Merrill, E.G., J. Lipski, L. Kubin, and L. Fedorko. Origin of the expiratory inhibition of nucleus tractus solitarius inspiratory neurons. *Brain Res.* 263:43-50, 1983.

21. Ni, H.F., J.X. Zhang, and R.M. Harper. Respiratory-related discharge of Periaqueductal neurons during sleep-waking states. *Brain Res.* 511:319-325, 1990.

22. Orem, J. Medullary respiratory neuron activity: Relationship to tonic and phasic REM sleep. *J. Appl. Physiol.* 48:54-65, 1980.

23. Orem, J. Inspiratory neurons that are activated when inspiration is inhibited behaviorally. *Neurosci. Lett.* 83:282-286, 1987.

24. Orem, J. Behavioral inspiratory inhibition: inactivated and activated respiratory cells. *J. Neurophysiol.* 62:1069-1078, 1989.

25. Orem, J., and E. Brooks. The activity of retrofacial expiratory cells during behavioral respiratory responses and active expiration. *Brain Res.* 374:409-412, 1986.

26. Orem, J., and W. Dement. Spontaneous eyelid behavior in the sleeping cat. *Exp. Neurol.* 44:145-159, 1974.

27. Orem, J., and R. Lydic. Upper airway function during sleep and wakefulness: Experimental studies on normal and anesthetized cats. *Sleep* 1:49-57, 1978.

28. Orem, J., and A. Netick. Characteristics of midbrain respiratory neurons in sleep and wakefulness in the cat. *Brain Res.* 244:231-241, 1982.

29. Orem J., and A. Netick. Behavioral control of breathing in the cat. *Brain Res.* 366:238-253, 1986.

30. Orem, J., A. Netick, and W.C. Dement. Breathing during sleep and wakefulness in the cat. *Resp. Physiol.* 30:265-289, 1977.

31. Orem, J., I. Osorio, E. Brooks, and T. Dick. Activity of respiratory neurons during NREM sleep. *J. Neurophysiol.* 54:1144-1156, 1985.

32. Phillipson, E.A., and G. Bowes. Control of breathing during sleep. In *Handbook of Physiology,* Section 3, vol. 2, ed. N.S. Cherniack and J.G. Widdicombe, 649-689. Bethesda, Md.: American Physiological Society, 1986.

33. Priano, L.L., D.L. Traberand, and R.D. Wilson. Barbiturate anesthesia: An abnormal physiologic situation. *J. Pharm. Exp. Ther.* 165:126-135, 1969.

34. Robson, J.G., M.A. Housely, and O.H. Solis-Quiroga. The mechanism of respiratory arrest with sodium pentobarbital and thiopental. *Ann. NY Acad. Sci.* 109:494-502, 1963.

35. Sieck, G.C., and R.M. Harper. Pneumotaxic area neuronal discharge during sleep waking states in the cat. *Exp. Neurol.* 67:79-102, 1980.

36. Sieck, G.C., and R.M. Harper. Discharge of neurons in the parabrachial pons related to the cardiac cycle: Changes during different sleep-waking states. *Brain Res.* 199:385-399, 1980.

37. Steiner, S.H., and J.R. Calvin. The effects of anesthesia with pentobarbital on hemodynamics and arterial blood gases in splenectomized dogs. *J. Thorac. Cardiovasc. Surg.* 54:592-598, 1967.

38. Trelease, R.B., R.M. Harper, and G.C. Sieck. Respiratory-related heart rate variation during sleep and waking states in cats. *Exp. Neurol.* 72:195-203, 1981.

39. Szereda-Przestaszewska, M., D. Bartlett, and J.C.M. Wise. Changes in respiratory frequency and end-expiratory volume accompanying augmented breaths in cats. *Pflügers Arch.* 364:29-33, 1976.

40. Zhang, J.X., R.M. Harper, and R.C. Frysinger. Respiratory modulation of neuronal discharge in the central nucleus of the amygdala during sleep and waking states. *Exp. Neurol.* 91:193-207, 1986.

42

Vomiting: Its Respiratory Components

Alan D. Miller

Vomiting is produced primarily by changes in intrathoracic and intraabdominal pressures that are generated by the coordinated action of the major respiratory muscles (25, 26). This article reviews the pattern of activation and current state of knowledge concerning the control of these muscles during the retching and expulsion phases of vomiting. The reader is referred to other recent reviews for more general considerations regarding vomiting (4, 9, 10), the gastrointestinal correlates of vomiting (21), motion and space sickness (7), pregnancy sickness (1), and vomiting associated with cancer chemotherapy and radiation (9, 10).

Respiratory muscle control is likely to be complex since these muscles are activated differently during vomiting and respiration. Numerous studies have shown that during vomiting the diaphragm and abdominal muscles, which are muscles of inspiration and expiration respectively, co-contract in a series of bursts of activity that culminates in expulsion (e.g., 18, 25, 36, 37). Abdominal muscle activity is prolonged during expulsion, both with respect to diaphragmatic activity and to abdominal discharge during the preceding retching phase (fig. 42.1). The external oblique abdominal muscle contracts phasically during vomiting while the rectus abdominis usually displays a variable tonic increase in activity as well as phasic bursts (36). The external intercostal (inspiratory) muscles also co-contract with the diaphragm and abdominal muscles during vomiting. In contrast, the internal intercostal (expiratory) muscles contract out of phase with these muscles during retching, are inactive during expulsion, and generate little or no positive thoracic pressure during either phase of vomiting (25). There is a marked increase in the activity of the major respiratory muscles during vomiting compared to normal respiration.

The portion of the diaphragm that surrounds the esophagus relaxes during vomiting, presumably facilitating rostral movement of gastric contents (32, 37). This relaxation is greatest during expulsion; however, some reduction in activity also occurs during retching. Peri-esophageal relaxation during vomiting is part of the central motor program for vomiting and does not depend on a reflex arising from movement of vomitus within the esophagus (32).

The muscles of the upper airway act to protect the nasopharynx and trachea during vomiting by raising the soft palate and closing the glottis, respectively (15, 18, 22). Closure muscles of the glottis (thyroarytenoid and lateral cricoarytenoid) discharge in phase with bursts of diaphragmatic and abdominal coactivation during vomiting, while the glottis opener (posterior cricoarytenoid) remains silent (15, 18). Also active during these bursts are the motor nerves to the genioglossus, a protrusor of the tongue, and the stylopharyngeus, which dilates and elevates the pharynx. The digastricus, which depresses the lower jaw, is active throughout the retching and expulsion phases (15). Following the expulsion phase, there are bursts of oropharyngeal nerve discharge that correspond to the buccopharyngeal stage of swallowing (15).

The discharge patterns of individual brainstem and upper cervical respiratory neurons have recently been studied during "fictive vomiting" in decerebrate, paralyzed cats. Fictive vomiting is identified by the same characteristic pattern of bursts of coactivation of diaphragmatic (phrenic) and abdominal muscle nerves, elicited by emetic agents, that would be expected to culminate in expulsion if the animals were not paralyzed (36). Using this preparation, we first recorded from bulbospinal expiratory (E) neurons located in the portion of the ventral respiratory group (VRG) caudal to the obex (nucleus retroambigualis) (36). These neurons make mono- or oligosynaptic excitatory connections with abdominal and internal intercostal motoneurons (20, 27, 29, 31). Two major response patterns are observed during vomiting (fig. 42.1). One-third of these neurons fire mainly during periods of abdominal nerve activity and thus could contribute to abdominal muscle activation during vomiting. Virtually all of the remaining neurons fire mainly between bursts of phrenic and abdominal nerve coactivation during the retching phase and thus have the appropriate firing pattern to activate internal intercostal motoneurons, which are known to discharge between bursts of abdominal and diaphragmatic activity during vomiting (25). Most of this latter group of VRG E neurons, however, are also active during the expulsion phase when internal intercostal muscles are reported to be silent. Cutting the axons of caudal VRG E neurons by a midsagittal section between C1 and the obex abolishes abdominal muscles nerve discharge during both expiration and fictive vomiting (34). Possible effects on internal intercostal activity were not tested. These observations from both cell-recording and lesion studies are consistent with abdominal muscle activation during vomiting being mediated by caudal VRG E neurons.

The pathways that activate phrenic motoneurons during vomiting, in contrast, remain uncertain. During res-

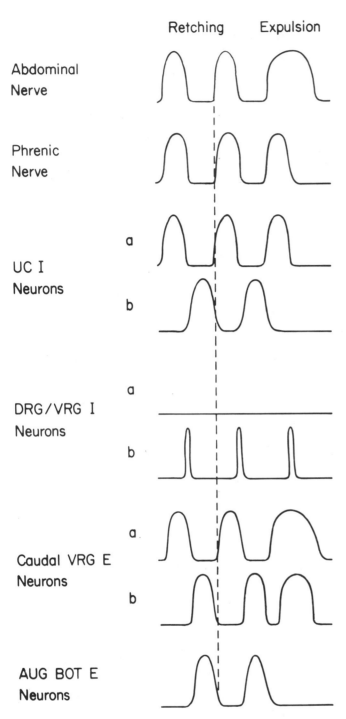

Retching   Expulsion

Abdominal
Nerve

Phrenic
Nerve

UC I
Neurons

a

b

DRG / VRG I
Neurons

a

b

Caudal VRG E
Neurons

a

b

AUG BOT E
Neurons

FIG. 42.1 Schematic representation of the activity of brainstem and upper cervical respiratory neurons during fictive vomiting. Vertical dashed line added for visual reference. Records in *a* and *b* represent different responses seen in different neurons. Some Bötzinger Complex expiratory (BOT E) neurons also fire during the expulsion phase. Sources: upper cervical (UC) inspiratory (I) neurons (38), dorsal respiratory group (DRG) and ventral respiratory group (VRG) I neurons (3, 35), caudal VRG E neurons (34, 36), augmenting (AUG) BOT E neurons (33).

piration, the inspiratory pattern generator produces high-frequency (50–100 Hz) oscillations (HFO) in phrenic discharge that are absent during vomiting, indicating that inputs from this pattern generator to phrenic motoneurons are shut off during vomiting (5). Bulbospinal inspiratory (I) neurons in the dorsal respiratory group (DRG, corresponding to the ventrolateral nucleus of the solitary tract) and in the VRG rostral to the obex (nucleus paraambiguus), which make mono- or oligosynaptic connections with motoneurons innervating the diaphragm and external intercostal muscles (6, 8, 11, 13, 16, 29), do not have the appropriate response pattern to initiate activation of these motoneurons during fictive vomiting (3, 35). Most (≥90%) of these bulbospinal I neurons are inhibited during vomiting and either are silent throughout the entire episode or fire only near the end of phrenic discharge. Only a few neurons start firing soon after the onset of phrenic discharge. This suggests that other brainstem neurons are important for the control of the diaphragm and the coactive external intercostal muscles during vomiting. In contrast to these bulbospinal I neurons, more than one-half of upper cervical (C1–3) propriospinal I neurons are active in phase with bursts of phrenic discharge during fictive vomiting (38). Many of these neurons start firing prior to the onset of phrenic discharge. Another 20% of upper cervical I neurons fire mainly between phrenic bursts during vomiting. Upper cervical propriospinal I neurons may affect spinal respiratory motoneurons via oligosynaptic, as opposed to monosynaptic, pathways (17, 23).

Expiratory neurons in the rostral portion of the VRG (Bötzinger [BOT] complex) make monosynaptic inhibitory connections with DRG (30) and VRG (12) I neurons, caudal VRG bulbospinal E neurons (19), laryngeal motoneurons (19), phrenic motoneurons (28), and perhaps some upper cervical I neurons (24). During fictive vomiting, augmenting BOT E neurons discharge between phrenic bursts and thus serve as a source of inhibitory input during that phase of the vomiting episode (33). Other brainstem neurons must also be involved in inhibiting bulbospinal I neurons which receive maximum hyperpolarization near the onset and during bursts of phrenic discharge during vomiting (5) while augmenting BOT E neurons are silent during most of the phrenic burst.

CONCLUSION

Based on the firing patterns of brainstem and upper cervical respiratory neurons during fictive vomiting and on their known or possible neuronal connections, it is possible to formulate a partial working hypothesis regarding the neural control of the major respiratory muscles during vomiting (fig. 42.2). Abdominal and internal intercostal motoneurons are probably driven by caudal VRG E neurons. In contrast, the pathways that drive phrenic and external intercostal motoneurons remain unknown, although some up-

Neural Network during Vomiting ?

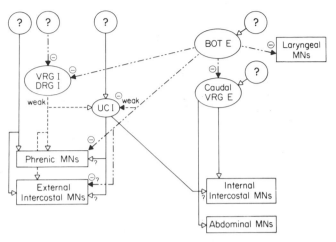

FIG. 42.2 Working hypothesis of the possible role of brainstem and upper cervical respiratory neurons in the control of the major respiratory muscles during vomiting. This hypothesis is based on patterns of single-cell activity during fictive vomiting and on known or possible neuronal connections. Arrows do not distinguish between mono- or oligosynaptic connections. Excitatory connections are indicated by open arrowheads, and inhibitory connections are shown using closed arrowheads and lines consisting of alternating dashes and dots. Dashed lines indicate weak inputs. MNs, motor neurons. (See figure 42.1 for descriptions of other abbreviations.)

per cervical I neurons may be involved via oligosynaptic pathways. Upper cervical I neurons that fire between phrenic bursts may provide excitation to internal intercostal motoneurons. Augmenting BOT E neurons provide extensive inhibitory inputs during periods between phrenic bursts. The relaxation of the periesophageal portion of the diaphragm that occurs during expulsion may be brought about, at least in part, by some BOT E neurons that fire during the expulsion phase (33).

Studies of central respiratory neurons during fictive vomiting have also led to more general observations regarding the respiratory neuronal circuitry. First, E neurons in the caudal VRG are not a homogeneous population but discharge in one of two distinct patterns during vomiting. Second, phrenic motoneurons do not appear to be activated primarily by DRG and VRG bulbospinal I neurons during vomiting and therefore probably receive important inputs from other sources. Similar observations have been made during rhythmic straining (14). In addition, bulbospinal I neurons are not a necessary relay for cortical activation of phrenic and inspiratory intercostal motoneurons (2). Third, the discharge patterns of propriospinal I neurons in the cervical cord are markedly different from bulbospinal DRG and VRG I neurons, implying that upper cervical I neurons receive important additional inputs.

The brainstem neurons that control the activity of the major respiratory muscles during vomiting are an essential

part of the pre-motor output pathways for vomiting. Better knowledge of these neural circuits would be an important step for determining how various inputs, for example from abdominal vagal afferents, the area postrema, and the vestibular system, can lead to vomiting under different conditions. Increased understanding of the pathways that produce vomiting and of their neurotransmitters and receptor subtypes may be expected to lead to more effective antiemetic drugs or drug combinations.

ACKNOWLEDGMENTS

I wish to thank my colleague Dr. Satoshi Nonaka for helpful discussions. This work is supported by grant NS20585 from the National Institutes of Health.

REFERENCES

1. Andrew, P., and S. Whitehead. Pregnancy sickness. *News in Physiol. Sci.* 5:5-10, 1990.

2. Bassal, M., A.L. Bianchi, and M. Dussardier. Effets de la stimulation des structures nerveuses centrales sur l'activité des neurones respiratoires chez le chat. *J. Physiol.* (Paris) 77:779-795, 1981.

3. Bianchi, A.L., and L. Grélot. Converse motor output of inspiratory bulbospinal premotoneurons during vomiting. *Neurosci. Lett.* 104:298-302, 1989.

4. Carpenter, D.O. Central nervous system mechanisms in deglutition and emesis. In *Handbook of Physiology,* Section 6, vol. 1, ed. J.D. Wood, 685-714. Bethesda, Md.:American Physiological Society, 1989.

5. Cohen, M.I., A.D. Miller, R. Barnhardt, and C.F. Shaw. High-frequency oscillations (HFO) of phrenic (PHR) discharge are absent during fictive vomiting (VOM). *Soc. Neurosci. Abstr.* 15:1192, 1989.

6. Cohen, M.I., M.F. Piercey, P.M. Gootman, and P. Wolotsky. Synaptic connections between medullary inspiratory neurons and phrenic motoneurons as revealed by cross-correlation. *Brain Res.* 81:319-324, 1974.

7. Crampton, G.H., ed. *Motion and space sickness.* Boca Raton, Fla: CRC Press, 1990.

8. Davies, J.G.McF., P.A. Kirkwood, and T.A. Sears. The distribution of monosynaptic connexions from inspiratory bulbospinal neurones to inspiratory motoneurones in the cat. *J. Physiol.* (London) 368:63-87, 1985.

9. Davies, C.J., G.V. Lake-Bakaar, and D.G. Grahame-Smith, eds. *Nausea and vomiting: mechanisms and treatment.* Berlin: Springer-Verlag, 1986.

10. Davison, J.S., and R.K. Harding, eds. Proceedings of the symposium on nausea and vomiting: A multidisciplinary perspective. *Can. J. Physiol. Pharmacol.* 68:217-345, 1990.

11. Duffin, J., and J. Lipski. Monosynaptic excitation of thoracic motoneurones by inspiratory neurons of the nucleus tractus solitarius in the cat. *J. Physiol.* (London) 390:415-431, 1987.

12. Fedorko, L., J. Duffin, and S. England. Inhibition of inspiratory neurons of the nucleus retroambigualis by expiratory neurons of the Bötzinger complex in the cat. *Exp. Neurol.* 106:74-77, 1989.

13. Fedorko, L., E.G. Merrill, and J. Lipski. Two descending medullary inspiratory pathways to phrenic motoneurons. *Neurosci. Lett.* 43:285-291, 1983.

14. Fukuda, H., and K. Fukai. Discharges of bulbar respiratory neurons during rhythmic straining evoked by activation of pelvic afferent fibers in dogs. *Brain Res.* 449:157-166, 1988.

15. Grélot, L., J.C. Barillot, and A.L. Bianchi. Activity of respiratory-related oropharyngeal and laryngeal motoneurones during fictive vomiting in the decerebrate cat. *Brain Res.* 513:101-105, 1990.

16. Hilaire, G., and R. Monteau. Connexions entre les neurones inspiratoires bulbaires et les motoneurones phréniques et intercostaux. *J. Physiol.* (Paris). 72:987-1000, 1976.

17. Hoskin, R.W., L.M. Fedorko, and J. Duffin. Projections from upper cervical inspiratory neurons to thoracic and lumbar expiratory motor nuclei in the cat. *Exp. Neurol.* 99:544-555, 1988.

18. Hukuhara, T., H. Okada, and M. Yamagami. On the behavior of the respiratory muscles during vomiting. *Acta Med. Okayama* 11:117-125, 1957.

19. Jiang, C., and J. Lipski. Extensive monosynaptic inhibition of ventral respiratory group neurons by augmenting neurons in the Bötzinger complex in the cat. *Exp. Brain Res.* 81:639-648, 1990.

20. Kirkwood, P.A., and T.A. Sears. Monosynaptic excitation of thoracic expiratory motoneurones from lateral respiratory neurones in the medulla of the cat. *J. Physiol.* (London) 232:87P-89P, 1973.

21. Lang, I.M. and S.K. Sarna. Motor and myoelectric activity associated with vomiting, regurgitation, and nausea. In *Handbook of Physiology*, Section 6, vol. 1, ed. J.D. Wood, 1179-1198. Bethesda, Md.: American Physiology Society, 1989.

22. Laskiewicz, A. Vomiting and eructation with regard to the upper respiratory organs. *Acta Oto-laryng.* 46:27-34, 1956.

23. Lipski, J., and J. Duffin. An electrophysiological investigation of propriospinal inspiratory neurons in the upper cervical cord of the cat. *Exp. Brain Res.* 61:625-637, 1986.

24. Mateika, J.H., and J. Duffin. The connections from Bötzinger expiratory neurons to upper cervical inspiratory neurons in the cat. *Exp. Neurol.* 104:138-146, 1989.

25. McCarthy, L.E., and H.L. Borison. Respiratory mechanics of vomiting in decerebrate cats. *Am. J. Physiol.* 226:738-743, 1974.

26. McCarthy, L.E., H.L. Borison, P.K. Spiegel, and R.M. Friedlander. Vomiting: Radiographic and oscillographic correlates in the decerebrate cat. *Gastroenterology* 67:1126-1130, 1974.

27. Merrill, E.G. Finding a respiratory function for the medullary respiratory neurons. In *Essays on the nervous system*. R. Bellairs and E.G. Gray, ed., 451-486. Oxford, U.K.: Clarendon, 1974.

28. Merrill, E.G., and L. Fedorko. Monosynaptic inhibition of phrenic motoneurons: A long descending projection from Bötzinger neurons. *J. Neurosci.* 4:2350-2353, 1984.

29. Merrill, E.G., and J. Lipski. Inputs to intercostal motoneurons from ventrolateral respiratory neurons in the cat. *J. Neurophysiol.* 57:1837-1853, 1987.

30. Merrill, E.G., J. Lipski, L. Kubin, and L. Fedorko. Origin of the expiratory inhibition of nucleus tractus solitarius inspiratory neurones. *Brain Res.* 263:43-50, 1983.

31. Miller, A.D., K. Ezure, and I. Suzuki. Control of abdominal muscles by brain stem respiratory neurons in the cat. *J. Neurophysiol.* 54:155-167, 1985.

32. Miller, A.D., S.F. Lakos, and L.K. Tan. Central motor program for relaxation of periesophageal diaphragm during the expulsive phase of vomiting. *Brain Res.* 456:367-370, 1988.

33. Miller, A.D., and S. Nonaka. Bötzinger expiratory neurons may inhibit phrenic motoneurons and medullary inspiratory neurons during vomiting. *Brain Res.* 521:352-354, 1990.

34. Miller, A.D., and S. Nonaka. Mechanisms of abdominal muscle activation during vomiting. *J. Appl. Physiol.* 69:21-25, 1990.

35. Miller, A.D., S. Nonaka, S.F. Lakos, and L.K. Tan. Diaphragmatic and external intercostal muscle control during vomiting: behavior of inspiratory bulbospinal neurons. *J. Neurophysiol.* 63:31-36, 1990.

36. Miller, A.D., L.K. Tan, I. Suzuki. Control of abdominal and expiratory intercostal muscles activity during vomiting: role of ventral respiratory group expiratory neurons. *J. Neurophysiol.* 57:1854-1866, 1987.

37. Monges, H., J. Salducci, and B. Naudy. Dissociation between the electrical activity of the diaphragmatic dome and crura muscular fibers during esophageal distension, vomiting and eructation. *J. Physiol.* (Paris) 74:541-554, 1978.

38. Nonaka, S., and A.D. Miller. Behavior of upper cervical inspiratory propriospinal neurons during fictive vomiting. *J. Neurophysiol.* 65:1492-1500, 1991.

Part IX

Ventilatory Control in Humans

43

An Overview

Jerome A. Dempsey, N. Omar Suwarno, and Douglas R. Seals

The study of the control of breathing in the human has an illustrious and rich history. Many of the fundamental characteristics of ventilatory control such as chemoresponsiveness, the effects of state, and the regulation of exercise hyperpnea are attributable to the pioneering efforts of Krogh, Haldane, Asmussen, and others through their study of humans. Other work utilizing carefully documented lesions of specific neural pathways in human patients provided invaluable insights into mechanisms of load perception and compensation (Campbell), voluntary control of breathing via corticospinal tracts (Plum), and length-compensating reflexes arising from the diaphragm (Mead). There are many excellent reasons to continue the study of the regulation of breathing in humans. Certainly, most of the very fundamental questions remain unresolved, but, as in other types of basic biomedical research, the mechanisms easiest to study have already been elucidated. In the future, we must continue to seek innovative and daring approaches in humans and combine work in these fully integrative models with those in more reduced preparations if we are to ever fully understand human ventilatory control.

There continue to be many questions related to the species specificity of ventilatory control among mammals. In what respects is the regulation of breathing in the human unique? One major unresolved question concerns the sensitivity of vagally mediated mechanoreceptor feedback from the human lung in the regulation of breathing pattern, respiratory muscle recruitment, and cardiovascular function. The importance of this very fundamental feedback effect on cardiopulmonary function is well established in the anesthetized and to a lesser extent in awake mammals other than humans; however, it is commonly assumed that vagal feedback is of little consequence in the adult human. This question is far from resolved, as it is only very recently that these reflexes have even been quantified in an unanesthetized physiologic state (sleep) (1) and only one study has been made of the effects of phasic volume feedback in the human by withholding eupneic tidal volume in the anesthetized state (2). These studies suggest varying degrees of lung inflation effects on breath timing.

On the other hand, a highly significant effect of vagal feedback may occur on cardiovascular reflexes in the human including sympathetic efferent output to various vascular beds responsible for regulating blood flow distribution (see fig. 43.1A–C) (3). This association was shown by using the technique of microneurography to provide con-

tinuous recording of the sympathetic efferent nerve activity to resting human muscle (4). Clearly, this tight association of lung inflation and sympathetic nervous outflow, like the regulation of breathing pattern, has many potential mediators in addition to phasic volume feedback from the lung. These include systemic or cardiac baroreceptor feedback (note phasic blood pressure change in fig. 43.1B) and "central command" from a medullary sympathetic "oscillator network," which is presumably linked closely with the respiratory rhythm generator. Although it is difficult to differentiate these possibilities in an integrative model such as the awake, intact human, one may test these hypotheses by employing various models and manipulations, such as (1) causing systemic blood pressure changes within the breath to be out of phase with respiration, for example by using inspiratory resistive loads; (2) using active (voluntary) versus passive (mechanical) ventilation to test the role of central descending neural influences; and (3) taking advantage of the clinical model of vagal denervation in the otherwise healthy lung-transplant patient. The results of such studies confirm a significant contribution of vagal feedback from the lung in the regulation of muscle sympathetic efferent activity in the human. This fundamental role for mechanoreceptor feedback from the lung deserves further intense study in the human (and in the conscious "behaving" animal preparation) along with related questions concerning the role of vagal feedback in the regulation of heart rate, distribution of blood flow, and even control of respiratory sinus arrhythmia. Furthermore, it is time to gain a definitive understanding of the role of phasic vagal feedback in the regulation of breathing pattern and respiratory muscle recruitment in the human.

The human's upright posture presents another unique feature which may have significant consequences for the regulation of respiratory muscle function and for mechanical interactions among different segments of the chest wall during breathing. For example, we know very little of the pattern of respiratory muscle recruitment and its mechanical consequences in truly physiologic states, especially during the hyperpnea of muscular exercise in the human or the conscious animal. Recent findings point to an important role for expiratory muscle recruitment in the generation of hyperpnea in both quadrupedal and bipedal locomotion. These data have significant implications for the regulation of respiratory muscle length and in turn for feedback and feedforward regulation of respiratory motor output and its

A

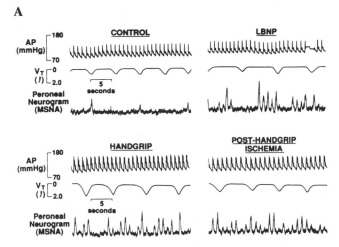

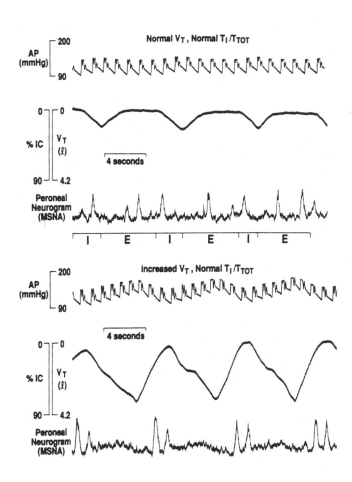

FIG. 43.1 Influence of lung inflation and breathing pattern on peroneal nerve sympathetic efferent activity in a resting limb in normal, intact humans. Sympathetic activity is recorded from a tungsten 0.2 mm electrode placed into the fascicle of the right peroneal nerve posterior to the fibular head. The amplified, filtered (band pass 700–2000 Hz), rectified, and integrated (100 msec time constant) mean voltage neurogram (MSNA) is shown. (A) Different means of stimulating background MSNA by lower body negative pressure (LBNP) (baroreceptor stimulation), sustained muscular contraction (handgrip), and local muscle ischemia immediately following handgrip. Note the increased frequency and amplitude of sympathetic bursts in each case. AP, arterial pressure; V_T, tidal volume. (B) V_T, inspiratory duration (T_I), and expiratory duration (T_E) were varied to determine the effect of lung inflation on sympathetic activity (inspiration is down on the volume signal) in a subject with heightened background sympathetic activity via LBNP. Note that sympathetic activity is completely inhibited during augmented inspiration and only appears during expiration. IC, inspiratory capacity; T_{TOT}, total cycle duration. (C) Effects of increased lung inflation in a subject with postexercise ischemia as the means of augmenting background sympathetic activity.

B

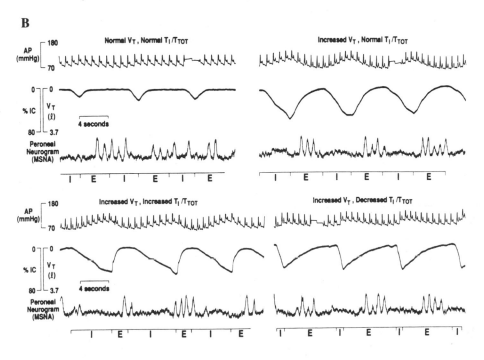

distribution. Certainly, something as fundamental as postural-locomotory-respiratory interactions must eventually receive some attention if we are to truly understand the regulation of breathing under natural conditions.

The human depends substantially less on breathing for temperature regulation than do other experimental mammals such as the dog, the sheep and the rat. This is especially true during the increased heat production of exercise, which may in part explain the greater dependence of these other mammals on breathing frequency responses and the fact that the human shows a more precise isocapnic hyperpnea than do other exercising mammals. Studies on even the very basic mechanisms of exercise hyperpnea must consider these fundamental questions of teleology in determining the relative contribution of various types of feedforward and feedback stimuli to the hyperpnea and most importantly in the extrapolation of findings in other animal preparations to the human.

Maturation effects on ventilatory regulation are probably quite different in the human given the markedly different rates of development among humans and other mammals in most types of motor control. Only very recently has the human infant been more fully utilized as a research subject. This remains a technically difficult but challenging and important area for research in the control of breathing. Of special interest is the maturation of mechanisms regulating distribution of respiratory motor output to upper-airway and chest-wall musculature and the age-dependent changes in the sensitivity of mechanoreceptor feedback effects from lung and chest wall. Often lost in the rush toward specific neurochemical mechanisms is the underlying change in metabolic rate in response to oxygen lack or temperature changes. How maturation influences this very basic, yet mysterious underpinning of the regulation of breathing is unknown (see Mortola, this volume). The development of animal models that truly mimic human development is also important to a more thorough understanding of human ventilatory regulation.

The use of the sleeping state has opened exciting avenues for human study that not only present the challenge to study ventilatory control in an entirely new physiologic state but also provide the opportunity to study many aspects of ventilatory regulation in the non-behaving, yet unanesthetized human. Some exciting, fundamental findings have emerged to date concerning the nature of the elusive "wakefulness drive" to breathe. The normal human sleeping subject shows (1) a critical dependence of rhythmic ventilation on very small changes in PCO_2; (2) the absence of immediate compensation to mechanical loads; (3) the selective redistribution of efferent respiratory motor output between upper-airway and pump-respiratory muscles; and (4) a remarkable sensitivity of ventilatory stability to even relatively small changes in cortical "state." Of course, an understanding of sleep obviates the use of the anesthetized state and requires that truly physiologic preparations be used. More recently, we have seen the development of uniquely instrumented animal models and imaginative uses of pharmacologic agents that it is hoped, will mimic normal REM sleep. The use of these approaches in concert with more in-depth investigations of the sleeping human promises an exciting future for research into the integrative complexity of neural-chemical-mechanical aspects of ventilatory regulation in the different physiologic states.

Parenthetically, it may be worthwhile to be reminded from time to time that anesthesia or decerebration is not one of the physiologic states in question. Anesthesia (type, duration, and depth) has marked and unpredictable effects on the gain of ventilatory responses to most ventilatory stimuli, on the level of background acid-base status, on the influence of mechanoreceptor feedback, and on the distribution of respiratory motor output to respiratory muscles. Some of those limitations must also apply to isolated, nonperfused preparations. Again, while such preparations are invaluable to further our understanding, the data they provide must be applied with caution. This is especially true if one wishes to determine the gain of responsivity inherent in a specific receptor or control network or the relative contribution of various types of primary and secondary afferent inputs to the final integrated response (i.e., respiratory motor output or breathing). When these answers are sought, the behaving, unanesthetized preparation must be incorporated at some point into the experimental design.

A traditional rationale for human study continues to be understanding the pathogenesis of human disease. Many of the classic questions remain unresolved in the pathophysiology of ventilatory control, such as the causes of respiratory failure and CO_2 retention; the chosen strategies to respond to internal loads which mimic the disease state; and the role of respiratory muscle fatigue in ventilatory control, that is, does it ever occur, and if so, how is it reversible? Why do some apneic infants show an apparent failure to arouse to restore rhythmic breathing? What precipitates the imbalance of respiratory motor output resulting in obstructive sleep apnea? How can we find better ways to artificially mimic the normal stimulation of the hypoglossal motor nerve (so that airways can open), or phrenic motor nerves (so that paralyzed diaphragms can contract)?

We have outlined just a few of the important problems and how they might be studied to yield basic information on some of the characteristics of ventilatory control which are especially relevant to the human. The message here is to bring new and inventive techniques, ideas, and experimental designs and new patient models to the study of ventilatory control. Of course, this appeal is not made to the exclusion of the need for more fundamental work at the level of the cell, slice, and reduced preparation in experimental animals. Indeed, while we refer to some of the above-mentioned findings in the human as "fundamental" in nature, we acknowledge that the basic neural elements, properties, and neurochemical mechanisms in ventilatory control, especially those within the central nervous system, must be studied at a subcellular level in greatly reduced preparations. Many of the exciting new findings reported in this volume came, of course, from the use of such preparations. It also remains clear that the important questions are the most difficult and complex; we must keep in perspective that the remaining "black boxes" in our control system come in many different sizes and levels of complexity. The best solution demands a truly comprehensive approach. The integrationist and reductionist would do well to strengthen their cooperative efforts.

ACKNOWLEDGMENTS

The original research reported here was supported by grants from NHLBI and NIA.

REFERENCES

1. Hamilton, R.A., A.J. Winning, R.L. Horner, and A. Guz. The effect of lung inflation on breathing in man during wakefulness and sleep. *Resp. Physiol.* 73:145-154, 1988.

2. Polacheck, J., E. Strong, J. Arens, C. Davies, I. Metcalf, and M. Younes. Phasic vagal influence on inspiratory motor output in anesthetized human subjects. *J. Appl. Physiol.* 49:609-619, 1980.

3. Seals, D.R., N.O. Suwarno, and J.A. Dempsey. Influence of lung volume on sympathetic nerve discharge in normal humans. *Circ. Res.* 67:130-141, 1990.

4. Valbo, A.B., K.E. Hagbarth, H.E. Torebjork, and B.G. Wallin. Somatosensory, proprioceptive, and sympathetic activity in human peripheral nerves. *Physiol. Rev.* 59:919-95, 1979.

44

The Effect of Increased Inspiratory Drive on the Sensory Activation of the Cerebral Cortex by Inspiratory Occlusion

Paul W. Davenport, Gregory A. Holt, and Paul McN. Hill

Respiratory sensations are common experiences that allow humans and animals to become aware of their breathing. Sensations elicited by increased inspiratory mechanical loads have been studied previously using psychophysical techniques. Yet very little is known about the sensory neural mechanisms mediating the sensation of mechanical loads. A prerequisite for understanding the mechanisms of respiratory sensations is identification of cerebral cortical activation by respiratory related stimuli. Sensory activation of the cerebral cortex in humans has been studied extensively in the auditory, visual, and somatosensory systems. Event-related potentials elicited by stimulation of afferents from these sensory modalities have been found using computer signal averaging techniques (3, 8). The evoked potential technique has been a useful tool in studying the neural mechanisms mediating these sensory systems. These techniques have been used recently to demonstrate the activation of somatosensory cortical regions by inspiratory loads.

Mechanical loads were applied while simultaneously recording from the somatosensory region in the adult human (5). The initial observation of a respiratory-related cortical evoked potential (RREP) was made using inspiratory occlusions applied at the onset of the breath. The electrodes were placed over the somatosensory region of the left hemisphere of the cerebral cortex. Mouth pressure (P_m) was the respiratory parameter that was used to trigger the signal averager. When P_m became negative the computer collected 800 msec of EEG activity. The EEG signals from 128 occlusions were averaged for each subject. An event-related potential was observed for occluded inspirations that was absent in unoccluded breaths. This respiratory related evoked potential had four peaks that were observed in all subjects. The first peak was positive with a mean latency of 60 msec. This was followed by a negative peak, a second positive peak, and another negative peak. When these results were compared to evoked potentials reported for other sensory modalities, a similar potential was found with mechanical stimulation of the foot and hand (9, 12, 13, 19). It was concluded that the RREP was similar to other somatosensory evoked potentials with a longer latency for the first positive peak (P_1) due to the time required for the inspiratory effort against the closed airway to stimulate the afferents mediating the RREP. More recent studies in normal subjects have demonstrated that this RREP can be elicited by occlusions presented either at the onset of inspiration or during mid-inspiration. The RREP was also

present bilaterally (14). These studies in adult humans demonstrate that inspiratory mechanical loads elicit cortical activity that can be recorded in the somatosensory region.

The P_1 latency with onset occlusions was found to correlate between subjects with their inspiratory drive as determined by the mouth pressure 0.1 sec after the onset of inspiration ($P_{0.1}$) (5). This observation suggested that the ventilatory status of the subject may be an important factor affecting the peak latency and waveform of the RREP. The present study was designed to investigate the role of increased inspiratory drive within the same subject on the latency and amplitude of the early portion of the RREP. The RREP was recorded in two separate trials with normal adult subjects breathing either room air or increased CO_2 (5% CO_2 and 95% O_2). The results of these experiments demonstrate that increased inspiratory drive decreases the latency but does not change the amplitude of the P_1 peak of the RREP.

METHODS

Five males and two females served as the subjects; three subjects had participated in previous RREP studies. The protocol was reviewed and approved by the Institutional Review Board at the University of Florida. The general methods were explained to each subject and signed consent was obtained.

The subjects were seated in a recliner that provided support for the head and neck. A two-way non-rebreathing valve was positioned to allow the subject to respire comfortably through the mouthpiece, maintain a tight seal around the lips, and relax the muscles of the head and mouth (fig. 44.1). Mouth pressure (P_m) was recorded with a differential pressure transducer connected to the center of the non-rebreathing valve. PCO_2 was recorded with an infrared analyzer (Puritan Bennet) connected to a separate port in the center of the valve. Reinforced tubing connected the balloon occluder to the inspiratory port of the breathing valve. Inflation of the balloon provided the occlusion of inspiration. A differential pressure transducer was connected to the pressure supply line for the balloon. It was the balloon pressure that served as the trigger signal for the signal processor (Cambridge Electronic Design, Model 1401). P_m and PCO_2 were displayed on a polygraph.

Surface-cup electrodes were placed bilaterally over the somatosensory region of the cerebral cortex: C_Z, C_3 and C_4 (International 10–20 system). The electrode impedances

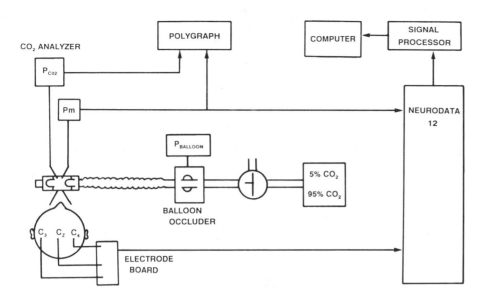

FIG. 44.1 Schematic representation of the experimental preparation. The subject was seated in a semi-reclining position. (See methods for explanation.)

were checked and the electrodes replaced if necessary. EEG activity was recorded from C_Z-C_3 and C_Z-C_4 electrode pairs, amplified (100K) and band pass filtered (0.3–3000 Hz, Grass Instruments, Neurodata 12). Balloon pressure, P_m, and the two EEG channels were connected to the signal processor. Experimental sounds were masked by headphones placed on the subject after the electrodes were in place. Music was played throughout the experiment.

Mid-inspiratory occlusion trials were presented with the subject breathing room air. The occlusion trial began with the subject respiring through the apparatus for 2–5 min of unobstructed breathing. The occlusions were presented by inflation of the balloon during an inspiration. The experimenter manually pressed the occlusion switch during the early portion of the inspiration. This interrupted the inspiratory air flow for about 400 msec and is referred to as a mid-inspiratory occlusion. Occlusions were presented every three to six breaths with the subject unaware of when an occlusion was to be presented. A minimum of eighty mid-inspiratory occlusions were presented. A series of ten occlusions presented at the onset of the breath was applied in the middle of the trial and recorded on the polygraph for the determination of $P_{0.1}$. The subject removed the mouthpiece when the trial was complete and was given a 10 min rest period.

A Douglas bag filled with 5% CO_2 and 95% O_2 served as a reservoir while the same gas mixture was continuously supplied from a cylinder. The bag was connected to a three-way valve in the inspiratory circuit. The subject began the trial with 2–5 min of unobstructed breathing of room air. The CO_2 gas mixture was then valved to the subject and 5 min were allowed for ventilation to increase and stabilize. Mid-inspiratory occlusions were then presented for a minimum of eighty occlusions. Ten onset occlusions were again presented in the middle of the trial to determine the $P_{0.1}$ with elevated CO_2. When all the occlusions had been presented, the subject was valved to room air and the mouthpiece was removed.

The computer (Dell 310) collected on-line 500 msec samples of P_m and EEG activity from the two electrode pairs (C_Z-C_3 and C_Z-C_4) with each occlusion. The increase in balloon pressure triggered the digital sampling (4 kHz) of the analog signals. The 500-msec digitized sample for each occlusion was stored individually for subsequent averaging and analysis. To generate the computer averages for each trial it is critically important that the trigger signal occur at the same time for each presentation to be included in the average. The P_m was used to determine synchronization of the stimuli. The P_m for the individual occlusion was displayed and inspected to determine when the occlusion occurred. The occlusion was included in the average only if it occurred at the same time in the 500 msec sample as the other presentations. The average for each trial was generated with only the P_m displayed. A minimum of sixty-four mid-inspiratory occlusions were averaged for each trial.

Zero time, the beginning of the occlusion, was defined as the point of intersection of two lines drawn on the averaged P_m trace as illustrated in figure 44.2. The P_1 latency of the RREP is the time from this point to the peak of the first positive potential. This latency was determined for each electrode pair in each trial. The zero-peak amplitude of P_1 was measured for each electrode pair and each trial. The pressure at which this peak occurred (ΔP_m) was also determined. End-tidal PCO_2 for room air and CO_2 trials were measured from the polygraph record. Inspiratory drive was estimated by determining the $P_{0.1}$ from the polygraph record of P_m for the onset occlusions presented in the middle of each trial. A multifactorial ANOVA and paired t-test were used for statistical comparison.

RESULTS

RREPs were recorded bilaterally in all subjects breathing room air (figure 44.3). The mean P_1 peak latency was 54.06 ± 5.44 msec and 52.95 ± 10.28 msec for C_Z-C_3 and C_Z-C_4 respectively (table 44.1). There was no significant

FIG. 44.2 Computer-averaged mouth pressure with mid-inspiratory occlusions. The bottom trace is the averaged mouth pressure (eighty occlusions) for one subject breathing room air. Negative pressure is plotted up the y-axis. Time (in milliseconds) is plotted on the x-axis. The point of zero time, when the occlusion began, was determined by drawing a line through the baseline pressure and a second line through the portion of the trace where pressure was decreasing rapidly. The point of intersection of these two lines was defined as zero time for the determination of RREP latencies. The top trace is the averaged mouth pressure (eighty occlusions) for the same subject breathing the elevated CO_2 gas.

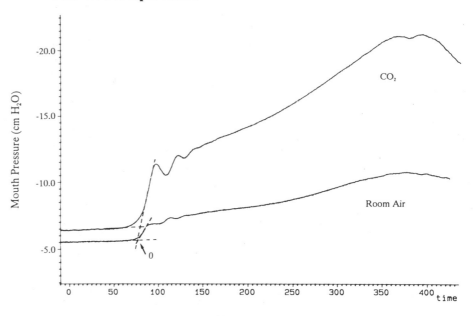

Table 44.1. Average Pressures and Peak Evoked Potential Data for Trials during Room Air and CO_2 Breathing.

	Room Air		CO_2[1]	
	C_Z-C_3	C_Z-C_4	C_Z-C_3	C_Z-C_4
P_1 Latency[2]	54.06[3]	52.95	41.82*	45.56*
	(5.44)	(10.28)	(6.92)	(9.02)
P_1 Amplitude[4]	2.18	1.52	2.28	2.07
	(0.76)	(0.54)	(0.87)	(1.41)

	Room Air	CO_2	
$P_{0.1}$[5]	1.68	4.21*	
	(0.61)	(1.97)	
ΔP_m	1.63	5.20*	
	(0.18)	(0.66)	

[1] Inspired gas was 5% CO_2/95% O_2.
[2] In milliseconds.
[3] Mean (SD).
[4] In microvolts.
[5] $P_{0.1}$ and ΔP_{mM} in cm H_2O.
* $P < 0.05$

difference between these latencies. The mean $P_{0.1}$ for room-air breathing was 1.68 ± 0.61 cm H_2O. Breathing 5% CO_2 and 95% O_2 significantly increased end-tidal PCO_2 by 4.57 ± 2.26 mmHg. The mean $P_{0.1}$ was significantly increased to 4.21 ± 1.97 cm H_2O. RREPs were again recorded bilaterally (fig. 44.4). The mean P_1 peak latencies were 41.82 ± 6.92 msec and 45.56 ± 9.08 msec, respectively, and were significantly ($p<0.05$) shorter than room-air trials. The zero-peak amplitude of P_1 from both electrode pairs during CO_2 breathing was not significantly different from the room-air trials. The ΔP_m from zero time to the P_1 peak latency was significantly increased from 1.63 ± 0.18 cm H_2O for the room air trials to 5.20 ± 0.66 cm H_2O during CO_2 stimulation (table 44.1).

DISCUSSION

Interruption of inspiration with a transient occlusion produces bilateral cerebral cortical neural activity within 55 msec from the application of the occlusion. This result with subjects breathing room air is similar to previous reports using mid-inspiratory occlusions (14). Stimulation of the afferents (as yet unknown) that elicit the RREP is the result of the subject inspiring against the occluded airway. This is a unique aspect in the recording of RREP. In other sensory systems, the experimenter controls the stimulus parameters. With respiratory loads, the experimenter presents the subject with a load to inspiration, but stimulation does not occur until the subject acts on the load. The activation of the afferents mediating the RREP is therefore dependent on self-stimulation by the subject. This makes the ventilatory status of the subject an important factor in the generation of the sensory signal that elicits the RREP. Changing the inspiratory drive will alter the rate at which the load dependent mechanical changes occur and will similarly affect the afferents that transduce those mechanical parameters. It was shown previously with occlusions presented at the onset of the inspiration, that the latency of the first positive peak decreased with increasing inspiratory drive (5). This correlation was found by comparing intersubject variation of $P_{0.1}$ breathing room air with their corresponding RREP P_1 latency. Using mid-inspiratory occlusions, the present study found that intrasubject increases in inspiratory drive were also associated with decreases in the latency of the P_1 peak.

Mid-inspiratory occlusions were found previously to produce shorter-latency and larger-amplitude RREP than occlusions presented at the onset of the inspiration which have a slower rate of change in P_m (14). Increasing inspiratory drive will increase the rate of change in P_m during an occlusion. The afferents under these conditions will reach

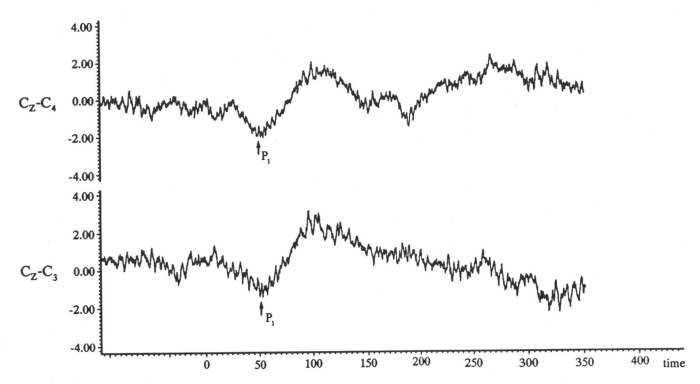

FIG. 44.3 Computer averaged EEG response to mid-inspiratory occlusions presented during room air breathing. These data are for the same subject as in figure 44.2. Voltage (in microvolts) is plotted as a function of time (in milliseconds). Eighty mid-inspiratory occlusions were averaged. C_z-C_3 was the electrode pair over the left and C_z-C_4 was the electrode pair over the right somatosensory cortex. The P_1 peak is indicated. The P_1 latencies were 52.0 msec for both electrode pairs.

threshold sooner and be activated more simultaneously. This should result in a decrease in the time necessary for afferent activation of the cerebral cortex, and the corresponding latencies of the cortical evoked potentials should be decreased. Thus, the effect of increased inspiratory drive was a decreased RREP P_1 latency. Therefore, the ventilatory status of the subject must be considered when interpreting variations in RREP latencies.

The peak referred to as P_1 with RREP is believed to be the same peak found with mechanical stimulation in other somatosensory systems with a latency of 40–50 msec (10). This peak has been found with a variety of mechanical stimulation paradigms (9, 10, 12, 13, 18, 19). The origin of this peak has been interpreted as reflecting the initial activation of the sensory cortex (10). With tactile stimulation, the amplitude of this peak has been shown to be related to stimulus magnitude by a power function (9). Increased inspiratory drive more than doubled the change in P_m coincident with the P_1. The P_1 latency decreased but the peak amplitudes did not change. This suggests that, while P_m is a useful signal averaging parameter for observing the RREP, the magnitude of the P_m is not the stimulus for the occlusion dependent RREP.

In an attempt to identify the afferents mediating respiratory sensations, conscious dogs were behaviorally conditioned to signal the detection of inspiratory occlusion and graded resistive loads (7). The loads were presented

through a tracheostomy that excluded the larynx, pharynx, mouth, and nose. The dogs could signal the detection of an inspiratory occlusion within the first inspiratory effort. Their resistive load detection threshold was similar to humans. Thus, dogs can signal the sensation of inspiratory mechanical loads, and the detection of these loads was mediated by afferents distal to the tracheostomy. Experiments performed with cats have shown that electrical stimulation of phrenic nerve afferents elicits neural activity in the somatosensory cortex (4). It has also been shown that the mechanical stimulation of intercostal muscle afferents can activate neurons in this same region (6). Projection of vagal and superior laryngeal nerve afferents to the somatosensory cortex has been reported in cats (1, 2, 17). Trigeminal and facial nerve afferents have similarly been demonstrated to elicit neural activity in the somatosensory cortex in humans (11, 15). Thus, the neural pathways to the somatosensory region of the cerebral cortex are present for respiratory related afferents from the mouth, airways, lung, and respiratory muscles.

Mechanoreceptors in the mouth and pharynx are one potential population of afferents that may be activated by the rapid decrease in P_m that occurs with mid-inspiratory occlusions. Williams et al. (20) reported the detection threshold for positive pressures in the mouth to be approximately 1.0 cm H_2O. Mechanical stimulation of the face has been reported to elicit an evoked potential with the first

FIG. 44.4 Computer averaged EEG response to mid-inspiratory occlusions presented during CO_2 breathing. These data are for the same subject as in figures 44.2 and 44.3. Voltage (in microvolts) is plotted as a function of time (in milliseconds). Eighty mid-inspiratory occlusions were averaged. The P_1 latencies were 50.0 and 43.8 msec for C_z-C_3 and C_z-C_4, respectively.

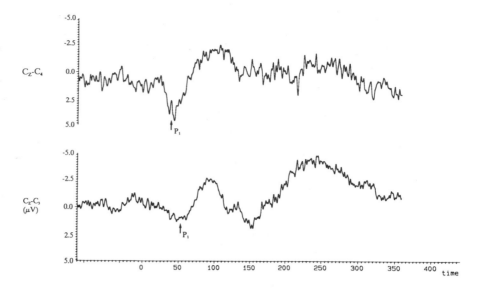

positive peak occurring at a latency of 10.37 msec (16). Schieppati and Ducati (15) found that the latency of the first positive peak of the evoked potential elicited by mechanical stimulation by air puffs on the face and tongue (innervated by branches of the trigeminal nerve) was 21–22 msec. The latencies for similar stimulation of the hand and toe were 30 and 56 msec, respectively. The trials with subjects inspiring increased CO_2 resulted in P_1 latencies greater than 40 msec. This is the shortest P_1 latency reported to date for RREP and is in the same range as found with mechanical stimulation of the limbs (9, 10, 12, 13, 18, 19). This latency is nearly twice that for air pressure stimulation of the tongue. This large disparity in evoked potential latency would suggest that afferents in the mouth and pharynx may not be mediating the RREP. It remains unknown, however, which population of receptors are mediating the RREP.

This study demonstrates that increases in inspiratory drive decrease the latency of the RREP. It will be important in future studies to also determine the role of lung volume, air flow rates, and intrinsic loads on the RREP. Additional studies will be needed to identify the cortical neural generators of the component peaks of the RREP. This will aid in understanding the neural processing of this respiratory-related sensory information. It will also be important for future experiments to correlate these neural measures of cortical sensory processes with psychophysical ratings of respiratory sensation. The results of these studies should provide new insight into the physiological mechanisms mediating the sensation of respiratory stimuli.

REFERENCES

1. Aubert, M., and J. Legros. Topographie des projections de la sensibilite viscérale sur l'écorce cérébrale du chat. I. Étude des projections corticales du vague cervical chez le chat anesthésié au nembutal. *Arch. Ital. Biol.* 108:423-446, 1970.

2. Aubert, M., and C. Guilhen. Topographie des projections de la sensibilité viscérale sur l'écorce cerebrale du chat. III. Étude des projections corticales du nerf larynge superieur. *Arch. Ital. Biol.*, 109:236-252, 1971.

3. Clark, W.A., M.H. Goldstein, Jr., B.M. Brown, D.F. O'Brien, and H. Zieman. The average response computer (ARC): A digital device for computing averages and amplitude and time histograms of electrophysiological responses. *Trans. IRE*, BME-8(1):46-51, 1961.

4. Davenport, P.W., F.J. Thompson, R.L. Reep, and A.N. Freed. Projection of phrenic nerve afferents to the cat sensorimotor cortex. *Brain Res.* 328:150-153, 1985.

5. Davenport, P.W., W.A. Friedman, F.J. Thompson and O. Franzen. Respiratory-related cortical potentials evoked by inspiratory occlusion in humans. *J. Appl. Physiol.* 60(6):1843-1848, 1986.

6. Davenport, P.W., A. Mercack, R. Shannon, and B.G. Lindsey. Sensorimotor cortical evoked potentials (CEP) elicited by intercostal muscle vibration. *Fed. Proc.* 46:1103, 1987.

7. Davenport, P.W., D.J. Dalziel, B. Webb, J.R. Bellah, and C.J. Vierck, Jr. Inspiratory resistive load detection in conscious dogs. *J. Appl. Physiol.* 70:1284-1289, 1991.

8. Dawson, G.D. A summation technique for the detection of small evoked potentials. *Electroenceph. Clin. Neurophysiol.* 6:65-84, 1954.

9. Franzen, O., and K. Offenloch. Evoked response correlates of psychophysical magnitude estimates for tactile stimulation in man. *Exp. Brain Res.* 8:1-18, 1969.

10. Hämäläinen, H., J. Kekoni, M. Sams, K. Reinikainen, and R. Näätänen. Human somatosensory evoked potentials to mechanical pulses and vibration: Contributions of SI and SII somatosensory cortices to P50 and P100 components. *Electroenceph. Clin. Neurophysiol.* 75:13-21, 1990.

11. Hashumoto, I. Somatosensory evoked potentials elicited by air-puff stimuli generated by a new high-speed air control system. *Electroenceph. Clin. Neurophysiol.* 67:231-237, 1987.

12. Larsson, L.-E., and T.S. Prevec. Somato-sensory response to mechanical stimulation as recorded in the human EEG. *Electroenceph. Clin. Neurophysiol.* 28:162-172, 1970.

13. Pratt, H., R.N. Amlie, and A. Starr. Short latency mechanically evoked somatosensory potentials in humans. *Electroenceph. Clin. Neurophysiol.* 47:524-531, 1979.

14. Revelette, W.R., and P.W. Davenport. Effects of timing of inspiratory occlusion on cerebral evoked potentials in humans. *J. Appl. Physiol.* 68:282-288, 1990.

15. Schieppati, M., and A. Ducati. Short-latency potentials evoked by tactile air-jet stimulation of body and face in man. *Electroenceph. Clin. Neurophysiol.* 58:418-425, 1984.

16. Seyal, M., and J.K. Browne. Short latency somatosensory evoked potentials following mechanical taps to the face: Scalp recordings with a non-cephalic reference. *Electroenceph. Clin. Neurophysiol.* 74:271-276, 1989.

17. Siegfried, J. Topographie des projections corticales du nerf vague chez le chat. *Helv. Physiol. Acta* 19:269-278, 1961.

18. Soininen, K., and T. Jarvilehto. Somatosensory evoked potentials associated with tactile stimulation at detection threshold in man. *Electroenceph. Clin. Neurophysiol.* 56:494-500, 1983.

19. Starr, A., B. McKeon, N. Skuse, and D. Burke. Cerebral potentials evoked by muscle stretch in man. *Brain* 104:149-166, 1981.

20. Williams, W.N., W.S. Brown, Jr., and G.E. Turner. Intraoral air pressure discrimination by normal-speaking subjects. *Folia Phoniat.* 39:196-203, 1987.

45

Control of Respiratory Cycle Timing in Newborn Infants

Ann R. Stark

This chapter discusses several aspects of our work on respiratory cycle timing in infants and focuses on developmental differences that occur between infants and adults. First, infants differ from adults in the control of end-expiratory lung volume (EEV) and in the response to changes in lung volume. Second, infants have potent volume-sensitive timing reflexes similar to those described in animals. Third, infants have frequent disruptions in the expected sequential activation of the upper airway and inspiratory pump muscles. Some of these observations may be of clinical significance.

Compared to adults, infants·have a mechanical disadvantage in breathing due to their highly compliant chest wall. Although this is important for the birth process, it results in a relatively small relaxation volume determined by the opposing recoils of the lungs and chest wall. To compensate, newborns, unlike adults, breathe at rest from an EEV that is higher than the relaxation volume (12). Breathing from an elevated EEV avoids the potential risks of hypoxemia and atelectasis that might occur at low lung volume. This newborn breathing strategy is accomplished by the interactions of the inspiratory pump muscles, the upper airway muscles, and respiratory cycle timing.

The effect on breathing of a shift from the supine to the upright posture illustrates the difference in breathing strategy between infants and adults. When adults move from the supine to the upright posture, lung volume increases substantially. This volume increase is accompanied by the substantial increase in activation of the inspiratory muscles seen when they act at shorter operating length (4). Thus, in spite of the decreased mechanical advantage of the inspiratory muscles at higher lung volume, ventilation is not adversely affected (2). In contrast, when sleeping newborn infants were tilted from the supine to the upright posture, the effect on breathing was quite different (16). First, the changes in EEV were small and variable. They ranged from occasional decreases to increases of slightly less than one average tidal volume. Second, there were significant changes in timing. Expiratory (Te) and inspiratory (Ti) duration increased by 24% and 9%, respectively. This corresponded to a decrease in breathing frequency from 51 to 41 breaths per minute. Tidal volume increased slightly. Ventilation decreased by 12%, and this was accompanied by a small increase (about 0.5 torr) in mean end-tidal PCO_2. Our interpretation of these findings is that the prolonged Te seen when infants are tilted upright acts to minimize any

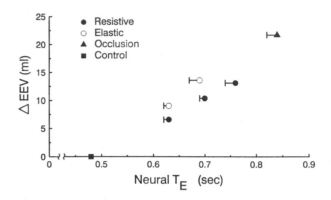

INCREASE IN EEV VERSUS NEURAL EXPIRATORY TIME

FIG. 45.1 Relationship of neural expiratory duration (T_E) and increase in end-expiratory volume (EEV) for loaded expirations in nine infants. Values are the mean ± S.E. (10).

change in EEV. This would avoid the need for a compensatory muscle response. At some point during development, infants must switch from this strategy of defending lung volume by altering timing to the adult strategy of responding to a change in lung volume by altering inspiratory muscle activation.

These observations prompted further investigation of the control of respiratory cycle timing in infants. These studies were based on observations that had been made in animals of the effect on timing of changes in lung volume. As in the animal studies, applications of mechanical loads were used to examine the modulation of timing (12). By using either resistive or elastic loads, the trajectory of inflation or deflation was altered. To better reflect neural control, timing was measured from the diaphragm EMG as well as from the volume recording. Unlike the animals, the infants were not anesthetized, but were studied during natural sleep.

The relationship between expired volume and expiratory timing in infants is similar to that found in cats (fig. 45.1) (10). Te was longer in the loaded breaths than in the preceding control breaths. Even though Te was longer, expired volume was less than in control breaths, resulting in an EEV that was higher in the loaded breaths. As the loads increased, the change in EEV from control increased and Te was progressively longer.

INSPIRED VOLUME VERSUS INSPIRATORY TIME

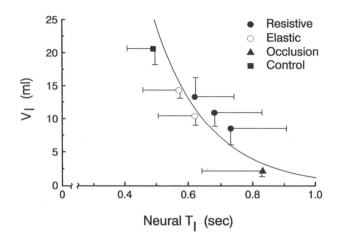

FIG. 45.2 Relationship of neural inspiratory duration (T_I and neural inspired volume (V_I) (volume corresponding to the termination of neural T_I) for loaded inspirations in six infants. Values are the mean ± S.E. (11)

The type of mechanical load changed the volume-timing profile of the loaded expiration and also affected the extent of change in Te. For similar increases in EEV, Te was longer for the resistive-loaded breaths than for the elastic-loaded ones. This finding supports the hypothesis that the accumulated expired volume history, including both EEV and the rate of lung deflation, is an important determinant of expiratory timing in infants (9).

The modulation of Ti was also investigated in infants using similar techniques. Although the relationship between inspired volume and Ti is well described in animals, this work extended observations in infants in whom the technique of airway occlusion had been primarily used to demonstrate reflex changes in inspiratory timing. By using inspiratory loads, the effect on timing could be observed during changes induced within the normal tidal volume range.

When mechanical loads and airway occlusions were applied to single inspirations, inspired volume was decreased from control and decreased progressively with increasing loads (fig. 45.2) (11). The type of load changed the inspired volume-time profile of the loaded inspiration but did not alter the extent of change of Ti. At similar inspired volume achieved by either resistive or elastic loads, neural Ti was not significantly different. Unlike the results obtained with expiratory loading, the relationship between inspired volume and Ti appeared to be unique and did not depend on the inspired volume trajectory.

The similarity of these results to those described in animals suggests that in infants the phasic regulation of Ti depends on a central neural timing threshold with vagally mediated inspiratory inhibition in response to increases in volume (5, 15). This inspiratory inhibition is related to the phasic volume change, independent of the inspired volume trajectory.

Premature infants have even greater disadvantages in breathing than do full-term infants. These include a more compliant chest wall and frequent irregularities in their breathing pattern, including apneic spells. Also, during active sleep, the predominant state of premature infants, dynamic mechanisms to maintain an elevated EEV may be altered (14). We expected that the volume-timing relationship might be less well developed in premature infants. However, a comprehensive comparison, after normalizing for size differences, suggests that the strength of the timing response for similar decrements in inspired volume was comparable in premature and term infants (6). In contrast to previous studies that suggest that maturation influences the volume-timing relationship (7), the inspiratory timing response to external inspiratory loads appears to be intact at this point in gestation.

Although there do not appear to be developmental differences between premature and term infants in their inspiratory timing responses with loading, we have observed effects of maturation on the sequence of activation of the respiratory muscles. Studies in animals and adult humans have examined the coordinated activity of the diaphragm and the posterior cricoarytenoid (PCA), the laryngeal abductor, in the control of airflow (1, 13). These studies show a sequence of muscle activation with inspiration. Activation of the upper airway muscles, including the alae nasi, the genioglossus, and the PCA, precedes diaphragm inspiratory activity. This presumably stabilizes or dilates the upper airway in the face of negative pressures developed by the inspiratory pump muscles. Our unexpected observation was that this sequence appears to be disrupted in premature infants, and to a lesser extent, even in term infants (8).

We studied the coordination of PCA and diaphragm activity in healthy premature and full-term infants. Measurements of the relationship between the onset of diaphragm and PCA activity and the onset of inspiratory flow revealed two patterns of respiratory muscle sequence. In the expected and most common sequence, categorized as a "lead breath," the onset of PCA activity preceded that of the diaphragm. All infants, however, also had "lag breaths" in which the usual sequence was disrupted and onset of PCA activity followed that of the diaphragm.

The frequency of breaths with the disrupted sequence was compared in premature and term infants (fig. 45.3). In the premature infants, the frequency ranged from 16% to 61% of all breaths for each individual. In the term infants, the range was from 6% to 43%. Although there is substantial overlap, the mean frequency of these disrupted breaths in the premature infants was significantly greater than that in the term infants.

These different activation sequences affected respiratory timing intervals. When PCA onset followed that of the

PERCENT LAG BREATHS IN PREMATURE AND TERM INFANTS

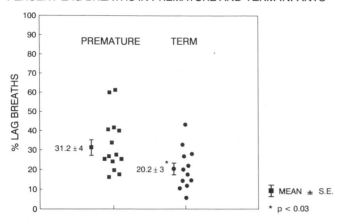

FIG. 45.3 Percent of breaths in which the onset of PCA EMG activity followed onset of diaphragm EMG activity for individual premature and full-term infants.

diaphragm, the interval between the start of diaphragm EMG activity and start of inspiratory air flow was longer than in the breaths with the expected sequence. This delayed onset of flow may result from delayed glottic opening. As expected, the lag breaths had a decreased delay between the onset of PCA and the start of flow. Lag breaths also had prolonged neural Ti. This longer Ti may be due to the delayed increase in inspired volume and is consistent with reflex control of Ti. In contrast, no differences were observed between the two sequences in mechanical Ti, tidal volume, or peak and mean inspiratory flows.

The effect of the different sequences on neural timing intervals was comparable in the term and premature infants, with one exception. This exception occurred in the comparison of the intervals between the onset of PCA and diaphragm EMG activity. In breaths with the expected sequence, the interval between PCA onset and diaphragm onset was similar in the premature and term infants. In contrast, when lag breaths occurred in term infants, the delay between PCA and diaphragm onset was significantly shorter than it was in the premature infants.

It is unclear why these disruptions in sequential activity occur. One possibility is that infants have a disturbance in central respiratory control, perhaps an alteration in central neuronal depolarization thresholds, that may change with maturation.

CLINICAL IMPLICATIONS

Some of these observations about the control of respiratory cycle timing in newborn infants may have implications of clinical significance. First, volume-sensitive reflexes contribute to the infant breathing strategy of dynamically maintaining an EEV above relaxation volume. Toward the end of the first year of life, this infant breathing strategy is replaced by the adult strategy of breathing from relaxation

volume (3). It is possible that some infants do not successfully maintain an elevated EEV, putting them at risk for hypoxemia or atelectasis. Second, the disruptions observed in sequential activation of the upper airway and diaphragm appeared to be well tolerated and resulted in no detectable change in airway resistance. The infants that were studied, however, were healthy. The increased delay between diaphragm onset and flow that occurs in the disrupted breaths may represent a period of ineffective diaphragm contraction. These periods of ineffective contraction might be inefficient and tax infants with limited inspiratory pump muscle reserve or increased respiratory demands. It is possible that these disruptions might promote muscle fatigue or respiratory decompensation in infants already at risk. Finally, many premature infants with severe respiratory disease are treated with endotracheal intubation and mechanical ventilation for prolonged periods. It is not known what the effects are of bypassing the larynx and artificially controlling lung volume on the development of volume-timing reflexes. This therapy might disrupt either breathing strategy or coordinated muscle activation. Future investigations may provide answers to these questions.

ACKNOWLEDGMENTS

This work was supported by the National Heart, Lung, and Blood Institute Specialized Center of Research Grant HL-34616.

REFERENCES

1. Brancatisano, T.P., D.S. Doss, and L.A. Engel. Respiratory activity of posterior cricoarytenoid muscle and vocal cords in humans. *J. Appl. Physiol.* 57:1143-1149, 1984.
2. Burki, N.K. The effects of changes in functional residual capacity with posture on mouth occlusion pressure and ventilatory pattern. *Am. Rev. Resp. Dis.* 116:895-900, 1977.
3. Colin, A.A., M.E.B. Wohl, J. Mead, F.A. Ratjen, G. Glass, and A.R. Stark. Transition from dynamically maintained to relaxed end-expiratory volume in human infants. *J. Appl. Physiol.* 67:2107-2111, 1989.
4. Druz, W.S., and J.T. Sharp. Activity of respiratory muscles in upright and recumbent humans. *J. Appl. Physiol.* 51:1552-1561, 1981.
5. Euler, C.V. On the central pattern generator for the basic breathing rhythmicity. *J. Appl. Physiol.* 55:1647-1659, 1983.
6. Fox, R.E., P.C. Kosch, H.A. Feldman, and A.R. Stark. Control of inspiratory duration in premature infants. *J. Appl. Physiol.* 64:2597-2604, 1988.
7. Gerhardt, T., and E. Bancalari. Maturational changes of reflexes influencing inspiratory timing in newborns. *J. Appl. Physiol.* 50:1282-1285, 1981.
8. Howell, R.G., L.E. Leszczynski, P.C. Kosch, and A.R. Stark. Uncoupling of laryngeal abduction and inspiratory effort in premature infants. *Pediatric Res.* 23:510A, 1988.
9. Koehler, R.C., and B. Bishop. Expiratory duration and abdominal muscle responses to elastic and resistive loading. *J. Appl. Physiol.* 46:730-737, 1979.

10. Kosch, P.C., P.W. Davenport, J.A. Wozniak, and A.R. Stark. Reflex control of expiratory duration in newborn infants. *J. Appl. Physiol.* 58:575-581, 1985.

11. Kosch, P.C., P.W. Davenport, J.A. Wozniak, and A.R. Stark. Reflex control of inspiratory duration in newborn infants. *J. Appl. Physiol.* 60:2007-2014, 1986.

12. Kosch, P.C., and A.R. Stark. Dynamic maintenance of end-expiratory lung volume in full-term infants. *J. Appl. Physiol.* 57:1126-1133, 1984.

13. Lunteren, E. van, and K.P. Strohl. The muscles of the upper airway. *Clin. in Chest Med.* 7:171-188, 1986.

14. Stark, A.R., B.A. Cohlan, T.B. Waggener, I.D. Frantz III, and P.C. Kosch. Regulation of end-expiratory lung volume during sleep in premature infants. *J. Appl. Physiol.* 62:1117-1123, 1987.

15. Miserocchi, G., and J. Milic-Emili. Effect of mechanical factors on the relation between rate and depth of breathing in cats. *J. Appl. Physiol.* 57:1126-1133, 1984.

16. Stark, A.R., T.B. Waggener, I.D. Frantz III, B.A. Cohlan, H.A. Feldman, and P.C. Kosch. Effect on ventilation of change to the upright posture in newborn infants. *J. Appl. Physiol.* 56:64-71, 1984.

17. Zechman, F.W., Jr., D.T. Frazier, and D.A. Lally. Respiratory volume-time relationships during resistive loading in the cat. *J. Appl. Physiol.* 40:177-183, 1976.

46

Modulation of Respiratory Pattern during NREM Sleep

James B. Skatrud, M. Safwan Badr, and Jerome A. Dempsey

During wakefulness, the ventilatory control system provides effective control of the overall level of alveolar ventilation and the relative stability of breathing pattern. Ventilatory compensation to mechanical loads or to low levels of chemical stimuli occurs quickly causing only transient changes in respiratory pattern. In contrast, withdrawal of wakefulness is associated with changes in mechanical and chemical influences which can result in periodic breathing, apnea, and upper airway obstruction. First, the sleeping state is directly linked to an increase in upper airway resistance. Lack of immediate compensation for this increased impedance can accentuate episodes of hypoventilation during fluctuating sleep states. Secondly, sleep unmasks a sensitive apneic threshold for CO_2 which will amplify any perturbation related to state or resistance. In addition to amplifying ventilatory changes in response to oscillation of sleep state, oscillations of airway resistance or chemical stimuli have been implicated in the periodic breathing of obstructive sleep apnea syndrome (9) and the periodic breathing at high altitude (2, 12), respectively. The purpose of this presentation is to discuss the contribution of fluctuating sleep state, upper airway resistance, and chemical stimuli in the genesis of breathing pattern instability.

The effect of sleep state on ventilation independent of changes in upper airway resistance has been difficult to determine in humans. In tracheotomized humans (12) and animals (11), the PCO_2 is usually 1–2 mmHg higher during sleep compared to wakefulness. In non-snorers who showed only a small increase in resistance between wakefulness and sleep, minute ventilation and tidal volume decreased 11% and 5%, respectively (13). When the sleep-related increase in upper airway resistance was minimized with either nasal continuous positive airway pressure (CPAP) (6) or helium (14), the PCO_2 still remained slightly elevated compared to wakefulness. These findings indicate that the sleep-related decrease in ventilation compared to wakefulness is present but is small when the state-related increase in resistance is minimized. Therefore, oscillation of sleep state alone would not be expected to produce large fluctuations in ventilation unless changes in resistance or chemical stimuli also occurred to amplify the instability.

Such changes in airway resistance occur frequently because of the close linkage between sleep state and resistance. A consistent increase in airway resistance is noted during sleep compared to wakefulness (8, 13). The increased resistance is sleep-stage dependent, with the highest resistance occurring in stage 3–4 sleep. These changes are especially prominent in snorers and, in the extreme form, can result in complete upper airway occlusion and apnea. Ventilation is decreased during these periods of high resistance, as indicated by the increase in ventilation when the mechanical impedance is reduced with nasal CPAP (6) or helium (14).

Oscillation of sleep state and chemical stimuli are important determinants of airway resistance. During periodic breathing, airway resistance is inversely related to the size of the tidal breath and the activity of genioglossus and diaphragmatic EMG, that is, resistance is higher during the nadir of the periodic cycles when the tidal volumes are smaller and the level of respiratory muscle activity is lower (1, 10, 15). Obstructed breaths have been noted during periods of low drive in subjects whose upper airways are susceptible to collapse as indicated by snoring (15). Thus, fluctuating resistance can act as a powerful sleep-linked destabilizer of the ventilatory control system. The magnitude of the resistance change with sleep state is an important determinant of the degree of ventilatory oscillation, which can range from mild hypopnea to frank obstructive apnea.

Another important effect of sleep in destabilizing rhythmic breathing is its unmasking of a sensitive apneic threshold for CO_2. During wakefulness, voluntary hyperventilation with hypocapnia to less than 25 mmHg is not consistently associated with posthyperventilation apnea (5, 12). In contrast, during NREM sleep, lowering of PCO_2 back to awake levels (−4 to −6 mmHg) with passive hyperventilation is associated with a prolonged apnea (fig. 46.1). The duration of the apnea is related to the magnitude of hypocapnia and the level of background ventilatory stimulation. Apnea was shorter for a given level of hypocapnia during hypoxia versus normoxia. Thus, the sleeping state removes the nonchemical tonic influences which prevent hypocapnic respiratory inhibition or disfacilitation. Consequently, rhythmic breathing during sleep is critically dependent on the level of CO_2.

A distinction between active and passive hyperventilation is important in evaluating the effect of hypocapnia on breathing pattern. Active hyperventilation has been associated with a poststimulus potentiation of ventilatory output or after-discharge that could serve as an important stabilizing influence (4). Once activated, this feedback process maintains the activity of respiratory neurons even after the

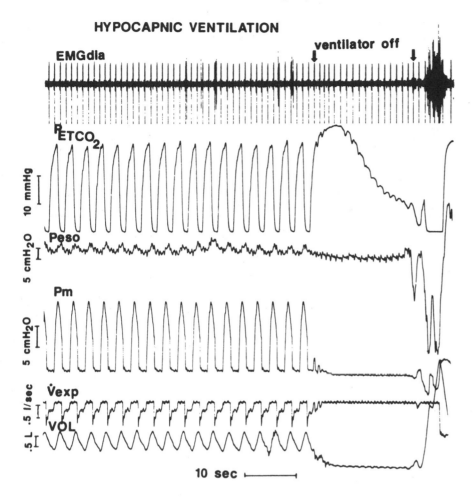

HYPOCAPNIC VENTILATION

ventilator off

EMGdia

$P_{ET}CO_2$

10 mmHg

Peso

5 cmH₂O

Pm

5 cmH₂O

Vexp

.5 l/sec

VOL

.5 L

10 sec

FIG. 46.1 Posthyperventilation apnea following passive hyperventilation during NREM sleep. At the first arrow, the ventilator was turned off and was followed by a 22 sec apnea. EMGdia, surface diaphragmatic EMG; $P_{ET}CO_2$, end-tidal PCO2; Peso, esophageal pressure; Pm, mouth pressure; Vexp, expiratory flow; vol, tidal volume.

primary stimulus has been removed. The slowly declining respiratory activity after stimulus removal reflects the gradual decay of activity within these reverberating neural circuits located in the brainstem. The after-discharge is activated by a variety of stimuli that increase respiratory output and are not impaired by anesthesia, decerebration, vagotomy, or paralysis. Thus, the after-discharge mechanism is presumed to be active during the sleeping state and would tend to limit the undershoot following an actively induced hypocapnia.

The ability of the after-discharge mechanism to prevent apnea following active hyperventilation was tested during NREM sleep (fig. 46.2). Active hyperventilation was produced in normal humans by inducing mild hypoxia (O_2 saturation 80%) for 5 min. The stimulus was abruptly removed by adding 100% oxygen. Apnea was consistently observed indicating that either the after-discharge mechanism was impaired during this experimental condition or that it was not sufficient to overcome the powerful inhibitory influence of hypocapnia. Impairment of the after-discharge by sleep state alone is unlikely because it has been shown to be active even in decerebrate animals. A more likely explanation is the development of hypoxic depression of the central nervous system directly involving the neurons

that generate the after-discharge or indirectly by acting on neurons that are normally activated by the after-discharge mechanism. Hypoxic depression of ventilation has been demonstrated in awake and sleeping humans (3, 7).

To determine the presence of the after-discharge phenomenon independent of hypoxic depression, hypoxia-induced active hyperventilation was produced for short periods of time (<1 min) which are unlikely to produce hypoxic depression. The isocapnic, active hyperventilation was abruptly stopped with hyperoxia, and the subsequent breaths were observed for evidence of after-discharge (fig. 46.3). As a control, the transition from room air to hyperoxia indicated the decrease in ventilation which occurred due to hyperoxia alone. The abrupt termination of active hyperventilation resulted in ventilation remaining elevated above the room air to hyperoxia transition control for six breaths. Based on a lung-chemoreceptor delay of 6 sec, chemoreceptor stimulation cannot account for the persistently elevated ventilation beyond the second or third breath. We concluded that the after-discharge phenomenon caused the small elevation in ventilation following removal of the chemoreceptor stimulus.

The relative strength of the after-discharge phenomenon in preventing hypocapnic-induced apnea was determined

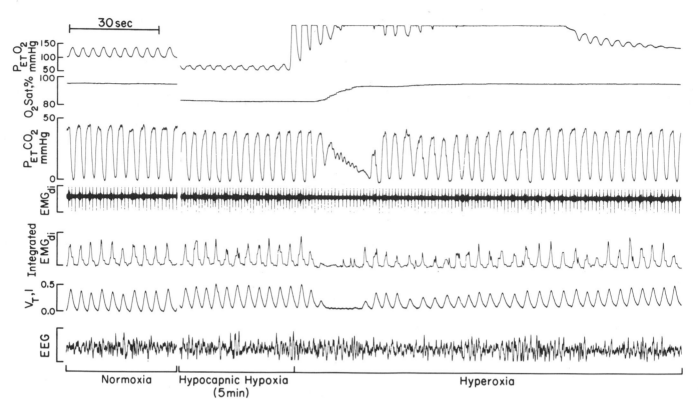

FIG. 46.2 Posthyperventilation apnea following active hyperventilation with 5 min of hypoxia. Hyperventilation was abruptly terminated with administration of hyperoxia. $P_{ET}O_2$, end-tidal PO_2; $P_{ET}CO_2$, end-tidal PCO_2; V_T, I, tidal volume.

(fig. 46.3). A short period (<1 min) of hypocapnic hypoxia-induced hyperventilation was abruptly stopped with hyperoxia and the subsequent breaths compared to the room air to hyperoxia transition. The minute ventilation was below the room air to hyperoxia transition and also below the post isocapnic hypoxia period. Thus, the after-discharge was insufficient to prevent the powerful inhibitory effect of hypocapnia on ventilation. The reduction in ventilation and prolongation of expiratory time (130% of room air) is a substantial destabilizer of breathing pattern that can cause hypopnea and apnea during NREM sleep.

The role of hypoxic depression on the manifestation of the after-discharge was investigated by comparing the ventilatory response following 1-min and 5-min periods of isocapnic hypoxia-induced hyperventilation (fig. 46.4). Ventilatory depression occurred after 5 min of hypoxia, but not after 1 min, indicating absence of the after-discharge phenomenon related to the length of hypoxic exposure. The administration of hyperoxia unmasked the central nervous system depression that was obscured by stimulation from the peripheral chemoreceptors.

The reduced after-discharge with relatively mild hypoxia compromises an important stabilizing influence on ventilatory control and may predispose to periodic breathing and apnea. For example, the effect of hypocapnia on ventilation is greater after 5 min than 1 min of hypoxia. The Te was prolonged 215% following hyperoxic cessation of 5 min of hypocapnic hypoxic hyperventilation ($P_{ET}CO_2$ 41 mmHg,

$P_{ET}O_2$ 64 mmHg) compared to only a 130% prolongation following 1 min of hypoxic hyperventilation ($P_{ET}CO_2$ 48 mmHg, $P_{ET}O_2$ 48 mmHg). In addition to its effect on after-discharge, 5 min of hypoxia may also affect neural mechanisms responsible for switching from expiration to inspiration, which would further prolong Te (16). The time-dependent onset of hypoxic depression may account for the observation that periodic breathing takes minutes to develop during NREM sleep. Therefore, hypoxic periodic breathing represents a complex interaction between stimulation of the peripheral chemoreceptor and depression of central neural stabilizing mechanisms.

SUMMARY

Several determinants of respiratory pattern stability during NREM sleep have been presented. Sleep state alone has only a small effect on the overall level of alveolar ventilation, and the ventilatory response to increased levels of chemical stimuli is only slightly reduced. However, the removal of nonchemical tonic influences associated with wakefulness causes an increase in upper airway resistance and an unmasking of an apneic threshold for PCO_2. Fluctuations in airway resistance and chemical stimuli will greatly exaggerate the ventilatory response to primary oscillation in sleep state. Periodic breathing, apnea, and even complete upper airway occlusion are frequent consequences.

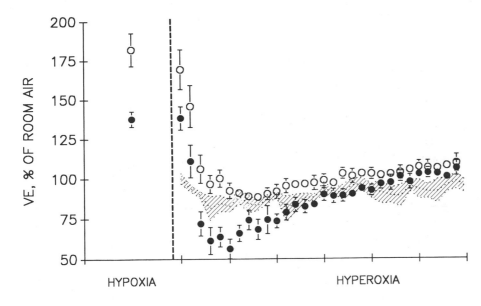

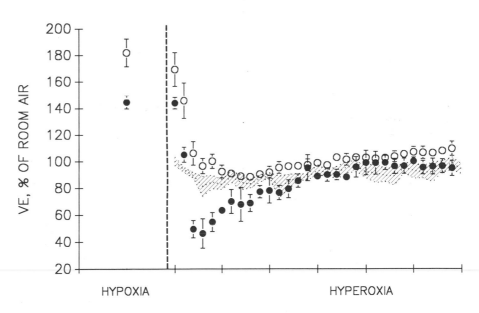

FIG. 46.3 Change in ventilation following hypoxia-induced hyperventilation. Active hyperventilation was induced with 1 min of isocapnic (O) or hypocapnic (●) hypoxia. At the dashed vertical line, hyperoxia abruptly terminated the hypoxic stimulus. The stippled area represents the mean ± SD of the change in ventilation during the transition from room air to hyperoxia that was used as the control condition. Following isocapnic hyperventilation, note that ventilation remains above the room air to hyperoxia range for six breaths, indicating the presence of the after-discharge phenomenon. Following hypocapnic hyperventilation, ventilation falls below the room air to hyperoxia range, indicating the ability of hypocapnia to override the stabilizing influence of the after-discharge. Isocapnic hypoxia trials: room air — $P_{ET}CO_2$ 47 mmHg, $P_{ET}O_2$ 106 mmHg; isocapnic hypoxia — $P_{ET}CO_2$ 47 mmHg, $P_{ET}O_2$ 63 mmHg. Hypocapnic hypoxia trials: room air—$P_{ET}CO_2$ 44 mmHg, $P_{ET}O_2$ 105 mmHg; hypocapnic hypoxia—$P_{ET}CO_2$ 40 mmHg, $P_{ET}O_2$ 50 mmHg. V_E, minute ventilation.

FIG. 46.4 Effect of hypoxic depression on ventilation following hypoxia-induced hyperventilation. Active isocapnic hyperventilation was induced with hypoxia for 1 (O) and 5 (●) min. Following 1 min of hyperventilation, after-discharge maintained ventilation above the room air to hyperoxia range. In contrast, 5 min of hypoxic hyperventilation caused ventilation to decrease below the room air to hyperoxia range, indicating the presence of hypoxic depression of the after-discharge phenomenon. Isocapnic hypoxia trials (1 min): same as above. Isocapnic hypoxia trials (5 min): room air — $P_{ET}CO_2$ 43 mmHg, $P_{ET}O_2$ 106 mmHg; isocapnic hypoxia — $P_{ET}CO_2$ 43 mmHg, $P_{ET}O_2$ 62 mmHg.

Hypoxia has a dual action in causing ventilatory instability via its peripheral effect on increasing controller gain and via its central effect of causing hypoxic depression of the central nervous system. Ventilation following a period of apnea or hypopnea is greatly augmented in the presence of hypoxia because of peripheral chemoreceptor stimulation. This ventilatory overshoot will lower the PCO_2 toward or below the apneic threshold and thereby accentuate the subsequent ventilatory undershoot. Hypoxia also interferes with the expression of the after-discharge phenomenon and thereby eliminates an important stabilizer of ventilatory pattern. Hypoxia may also prevent normal neural phase switching from expiration to inspiration, thereby prolonging periods of central apnea (16). Thus, hypoxia can be a potent initiator of periodic breathing and can serve as a powerful amplifier of other primary oscillations in ventilatory control.

ACKNOWLEDGMENTS

Supported by NIH SCOR and VA Medical Research Service.

REFERENCES

1. Aronson, R.M., E. Onal, D. Carley, and M. Lopata. Changes in upper airway and respiratory muscle activity and pulmonary resistance during sleep-induced periodic breathing. *Amer. Rev. Resp. Dis.* 137:126, 1988.

2. Berssenbrugger, A., J. Dempsey, C. Iber, J. Skatrud, and P. Wilson. Mechanisms of hypoxia-induced periodic breathing during sleep in humans. *J. Physiol.* (London) 343:507-524, 1983.

3. Chin, K., O. Motoharu, H. Masashi, K. Takanobu, S. Yanosuke, and K. Kenshi. Breathing during sleep with mild hypoxia. *J. Appl. Physiol.* 67:1198-1207, 1989.

4. Eldridge, F. Posthyperventilation breathing: Different effects of active and passive hyperventilation. *J. Appl. Physiol.* 34:422-430, 1973.

5. Henke, K., A. Arias, J.B. Skatrud, and J. Dempsey. Inhibition of inspiratory muscle activity during sleep. *Am. Rev. Resp. Dis.* 138:8-15, 1988.

6. Henke, K., J.A. Dempsey, J.M. Kowitz, and J.B. Skatrud. Effects of sleep-induced increases in upper airway resistance on ventilation. *J. Appl. Physiol.* 69:617-624, 1990.

7. Holtby, S.G., D.J. Berezanski, and N.R. Anthonisen. Effect of 100% O_2 on hypoxic eucapnic ventilation. *J. Appl. Physiol.* 65:1157-1162, 1988.

8. Hudgel, D.W., R.J. Martin, B. Johnson, and P. Hill. Mechanics of the respiratory system and breathing pattern during sleep in normal humans. *J. Appl. Physiol.* 56:133-137, 1984.

9. Onal, E., and M. Lopata. Periodic breathing and the pathogenesis of occlusive sleep apneas. *Am. Rev. Resp. Dis.* 126:676-688, 1982.

10. Onal, E., D.L. Burrows, R.H. Hart, and M. Lopata. Induction of periodic breathing during sleep causes upper airway obstruction in humans. *J. Appl. Physiol.* 61:1438-1443, 1986.

11. Phillipson, E.A., and G. Bowes. Control of breathing during sleep. In *Handbook of Physiology,* Section , vol. 2, 649-689. Bethesda, Md.: American Physiological Society, 1986.

12. Skatrud, J.B., and J.A. Dempsey. Interaction of sleep state and chemical stimuli in sustaining rhythmic ventilation. *J. Appl. Physiol.* 55:813-822, 1983.

13. Skatrud, J.B., and J.A. Dempsey. Airway resistance and respiratory muscle function in snorers during NREM sleep. *J. Appl. Physiol.* 59:328-335, 1985.

14. Skatrud, J.B., J.A. Dempsey, S. Badr, and R.L. Begle. Effect of airway impedance on CO_2 retention and respiratory muscle activity during NREM sleep. *J. Appl. Physiol.* 65:1676-1685, 1988.

15. Warner, G., J.B. Skatrud, and J.A. Dempsey. Effect of hypoxia-induced periodic breathing on upper airway obstruction during sleep. *J. Appl. Physiol.* 62:2201-2211, 1987.

16. Younes, M. The physiologic basis of central apnea and periodic breathing. *Curr. Pulmonol.* 10:265-326, 1989.

47

Exercise and the Respiratory Mechanical Load

Magdy Younes

The respiratory mechanical load can affect exercise performance in a variety of ways. Two of these will be reviewed here: the respiratory load and exercise ventilation and breathing pattern.

Respiratory elastance and resistance determine the level of ventilation and tidal volume for a given pattern of respiratory muscle activation. Ventilation and tidal volume, in turn, determine arterial blood gas tensions and, to some extent, pH at a given level of exercise. These are clearly of some importance to the exercising muscles. It is, therefore, reasonable to ask whether the respiratory load constrains exercise ventilation, thereby possibly contributing to fatigue of the exercising muscles. Although arterial PCO_2 during heavy exercise is lower than resting PCO_2, thereby technically excluding hypoventilation, it may be argued that had the respiratory load been less, ventilation would have been even greater, with improved blood gas tensions and acid-base homeostasis. In fact Dempsey et al. (4) have advocated this scenario based on the response of arterial gas tensions to helium breathing during heavy exercise.

The issue of whether the respiratory load constrains exercise ventilation has been investigated by observing the response of exercise ventilation to changes in load. If the normal load constrains ventilation, then an increase in load should cause a reduction in $\dot{V}_E$ at a given power output, and vice versa. Most of the work in this area has been done with resistive loading and unloading. The effect of added resistance has been studied extensively (2, 5, 7, 13). All have found that exercise ventilation, particularly at high levels of work, is depressed if the resistance is increased. The significance of this finding to the issue of whether the internal load constrains ventilation is, however, dubious. These studies indicate that an increase in load constrains ventilation but do not necessarily indicate that the native load is particularly constraining. It is for this reason that the results of unloading assume a greater significance with respect to the issue being addressed.

The respiratory control system can follow one of three courses in response to a decrease in load: (1) Respiratory muscle activation may be down-regulated such that the same ventilation is obtained. (2) Respiratory muscle activation is maintained unchanged, whereby an increase in ventilation will result. (3) There may be an intermediate response whereby incomplete downregulation results in higher ventilation at somewhat lesser levels of activity. The first type of response would clearly indicate that the native load was not constraining ventilation. Either of the other two responses would suggest that the internal load constrains ventilation.

Until very recently the only means available to unload the respiratory system during heavy exercise was through the use of helium-O_2 mixtures. Because the density of these mixtures is less than that of air, airway resistance is reduced. The magnitude of reduction in resistance would depend on the degree of turbulence, and hence density dependence of the native resistance. The response of exercise ventilation to helium breathing has been studied extensively and the results are fairly uniform in that exercise $\dot{V}_E$ is considerably larger, particularly at high levels of ventilation where turbulence is high (9, 10, 12). Although the most obvious interpretation of this finding is that the normal resistance constrains exercise ventilation, more recent observations make it necessary to consider alternate interpretations.

First, the degree of reduction in resistance by helium is very modest. According to the data of Hussain et al. (9) resistance decreased by less than 1 cm $H_2O/l/sec$ during heavy exercise. In a recent study, we calculated the ventilatory consequences of reducing the resistance by this amount in the absence of any down-regulation of neural output (6). This was done by first estimating the time course of muscle pressure (P_{mus}) development given temporal patterns of flow and volume observed during heavy exercise, and assuming normal values of respiratory system elastance and resistance. The procedure was then reversed to result in the temporal pattern of flow and volume if P_{mus} remained the same but resistance decreased by the amount observed during helium breathing. This analysis indicated that ventilation should increase by only 6% if P_{mus} did not change. Considering that ventilation increased much more with helium (ca. 30%), the increase in ventilation was not likely due to unloading.

Second, it has recently become possible to unload the respiratory muscles during heavy exercise to a much greater extent than is possible with helium. This is done using an apparatus that delivers positive pressure at the mouth in proportion to inspired flow, expired flow, or both (15). Using this apparatus, we studied the effect of a negative resistance of -2.2 cm $H_2O/l/sec$ at different levels of exercise. As far as the muscles are concerned this is three times as much muscle resistive unloading as the reduction produced by helium. To our surprise, we found that with inspiratory

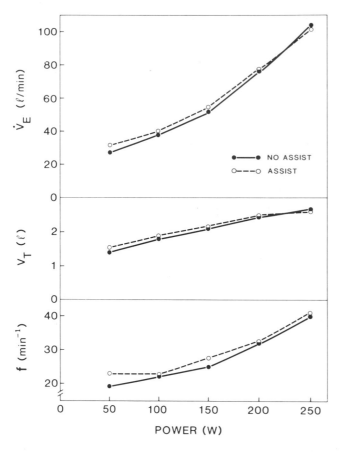

FIG. 47.1 Effect of inspiratory resistive unloading on ventilation ($\dot{V}_E$), tidal volume (V_T), and respiratory rate (f) during incremental exercise. (Drawn from 9.)

Table 47.1. Ventilatory and Pleural Pressure (P_{pl}) Responses to Pressure Assisted Ventilation (PAV) in Normals

	No Assist (±SEM)†		PAV (±SEM)		δ±(SEM)	
V_T (l)	2.02	(.17)	2.39	(.24)	.37	(.10)*
f (min^{-1})	28.0	(2.2)	27.5	(1.9)	−.5	(1.0)
$\dot{V}_E$ (l/min)	56.0	(4.3)	64.8	(3.6)	8.8	(1.3)***
P_{pl} 25 (cm H_2O)	−4.8	(.5)	−2.5	(.3)	.3	(.5)**
P_{pl} 50 (cm H_2O)	−10.2	(.7)	−4.5	(1.1)	5.7	(.9)***
P_{pl} 75 (cm H_2O)	−13.7	(.9)	−4.5	(1.6)	9.2	(1.5)***
P_{pl} EE (cm H_2O)	4.92	(.24)	4.81	(.13)	−.11	(.23)
IC (l)	2.97	(.46)	3.00	(.48)	.02	(.07)

V_T, tidal volume; f, respiratory rate; $\dot{V}_E$, minute ventilation; P_{pl} 25, P_{pl} 50, P_{pl} 75, pleural pressure at 25%, 50%, and 75% of T_i; P_{pl} EE, end-expiratory P_{pl}; IC, inspiratory capacity.

† Average of two bracketing controls.

*, **, *** Significant difference from "No assist" at $P \leq .05$, .02, and .01, respectively, using the paired t-test.

unloading alone ventilation increased only at very low levels of exercise with the difference decreasing as power output increased. At the highest level of exercise there was no difference in $\dot{V}_E$. (fig. 47.1). There were also no differences in breathing pattern (V_T and f).

We became concerned that the different responses to pressure and helium unloading may have been due to the expiratory unloading effect of helium. Additional experiments were, therefore, carried out where we unloaded expiration alone (negative pressure in proportion to expiratory flow) or both inspiration and expiration (positive pressure in proportion to inspiratory flow and negative pressure in proportion to expiratory flow). The changes in $\dot{V}_E$ with either type of unloading were again small and insignificant. In this latter study we also documented down-regulation of P_{mus} (6).

It follows that the ventilatory consequences of unloading depend on how unloading is done. There is no clear answer as to whether the native resistance constrains ventilation during heavy exercise. Because the increase in ventilation with helium is more than is expected on the basis of unloading alone (first interpretation above) and greater resistive unloading produced by pressure results in no hy-

perventilation, we speculate that the hyperventilatory response to helium is related to some other property of helium (6). It is of interest to note that in the only study in which the response to helium was documented breath by breath (9), the increase in ventilation was found to occur gradually over several breaths, whereas the reduction in resistance was complete within the first two breaths. Clearly, if unloading was the mechanism responsible for hyperventilation, the increase in ventilation should have been maximal within the first two breaths and may have abated somewhat later as a result of chemical negative feedback.

The apparatus referred to earlier (15) also permitted us to assess the effect of reducing the elastic as well as the resistive load in normal subjects during heavy exercise. In this experiment the pressure assist was such that the apparatus delivered half the resistive and half the elastic pressure (1.5 cm H_2O/l/sec + 5.0 cm H_2O/l) therefore assuming fully half the respiratory muscle work. Unlike the case with resistive loading alone, ventilation and tidal volume increased significantly but, despite massive unloading, the changes were small (table 47.1). Simultaneously, there was a reduction in P_{mus}. On average, down-regulation of P_{mus} canceled out 75% of the applied pressure assist, while only 25% of the extra pressure was used to increase ventilation.

In summary, when the respiratory system is given the option to increase ventilation during heavy exercise through pressure assist the tendency is for it to reduce its pressure output rather than increase ventilation. The case for the respiratory load constraining ventilation in normal subjects is, therefore, rather weak. Of course, the situation may be different in highly trained athletes who reach much greater levels of ventilation than the ones studied here (circa 90 l/min). This remains to be determined.

The respiratory load determines the level of pressure output during exercise. Should this be greater than the level that can be sustained indefinitely, a fatigue process is initiated. Because fatigue is a time-dependent process (14), the effect of fatigue, if it occurs, should be most evident near the end of exhaustive exercise. The development of respiratory muscle fatigue (RMF) could influence exercise in the following ways: (1) Producing unpleasant sensation that may contribute to the sense of exhaustion that usually terminates exercise in normal subjects, or to the dyspnea in patients with lung disease, (2) altering breathing pattern to a faster, shallower one with consequences to gas exchange and, hence, arterial blood gas tensions. Thus, one may speculate that RMF may be in part responsible for the tachypneic drift observed during long term exercise (3, 8, 11), (3) Inhibiting respiratory muscle activity through the process of central fatigue (1). Arterial blood gases may therefore be worse than they would have been in the absence of fatigue.

Although several laboratory methods have been described to identify RMF (e.g., maximum pressures, EMG power spectrum, twitch or sniff P_{di}, etc.), these are difficult to implement or interpret in the setting of heavy exercise. Furthermore, they lack functional significance. Thus, demonstration of RMF by one or more of these techniques need not reflect any impairment of function, and vice versa. For example, there is no compelling reason to believe that overworking muscles will influence respiratory control (motor output and pattern) or cause unpleasant sensation only when peripheral fatigue (identified by the above techniques) occurs.

To investigate the functional consequences of RMF on ventilation, breathing pattern and exercise endurance, we used the following protocol (figure 47.2, bottom) in seven healthy males. Each subject exercised three times at a submaximal level selected to result in an endurance time of 8–15 min (roughly 80% of $\dot{V}O_2$max determined in a separate incremental exercise test). In the first and third tests there was no respiratory muscle assist. In the second test, pressure assist was applied to offset half the resistance and elastance of the respiratory system (as described above). The assist was applied from the onset of exercise until a point roughly 3 min less than the endurance time of the first test. The assist was then removed. The rationale for this approach is that if there was an effect of RMF on $\dot{V}_E$ or breathing pattern near the end of the control test, there should be less of it in the assisted test at the same time (since the muscles were working at a lower level throughout most of the test). The fact that the actual load is the same near the end of exercise in both kinds of test would make it possible to attribute differences at this point to cumulative effects of respiratory muscle work. Should the assist be sustained throughout exercise, differences between control and assisted tests near the end may be related to the difference in actual load at the time of comparison and not to the cumulative aspect of respiratory muscle work (i.e. the fatiguing process).

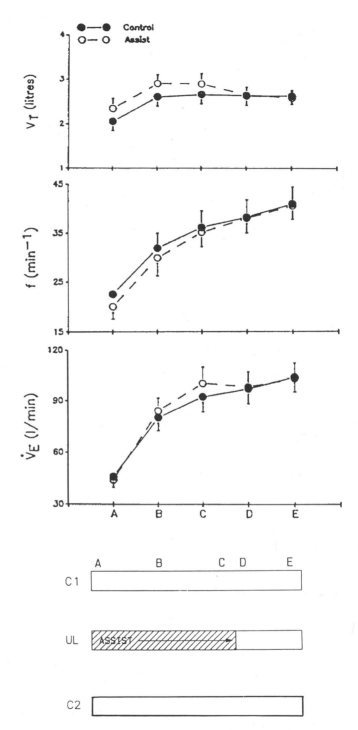

FIG. 47.2 Effect of elastic and resistive unloading (UL, shaded area) early during submaximal exercise on ventilation ($\dot{V}_E$), tidal volume (V_T), and frequency (f) during and following the period of assist. Points *A, B,* and *C* are data in early, mid, and late assist (open circles) compared with data at the same time in unassisted runs (solid circles, average of two control runs). Point *D* is 1 min after removal of assist and corresponding time of unassisted runs. Point *E* is the last minute of exercise. (For further details, see text.)

Figure 47.2 (top) shows the average results for the seven subjects. During the period of assist (points *A, B* and *C*) ventilation and tidal volume were higher and frequency was lower than at the same times in the control studies. Also, the Borg score for respiratory sensation was lower (not shown). Ventilation, breathing pattern, and Borg scores, however, were not different once the assist was removed (point *D,* 1 min after removal of assist), or at the end of exercise (point *E*). The endurance time was also not different (10.22 min versus 10.29 min). These results indicate that RMF, if any, does not affect ventilation, breathing pattern, respiratory sensation, or endurance time of exhaustive submaximal exercise.

A similar protocol applied to seven patients with severe chronic obstructive pulmonary disease (COPD) who were clearly ventilation-limited produced equally unimpressive results. The only significant difference at point D (1 min after removal of assist versus corresponding time of control tests) was a slightly lower frequency in the assisted test (22.8 versus 25.6 min^{-1}). There was also no difference in endurance time (10.1 min versus 10.1 min).

In summary, the respiratory load does not appear to provide an appreciable constraint to exercise ventilation or breathing pattern in normal subjects, and respiratory muscle fatigue does not seem to influence ventilation, breathing pattern, or submaximal endurance time. The consequences of RMF are minimal even in ventilation-limited patients with severe COPD.

REFERENCES

1. Bellemare, F., and B. Bigland-Ritchie. Central components of diaphragmatic fatigue assessed by phrenic nerve stimulation. *J. Appl. Physiol.* 62:1307-1316, 1987.

2. Demedts, M., and N.R. Anthonisen. Effects of increased external airway resistance during steady-state exercise. *J. Appl. Physiol.* 35:361-366, 1973.

3. Dempsey, J.A., N. Gledhill, W.G. Reddan, H.V. Forster, P.G. Hanson, and A.D. Claremont. Pulmonary adaptation to exercise: Effects of exercise type and duration, chronic hypoxia and physical training. *Ann. NY Acad. Sci.* 301:243-261, 1977.

4. Dempsey, J.A., P. Hanson, and K. Henderson. Exercise-induced arterial hypoxemia in healthy human subjects at sea-level. *J. Physiol.* (London) 355:161-175, 1984.

5. D'Urzo, A.D., K.R. Chapman, and A.S. Rebuck. Effect of inspiratory resistive loading on control of ventilation during progressive exercise. *J. Appl. Physiol.* 62:134-140, 1987.

6. Gallagher, C.G., and M. Younes. Effect of pressure assist on ventilation and respiratory mechanics in heavy exercise. *J. Appl. Physiol.* 66:1824-1837, 1989.

7. Gee, J.B.L., C. Burton, C. Vassallo, and J. Gregg. Effects of external airway obstruction on work capacity and pulmonary gas exchange. *Am. Rev. Resp. Dis.* 98:1003-1012, 1968.

8. Hanson, P., A. Claremont, J. Dempsey, and W. Reddan. Determinants and consequences of ventilatory responses to competitive endurance running. *J. Appl. Physiol.* 52:615-623, 1982.

9. Hussain, S.N.R., R.L. Pardy, and J.A. Dempsey. Mechanical impedance as determinant of inspiratory neural drive during exercise in humans. *J. Appl. Physiol.* 59:365-373, 1985.

10. Maio, D.A., and L.E. Farhi. Effect of gas density mechanics of breathing. *J. Appl. Physiol.* 23:687-693, 1967.

11. Martin, B.J., E.J. Morgan, C.W. Zwillich, and J.W. Weil. Control of breathing during prolonged exercise. *J. Appl. Physiol.* 50:27-31, 1981.

12. Nattie, E.E., and S.M. Tenney. The ventilatory response to resistance unloading during muscular exercise. *Resp. Physiol.* 10:249-262, 1970.

13. Silverman, L., G. Lee, T. Plotkin, L.A. Sawyers, and A.R. Yancey. Air flow measurements on human subjects with and without respiratory resistance at several work rates. *Ind. Hyg. Occupational Med.* 3:461-478, 1951.

14. Vollestad, N.K., O.M. Sejersted, R. Bahr, J.J. Woods, and B. Bigland-Ritchie. Motor drive and metabolic responses during repeated submaximal contractions in humans. *J. Appl. Physiol.* 64:1421-1427, 1988.

15. Younes, M., D. Bilan, and D. Jung. An apparatus for altering the mechanical load of the respiratory system. *J. Appl. Physiol.* 62:2491-2499, 1987.

Contributing Laboratories

Albert Berger
University of Washington
    School of Medicine
Department of Physiology
    and Biophysics, SJ-40
Room G424 HSB
Seattle, WA 98195

Gerald E. Bisgard
School of Veterinary Medicine
University of Wisconsin-Madison
2015 Linden Drive West
Room 2015
Madison, WI 53706

William E. Cameron
Department of Behavior Neuroscience
University of Pittsburgh
446 Crawford Hall
Pittsburgh, PA 15260

Jean Champagnat
Laboratoire de Physiologie Nerveuse
C.N.R.S.
91190 Gif-sur-Yvette
France

Fat-Chun T. Chang
Neurotox & Experimental Therapeutics
USAMRICD, SGRD-UV-YN/EA
Aberdeen Proving Ground, MD 21010

Neil S. Cherniack
Dean's Office, School of Medicine
Case Western Reserve University
10900 Euclid Avenue
Cleveland, OH 44106-4915

Morton I. Cohen
Department of Physiology
Albert Einstein College of Medicine
Room 303U
Bronx, NY 10461

Hazel Coleridge
University of California San Francisco
School of Medicine
Cardiovascular Research Institute
San Francisco, CA 94143

Paul W. Davenport
Department of Physiological Science
University of Florida
Health Science Center
Box J-144
Gainesville, FL 32610

Michael S. Dekin
Dept. of Biological Sciences
101 Morgan Building
University of Kentucky
Lexington, KY 40506

Jerome A. Dempsey
University of Wisconsin-Madison
    Medical School
Department of Preventive Medicine
504 North Walnut Street
Madison, WI 53706

Howard H. Ellenberger
Department of Kinesiology
University of California
405 Hilgard Avenue
Los Angeles, CA 90024

Sandra England
Department of Pediatrics
Robert Wood Johnson
    Medical School
New Brunswick, NJ 08903

Jay P. Farber
Department of Physiology
University of Oklahoma Health Science
    Center
P.O. Box 26901
Oklahoma City, OK 73190

Robert S. Fitzgerald
Johns Hopkins University
Department of Environmental Physiology
615 North Wolf Street
Baltimore, MD 21205

Donald T. Frazier
Department of Physiology
Chandler Medical Center
University of Kentucky
Lexington, KY 40536-0084

Gabriel G. Haddad
Yale University School of Medicine
Pediatric, Respiratory Medicine
333 Cedar Street
Fitkin Bldg. Rm 506
New Haven, CT 06510

Ronald M. Harper
Department of Anatomy
University of California
Room 73-235
Los Angeles, CA 90024

Gerard Hilaire
Department de Physiologie
    et Neurophysiologie
Faculte des Sciences et Techniques
St. Jerome, Marseille
France

Ikuo Homma
Dept. of Physiology
Showa University
School of Medicine
1-5-8 Hatanodai, Shinagawa-ku
Tokyo 142, Japan

Yves Jammes
Université d'Aix-Marselle II
UFR de Médecine-Secteur Nord
Laboratoire de Physiologie
et URA 1330 CNRS
Bd. Pierre Dramard
13326 Marseille Cedex 15
France

David M. Katz
Case Western
School of Medicine
2119 Abington Road
Cleveland, OH 44106

Marc P. Kaufman
Department of Internal Medicine
    and Human Physiology
University of California TB-172
Davis, CA 95616

Hugo Lagercrantz
Department of Pediatrics
Karolinska Institute
Box 60400
104 01 Stockholm Sweden

Sukhamay Lahiri
Department of Physiology
University of Pennsylvania
    School of Medicine
Richards Building A201
Philadelphia, PA 19104-6085

Edward E. Lawson
Department of Pediatrics
University of North Carolina
Burnett Womack Building, CB 7220
Chapel Hill, NC 27599-7220

Janusz Lipski
Department of Physiology Medical School
University of Auckland
Private Bag, Auckland
New Zealand

Guosong Liu
Department of Kinesiology
University of California
405 Hilgard Avenue
Los Angeles, CA 90024

Jan Lundberg
Department of Pharmacology
Karolinska Institute
Box 60400
S-104 01 Stockholm
Sweden

Donald R. McCrimmon
Department of Physiology
Northwestern University Medical School
303 East Chicago Avenue
Chicago, IL 60611

Alan D. Miller
Rockefeller University
1230 York Avenue
New York, NY 10021

David E. Millhorn
Dept. of Physiology
Univ. of North Carolina
58 Med. Res. Wing,
    CB # 7545
Chapel Hill, NC 27599

Gordon S. Mitchell
Dept. of Comparative Bioscience
University of Wisconsin
2015 Linden Dr. West
Madison, WI 53706

Jacopo P. Mortola
Department of Physiology
McGill University
McIntyre Medical Sciences Bldg.
3655 Drummond Street
Montreal, Quebec
Canada H3G 1Y6

Judith A. Neubauer
Department of Medicine
Robert Wood Johnson
    Medical School
New Brunswick, NJ 08903

Colin Nurse
Department of Biology
McMaster University
1280 Main Street West
Hamilton, Ontario
Canada

John Orem
Texas Tech University
    Health Sciences Center
School of Medicine
Department of Physiology
Lubbock, TX 79430

Allan I. Pack
Cardiovascular Pulmonary Division
University of Pennsylvania
975 Maloney Boulevard
Philadelphia, PA 19104

W. Robert Revelette
Department of Physiology
Chandler Medical Center
University of Kentucky
Lexington, KY 40536-0084

Diethelm W. Richter
Georg-August-Universitat Gottingen
Zentrum Physiologie
Humboldtallee 23,
    D-3400 Gottingen
Germany

Giuseppe Sant'Ambrogio
Dept. of Physiology and Biophysics
University of Texas Medical Branch
Galveston, Texas 77550

T.A. Sears
Sobell Department of
    Neurophysiology
Institute of Neurology
Queens Square, London
WCIN 3BG
England

James B. Skatrud
Department of Preventive Medicine
University of Wisconsin
Health Science Center
504 North Walnut Street
Madison, WI 53706

Jeffrey C. Smith
Department of Kinesiology
University of California
Slichter Hall
Los Angeles, CA 90024

Dexter F. Speck
Department of Physiology
Chandler Medical Center
University of Kentucky
Lexington, KY 40536-0084

K. Michael Spyer
Department of Physiology
Royal Free Hospital School of Medicine
University of London
Rowland Hill Street
London NW3 2PF
England

Ann R. Stark
Department of Pediatrics
Harvard Medical School
Boston, MA 02115

Magdy K. Younes
Department of Internal Medicine
Manitoba University
Health Science Center
700 Williams Avenue
Winnipeg, Manitoba
Canada R3E 0Z3

Index